The Ultimate Medical School Interview Guide

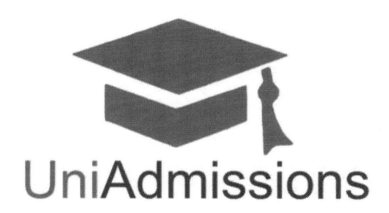

UniAdmissions

ISBN 978-0-9935711-0-7

Published by *RAR Medical Services Limited*
www.uniadmissions.co.uk
info@uniadmissions.co.uk
Tel: 0203 375 6294

The Ultimate Medical School Interview Guide

Dr Ranjna Garg

Dr Rohan Agarwal

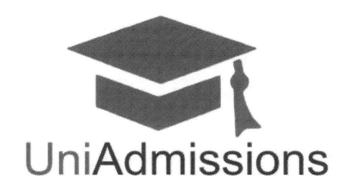

UniAdmissions

About the Authors

Ranjna is as a **Consultant Physician** at the Royal Free Trust London NHS Foundation Trust. Over the last decade, she has taught hundreds of junior doctors and prepared them through postgraduate examinations and job interviews. She enjoys helping students with their medical school preparation and has interviewed for London medical schools as well.

She has done significant research on the use of high strength insulin for patients with severe insulin resistance. In her spare time, she enjoys photography and running.

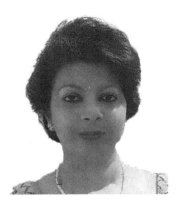

Rohan is **Director of Operations** at UniAdmissions and is responsible for its technical and commercial arms. He graduated from Gonville and Caius College, Cambridge, and is now a doctor in Leicester. Over the last five years, he has tutored hundreds of successful Oxbridge and Medical applicants. He has authored ten books on admissions tests and interviews.

He has taught physiology to undergraduates and interviewed medical school applicants for Cambridge. He has also published research on bone physiology and writes education articles for the Independent and Huffington Post. In his spare time, Rohan enjoys playing the piano and table tennis.

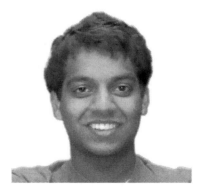

Foreword

Congratulations on taking the first step to medical interview success. If you are invited for an interview then that means the admissions tutors were interested in what you had to say in your personal statement and your test scores. The interview is not a place to recount all of this information; it is a place to showcase your knowledge, your integrity, and your ability to stay up to date on relevant medical news.

Different medical schools approach interviews in wildly different ways. Some may concentrate more on dissecting your personal statement, exploring your motivations and medical work experience so far. Others may try to test you primarily on your scientific grounding or your understanding of medical ethics. Some medical schools may question you on your BMAT essay. In most interviews, however, you are likely to face a combination of these. Similarly, some medical schools like to do a single long interview, while others like to do two (often one interview concentrates on science and the other on medical ethics / your motivations and work experience). Indeed, many medical schools now use MMIs.

Interviews require dedicated preparation - don't leave things to chance! Medical school interviews are extremely formulaic and you can predict the vast majority of questions that you're likely to be asked. Unsurprisingly, so can everyone else. Thus, you do yourself a great disservice if you don't have comprehensive answers prepared for these questions. Ensure you've done your research on the interview format, the pros/cons of that medical school and have answers lined up for the common interview questions, e.g. *"Why medicine?"* and *"Why this university?"* etc.

Ultimately, with fierce competition, there is no guarantee for success. With more than five applicants per place, it is now more important than ever to go the extra mile. Whilst there will undoubtedly be conflicting demands on your time – remember that a small amount of preparation has the potential to literally change your life. Don't take it lightly – work hard, put in the hours and do yourself justice.

Dr Rohan Agarwal

THE BASICS

Congratulations on securing a medical school interview! Getting this far is in itself a great accomplishment. Interviews for medical school can be a daunting prospect, but with the right preparation, there is every reason to be confident that you can present yourself in the best possible way.

This guide is aimed at giving you a comprehensive walkthrough of the entire interview process- from the very basics of your initial preparation to the moment you walk out of the interview room.

What is a Medical Interview?

A medical interview is a formal discussion between interviewer and interviewee. This is normally the *final* step in the medical school application process. Traditionally, interviews last around 20 – 30 minutes and take place from mid-October to April every year.

Why is there an Interview?

Medicine is competitive- the vast majority of applicants will already have outstanding grades at GCSE, fantastic predicted exam results, and a solid personal statement. As you can imagine, this makes many applicants look very similar on paper!

The interview process is designed to identify students that would be best suited for studying medicine at the university you've applied to. Thus, medical school interviews assess multiple qualities e.g. your motivation to study medicine, communication skills, team working and leadership skills etc.

Whilst the interview is not testing your knowledge and skills about a specific subject, it helps to have a good knowledge base. The interview process will assess candidates on their ability to learn. The universities are looking for candidates that have the ability and mindset to learn, i.e. can the candidate be taught. Universities recognise that the interviews can be stressful and may utilise this to assess candidates' reactions to stress; to see if they can cope with the pressure. It is a process where the candidates are judged on their quick thinking, logical approach, and ability to formulate a comprehensive, coherent, structured response. You will be guided through the process by your interviewer. The interview is not about tricking you. It's about testing your abilities to harp on your existing knowledge and use it to come up with a logical response. The interview is also about assessing your abilities to see if you can come up with plausible solutions, even if you don't know the answer.

Who gets an Interview?

Interviews are usually the last step in the application process. Each university has its own unique selection process and will value some parts of the admissions process more than others. However, most will only interview around 30-60% of applicants – the rest are rejected without interview (although there are some notable exceptions).

Whether or not you get an interview invite will depend on how well you satisfy each university's entrance criteria. This is normally a combination of predicted grades, your personal statement, school reference, UKCAT/BMAT scores, etc.

It is important to research your universities early on to get a better idea of their particular preferences. For example, Birmingham will generally only interview students who attain 8 or more A*s at GCSE; Kings will generally only students with very high UKCAT scores. Contrastingly, Cambridge tends to interview the great majority of applicants prior to making any decisions.

Who are the Interviewers?

Depending on the university, medical school interviews can be conducted by a host of different people:

➢ Dean of the Medical School
➢ Senior Doctors and Lecturers
➢ Nurses
➢ Other Allied Health Professionals
➢ Current Medical Students

When is the Interview?

This will vary depending on the university you've applied to. Generally, most universities will start interviewing in late October/early November and continue to do so until January. Some universities will carry on interviewing until early May. Oxbridge interviews are almost always between late November to mid-December. Cambridge may invite you to a second round of interviews in January should you get pooled.

Most universities will give you at least 2 weeks' notice prior to your interview. However, it's highly advisable to **begin preparing for your interview before you're officially invited**.

Can I Change the Interview Date?

It's generally not a good idea to change your interview date unless you absolutely have to and have a strong reason to do so, e.g. Family Bereavement. Rescheduling your interview for your friend's birthday or a sports match is unlikely to go down well!

If you do need to reschedule, give the medical school as much notice as possible and offer some alternative dates. Be aware that you may be putting yourself at a disadvantage by doing of this as your interview will likely be delayed.

Where is the Interview?

The interview will almost always take place at the medical school you've applied to. Logistically, it's worth booking an overnight hotel if you're travelling from far away.

Very rarely, interviews can be held via Skype at an exam centre- this normally only applies to international students or for UK students in extreme circumstances.

How long do I need to prepare for?

You will often hear the phrase "*You can't prepare for medical school interviews*" – this couldn't be further from the truth. You need to prepare both comprehensively and efficiently in order to cover all the material and acquire the skills you need to succeed. Thus, it's a generally a very good idea to start interview preparations as soon as you've applied through UCAS (although even earlier is better!). Don't leave your interview preparation until you've actually been invited to one as that won't give you enough time to shine on the day.

Remember, medical school interviews test a wide variety of skills that – unlike your Year 12/13 exams – you can't cram for, e.g. communication, analytical skills etc. Start preparing small amounts early on and increase this time the closer you get to your interview. Planning and practice will take you to perfection.

What Should I Wear?

When it comes to interviews, it's best to dress sharply and smartly.

Unless you're told otherwise by the medical school, this normally means a full suit for men and either a full suit or smart shirt + skirt for women.

Things to avoid:
➤ Excessively shiny or intricate jewellery
➤ Bold and controversial dress colours, e.g. orange ties
➤ Excessive amounts of makeup – it's not a beauty pageant
➤ Flashy nails or eyelashes
➤ Unnecessarily large bags – leave your overnight bags at a hotel or at the medical school reception
➤ Wearing your 'school prefect' or 'head boy' badges

Things to do:
➤ Carry an extra pair of contact lenses or glasses if appropriate
➤ Turn your phone off completely – you don't want any distractions
➤ Polish your shoes

Top Tip! Read! If you're genuinely interested in medicine then you should love reading around it. Read something accessible to you (i.e. NOT Grey's anatomy) and make some notes on it that you can easily discuss at your interview.

Body Language

First impressions last; body language contributes to a significant part of this. However, don't make the mistake of obsessing over body language at the expense of the quality answers you give.

Most people will only need to make some minor adjustments to remove some "bad habits", so don't worry about body language till fairly late in your preparation.

Once you're confident that you know the relevant material and have good answers prepared for common questions, allow your body language to show that you have what it takes to be a doctor by conveying maturity and confidence.

Posture
➢ When walking into the room, walk in with your head held high and back straight.
➢ When sitting down, look alert and sit up straight.
➢ Avoid crossing your arms – this can appear to be defensive.
➢ Don't slouch- instead, lean forward slightly to show that you're engaged with the interview.
➢ If there is a table, then ensure you sit around four to six inches away.
   ❖ Too close and you'll appear like you're invading the interviewers' space
   ❖ Too far and you'll appear too casual

Eyes
➢ Good eye contact is a sign of confidence and good communication skills.
➢ Look at the interviewer when they are speaking to you and when you are speaking.
➢ If there are multiple interviewers, look at the interviewer who is speaking to you or asked you the question. However, make sure you do look around at the other interviewers to acknowledge them.

Hands
➢ At the start, offer a handshake or accept if offered: make sure you don't have sweaty or cold hands.
➢ A firm handshake is generally preferable to a limp one.
➢ During the interview, keep your hands still unless you are using them to illustrate your point.
➢ Avoid excessive hand movements – your hands should go no higher than your neck.
➢ If you fidget when you're nervous, hold your hands firmly together in your lap to stop this from happening.

> *Top Tip!* Make sure you practise speaking articulately about the topics that interest you. Join your school's debating society (or set one up!), discuss it with friends & family, challenge your biology teacher regarding a point you don't quite understand or would like to know more about!

PREPARING FOR INTERVIEWS

How do I Prepare?

Many applicants will jump straight to the questions part of this book and attempt to learn the "good answers" by rote. Whilst this is psychologically comforting, it is of minimal value in actually preparing you for the interview. Use this book as guidance. Develop the skills to construct logical and structured answers so that you are familiar with the format. Cramming for your interview by rote learning the answers provided in this book will make your responses clichéd.

You are almost guaranteed to be asked certain questions at your interview, e.g. "Why Medicine?". So it's well worth preparing answers for these frequently asked questions. However, it's critical that you don't simply recite pre-prepared answers as this will appear unnatural and, therefore, rehearsed.

Step One: Do your Research
Start off by finding out exactly what is required of you for the interview, e.g. interview type, who your interviewers will be, commonly asked questions, etc.

Step Two: Acquire the pre-requisite Knowledge
Next, focus on learning the basics of interview technique and understanding the core healthcare topics that you'll be expected to know about. Once you're happy with this, go through the questions + answers in this book – don't try to rote learn answers. Instead, try to understand what makes each answer good/bad and then use this to come up with your own unique answer. Don't be afraid of using other resources, e.g. YouTube videos on medical ethics, etc.

When you've got this down, practice answering questions in front of a mirror and consider recording yourself to iron out any body language issues.

Step Three: Practice with People
It's absolutely paramount that you practice with a real person before your first interview. Whilst you might be able to provide fantastic answers to common questions with no one observing you, this may not be the case with the added pressure of a mock interviewer.

Practice interviews are best with someone you do not know very well - even easy questions may be harder to articulate out loud and on the spot to a stranger. MMIs, in particular, are worth practising beforehand, so you can work on using the time available as efficiently as possible. During your practice, try to eliminate hesitant words like "Errrr…." and "Ummm…" as these will make you appear less confident. Ask for feedback on the speed, volume, and tone of your voice.

Many schools will be able to arrange a mock interview for you. If you're struggling, you can book private mock interviews at www.uniadmissions.co.uk/mock-medical-interviews.

Top Tip! Practise structuring arguments in your head so that you can present them in a logical and easy-to-follow way. This will show that you have previously thought carefully about the topic in hand.

Types of Interviews

The first thing to understand is that there are several different formats of an interview. They can broadly be categorised into:

➤ Panel-Based Interview:
  o Multiple interviewers
  o Normally twenty – forty minutes
  o May have two long panel interviews
➤ Multiple Mini Interview (MMI):
  o There are normally five to twelve stations
  o Each station is five to ten minutes long and will focus on different topic
  o There is normally an interviewer at each station
  o You physically move from one station to another

Different medical schools approach interviews in different ways. Some may concentrate more on dissecting your personal statement, exploring your motivations and medical work experience. Others may try to test you primarily on medical ethics whilst the BMAT medical schools may question you on your BMAT essay. Hence, it's extremely important that you know what type of interview you will be going through as that determines how you prepare.

Medical schools will let you know the exact interview format in advance; some will also tell you who your interviewers will be. It can be useful to **look at your interviewers' teaching backgrounds and published work** as this can potentially shed some light on the topics they might choose to discuss during the interview. However, there is absolutely no need to know the intricacies of their research work so don't get bogged down in it. It can be useful to know their views on their areas of interest so that you are prepared and can offer both sides of the argument in a balanced manner.

Interviews tend to open with easier and more general questions and become more detailed and complicated as you are pushed to explore topics in greater depth. Remember, if the questions are getting harder, you are probably doing well!

The whole point of interviews is to identify individuals who will fit in at that institution, so your grades, interest, hobbies, and experiences are all important and you may be asked on any of these. Also, be prepared to discuss your personal statement, current affairs, and your BMAT essay if your university requires it.

Generally, MMIs tend to be highly scripted with each interviewer having a certain number of questions that they need to ask in the time limit. Contrastingly, traditional interviews are more free flowing – there are usually lots of follow-up questions based on your previous responses as there is more time to explore more complex issues. An example of that is a discussion that starts with a simple question like: *What did you enjoy in your work experience in the cardiology department and can go into detailed discussions about heart transplant ethics or cardiac physiology?*

Although the format of medical school interviews can vary considerably, the qualities which interviewers are looking for in applicants remain consistent. It's well worth your time to understand these qualities and exhibit them as much as possible when answering questions.

What Are the Interviewers Looking For?

Many applicants think that the most 'obvious' thing interviewers are looking for is excellent factual knowledge. This simply isn't true.

Interviewers are looking for an applicant that is **best** suited to study medicine at **their** university. They are looking for your **motivation** to be a doctor. Standard medical school interviews generally don't test your innate recall knowledge of facts. For example, you are unlikely to be asked, "What is the normal value of serum calcium?". Whilst having an excellent depth of knowledge may help you perform better during an interview- **you're very unlikely to be chosen based solely on your knowledge**.

The 'Outcomes for Graduates' section of the GMC's document "Tomorrow's Doctors" is useful for gaining an appreciation of what medical schools are looking for in prospective applicants. Remember that the ultimate aim of this long selection process is to choose students who will go on to make good doctors in the years to come. When preparing for the interview and answering interview questions, it's very useful to think about how any of the qualities below could be shown in your answer.

Diligence
Medicine is a very demanding profession and will require hard work throughout your whole career. Interviewers are looking not only for your ability to work hard (diligence) but also for an understanding that there will be times where you will have a responsibility to prioritise your medical work over other personal and social concerns (conscientiousness). This means that when you are a doctor and have just finished a twelve-hour shift and the night doctor is running late, you stay behind until they arrive so the ward isn't left without a doctor.

Professional Integrity
Medicine is a profession where lives could be at risk if something goes wrong. Being honest and having strong moral principles is critical for doctors. The public trusts the medical profession and this can only be maintained if there is complete honesty between both parties. Interviewers need to see that you are an honest person, can accept your mistakes and are learn from them.

Empathy
Empathy is the ability to recognise and relate to other peoples' emotional needs. It is important that you understand and respond to how others may be feeling when you're a doctor. The easiest way to demonstrate this is by recalling situations from your work experience (one of the many reasons why it's so important). However, it's important to not exaggerate how much an incident has affected you - experienced interviewers will quickly pick up on anything that doesn't sound sincere.

Resilience to Stress
There is no denying the fact that medical school can be stressful due to the extreme pressure you'll be put under. Medical schools understand that you are likely to become stressed during your studies, however, it's important that you have a way of dealing with it in a healthy manner. Interviewers are looking to see if you are able to make logical decisions when put under pressure (something doctors encounter on a daily basis). Pursuing interests outside of medicine, such as sport, music or drama is often a good way of de-stressing and gives you an opportunity to talk about your extra-curricular interests as well as team-working skills.

Scientific Aptitude
Medicine is undoubtedly a science; whilst your grades will demonstrate your scientific aptitude, you'll need to offer something, in addition, to make yourself stand out. The easiest way to do this is by referencing examples of where you have gone beyond the confines of your school syllabus, e.g. Science Olympiads, Science Clubs, extra reading (hopefully you mentioned these in your personal statement).

Self-Awareness

You need to show that you have the maturity required to deal with complex issues that you will face as a doctor. The vast majority of students will undergo changes in personality throughout medical school and you need to have a good understanding of yourself to ensure these changes are positive ones.

Firstly, it's important to be able to recognise your own strengths and weaknesses. In addition, you need to be able to recognise and reflect on your mistakes so that you can learn from them for the future. A person with good self-awareness can work on their weakness to avoid mistakes from happening again. Questions like, "What are your strengths?" or "What is your biggest weakness?" are common and fantastic opportunities to let your maturity and personal insight shine through.

Teamwork and Leadership

Working as a doctor requires working in a multidisciplinary team (MDT) – a group of individuals with a wide variety of skills that work to help patients. The MDT is a cornerstone of how modern healthcare functions. Thus, you need to be able to show that you're a team player. One of the best ways of doing this is by giving examples from your extracurricular activities, e.g. sports, music, duke of Edinburgh, other school projects.

> *Top Tip!* If you've got a bit of time before the interview then do something that shows your love and devotion to medicine. For example, set up a mini medical journal club at your school where people can submit pieces on interesting aspects of science.

Realistic Expectations

Interviewers are looking for individuals that are committed to medicine and have a realistic idea of what life as a doctor will entail. This is why it's extremely important to display your motivation to study medicine clearly during the interview. A common way to do this is to reflect on your work experience and have examples ready of common challenges that you will likely face. Examples include:

➢ Long hours and stress
➢ Repetitiveness. A career in medicine can sometimes demand great patience. Doing the same operation day-in-day-out, seeing the same diseases, sitting through endless clinics
➢ The balance between being empathetic, yet remaining objective
➢ **Ethical dilemmas** – these will be discussed in detail in the 'Medical Ethics' section

Interviewer Styles

Although interviewers have wildly different styles, it is helpful to remember that none of them are trying to catch you out. They are there to help you. You may come across an interviewer that is very polite and 'noddy' while others may have a 'poker face'. Do not be put off by their expressions or reactions. Sometimes what you thought was a negative facial response to your reply may just be a twitch. Contrastingly, a very helpful appearing interviewer may lull you into a false sense of security. Rarely, you may get an interviewer who likes playing 'Devil's advocate' and will challenge your every statement. In these cases, it's important not to take things personally and avoid getting worked up.

You don't know what type of interviewer you will get so it's important to practice mock interviews with as many people as possible so that you're prepared for a wider variety of interviewer styles.

Communicating your Answers

Many applicants don't secure places as they don't spend enough time preparing for their interviews. A common reason is that they feel that they "already know what to say". Whilst this may be true, it is not always **what** you say but **how** you say it. Interviews are a great test of your communication skills and should be taken seriously. A good way to ensure you consistently deliver effective answers is to adhere to the principles below:

Keep it Short:

In general, most your responses should be approximately one to two minutes long. They should convey the important information but be focussed on the question and avoid rambling. Remember, you are providing a direct response to the question, not writing an English essay! With practice, you should be able to identify the main issues being asked, plan a structured response, and communicate them succinctly. It's important to practice your answers to common questions, e.g. *'Why Medicine?'* so that you can start to get a feel for what is the correct response duration.

Some questions may require more time, e.g. questions that ask you to compare and contrast. Similarly, questions in MMIs are generally targeted so don't be shy to give slightly shorter (but still detailed) responses to them.

Give Examples:

Generic statements don't carry much weight without evidence to back them up. As a general rule, every statement that you make should be evidenced using examples. Consider the following statements:

Statement 1: "I am good at biology."
Statement 2: "I am good at biology as evidenced by my A* in biology AS and a gold medal in the UK biology Olympiad. I am an avid reader of 'Biology Review' as this allows me to keep up to date with new developments in the field."

Focus on Yourself:

It's not uncommon for candidates to go off on a tangent and start describing, for example, the many hurdles their young enterprise team faced. Remember, interviews are all about you - your skills, ability, and motivation to be a doctor. Thus, it's important that you spend as much time talking about yourself rather than others (unless absolutely necessary). Many students find it difficult to do this because they are afraid of being interpreted as 'arrogant' or 'a show-off'. Whilst this is definitely something to be aware of, it's important you do yourself justice and not undersell yourself.

Answer the Question:

This cannot be stressed enough – there are few things more frustrating than students that ignore the interviewer's questions. Remember, you need to **answer the question**; **don't answer the topic**. If a question consists of two parts – remember to answer both, e.g. *'Should we legalise euthanasia? Why?'*

Ending the Interview

At the end of the interview, the interviewers are likely to ask you if you have any questions for them. You should have gleaned enough information from the open days, school website, prospectus etc., that you do not have many questions. Unless the question is crucial, this may not be the right time to ask questions about the course, school or activities within the school as it will show your ignorance about the course/school. You can use this as an opportunity to show your interest in the course and medical school. Don't be perturbed that you do not have a question to ask.

MMIs may well end abruptly and you may be asked to stop when the end of time is signalled (bell rings or knock on the door). Avoid the temptation to linger on to answer the question that is half-answered unless you are asked to - extra time taken at one station means less time for the next one.

Dealing with Unexpected Questions

Although you can normally predict at least 90% of questions that you're likely to get asked, there will be some questions that you won't have prepared for. These assess your ability to handle difficult situations to see how you react to pressure and how you deal with the unknown.

Completely abstract questions are rare in traditional medical school interviews. Unless you're applying to Oxbridge, it's unlucky to be asked a question that you don't have a clue about. If you do find yourself in this situation, do not panic. Pause and think. Have you come across something at school? Have you read something about it? Can you see/apply the basic principles? Can you these to start a discussion?

Good applicants will endeavour to engage with the topic and try to link in their knowledge to the question, e.g. *"I have not come across this before but it seems that…"*. Weaker applicants would be perturbed by the question or not consider it seriously, e.g. *"I don't know."*

Consider the example: *"Is there is life on Mars?"*

You may not have read about this specific topic. However, you may know about different space missions.

"As far as I know, there is not life on mars. However, given that there is some water on Mars, it would not be altogether impossible for there to be life."

Of course, this relies on you having a basal level of general knowledge. If you really have no clue at all and have not come across anything about this topic then it is better to acknowledge the gap in your knowledge.

"Unfortunately, I have limited information about this topic but it is an interesting question. I did read about NASA's mission to Mars but I'm unable to say if they have found life. I will endeavour to look this up."

Dealing with difficult questions like this gives you the opportunity to show that you are a motivated and enthusiastic student.

Interview Myths

1. Your interviewer is only interested in catching you out.
The interviewer is there to help you and to encourage you. It is best to think of the interview as a conversation between you and the interviewer. It is nothing more than an opportunity for you and the interviewer to get to know one another and see if you would be a good fit at that university.

2. The interview is the only important part of the admissions process.
Although the interview can be the final hurdle in some medical schools, many will also take your personal statement, academic grades and UKCAT/BMAT scores when making offers. Most medical schools will shortlist for interviews based on these so you cannot just focus purely on interview preparation from the outset.

3. You need to have immaculate knowledge of recent medical developments.
Many students claim that they are vicarious readers of Student BMJ and New Scientist on their personal statements, and then panic 'cram learn' the latest editions of these journals before their interview. Relax. You are not expected to be able to recite the articles from them. However, **you will be** expected to be familiar with current affairs and have a basic understanding of recent healthcare news.

4. All of the other interview candidates will know far more than you.
Whilst some students may give the impression that they have swallowed several encyclopaedias - don't let this put you off. Interviews are an opportunity to focus on yourself, expand your knowledge, and most importantly, show yourself as a potential doctor for tomorrow – not worry about whether you have read Grey's Anatomy back-to-back.

Structuring your Answers

You can approach questions in both MMIs and traditional interviews by using a simple framework:

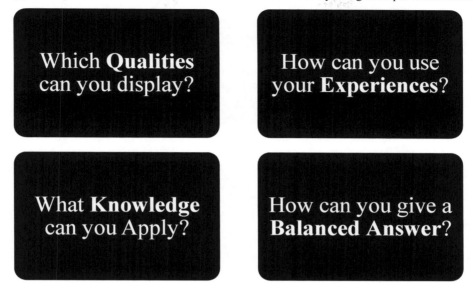

A good trick in MMIs can be to try and tick off each of these in an answer where applicable. This is a good way to ensure that you are not spending too long talking about one thing and so leaving yourself no time to talk about other things. There is little point in reeling off a list of unrelated facts when that would leave no time to show how your experiences apply.

It is better to demonstrate good knowledge and then move on to describe how insights from your work experience have also influenced you to give a more well-rounded answer. It's worth practising answering questions using this framework.

For example, consider: *'What do you think is the greatest challenge of being an FY1 doctor?'*

1.   What knowledge can I apply?
I know FY1 doctors have very long hours, including regular night shifts. I know they suddenly progress from a position of little responsibility as medical students to one of great responsibility. I know the structure of medical training after medical school, which I might be able to work into the answer.

2.   What experiences can I use?
I remember seeing a lot of FY1s looking exhausted on my work experience. I remember one FY1 complaining that he was not getting to apply much of his medical knowledge, but instead felt like a secretary. I remember another FY1 saying how scary it is to suddenly go from being a student to being responsible for people's lives and expected to be able to practice relatively independently.

3.   What positive qualities can I display?
I can show a realistic understanding of the challenges of medicine. I can show a diligent and conscientious attitude towards the challenge of hard work and long hours. I can show an ability to handle stress.

4.   How can I give a balanced answer?
I should recognise that there are multiple factors that make FY1 a challenge in order to balance the answer.

You can go through a thought process like this in a few seconds and continue to think about it as you begin to answer the question. Thus, your answer may be along the lines of:

"There are clearly lots of different factors that are challenging for an FY1 doctor. For a start, the long hours and regular night shifts must be quite draining. Though FY1s will be used to hard work from medical school, this may still require a step up and even more sacrifices to be made in terms of a social life. However, whilst I was on my work experience I remember an FY1 doctor telling me that the thing she found most challenging was the sudden jump in responsibility and expectations between being a medical student and being an FY1 doctor. It was this that she and her peers found most stressful."

You can see how you have to be very picky about what you include in your answer to make sure you give a well-rounded answer in the tight time limit of the MMI. For the same question, another response could focus on striking a work-life balance as being most challenging:

"Whilst doing my work experience, I saw FY1 doctors working long hours and busy shifts. In addition, they had to study for additional exams to ensure their career progression. This meant that the weekends were spent either on calls or attending courses. All this limited their social life. Thus, I think striking a good work-life balance could be challenging albeit possible with forward planning."

The STARR Framework

You may be asked questions where you need to give examples, e.g. *"Tell me about a time when you showed leadership?"*

It's very useful to **prepare examples in advance** for these types of questions as it's very difficult to generate them on the spot. Try to **prepare at least three examples** that you can use to answer a variety of questions. Generally, more complex examples can be used to demonstrate multiple skills, e.g. communication, leadership, team-working, etc.

In the initial stages, it's helpful to use a framework to structure your answers, e.g. the STARR Framework shown below:

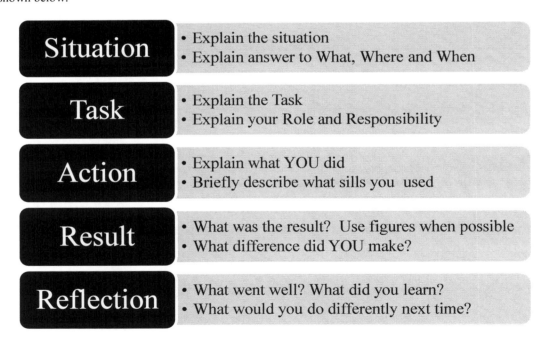

Situation
- Explain the situation
- Explain answer to What, Where and When

Task
- Explain the Task
- Explain your Role and Responsibility

Action
- Explain what YOU did
- Briefly describe what sills you used

Result
- What was the result? Use figures when possible
- What difference did YOU make?

Reflection
- What went well? What did you learn?
- What would you do differently next time?

MULTIPLE MINI INTERVIEWS

A Multiple Mini Interview (MMIs) is a series of short interviews. There are normally five to twelve stations and each station is five to ten minutes long. There is a new challenge and a new interviewer at each station. Most MMIs are one to two hours in total duration. All candidates must go through every station and will be asked the same questions. The major implications of this arrangement are:

1) You have a lot less time to make your points & build a rapport with the interviewer
2) There is a greater diversity of topics you can be tested on
3) You have a 'fresh start' at each station so can recover from poor previous stations
4) MMIs are fairer as everyone will get asked the same questions

The time pressure in MMIs makes communication challenging because there is less time to make a good impression on your interviewer and less time for them to judge you. This means that unlike traditional interviews, there is little time for ice-breakers; you'll need to give focussed yet comprehensive answers to ensure success.

What will I be asked?

Each MMI station will test different skills and topics like:

➢ One-To-One interviews on commonly asked topics, e.g. medical ethics, motivation to study medicine, work experience, situational questions
➢ Writing Task where you're required to write answers to common questions. Normally, there are no interviewers
➢ Role Play where you need to interact with an actor, e.g. convince a patient to stop smoking
➢ Video Analysis where you need to comment on a video, e.g. of a doctor-patient consultation
➢ Calculations, e.g. calculate drug doses
➢ Rarely, there may be a rest station where there are sometimes drinks and snacks

A typical MMI circuit could involve:

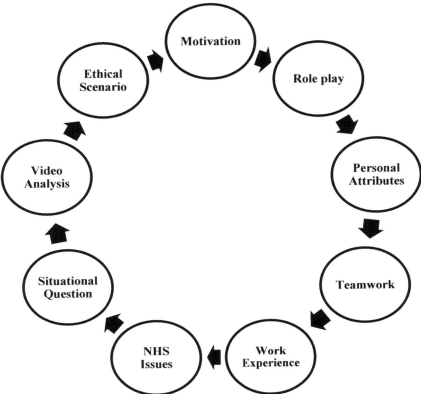

How to Tackle MMIs

Step One: Do your Research

Start off by finding out exactly how many stations there are and what duration. Then try to establish what topics are frequently asked and which topics have come up in the past. Are there any non-standard stations like maths or practical skills stations? Don't rely on your seniors – universities frequently change their MMI structures, so ensure you get the information from the university website or email the admissions office if you're unsure.

Step Two: Acquire the pre-requisite Knowledge

Once you have an idea about timings, you can start to tailor your preparation. For example, there is little point in practicing extensive thirty-minute ethical arguments when the stations are only five minutes. Nevertheless, it's important to ensure you're familiar with the commonly asked questions. Again, don't spend extensive time trying to rote learn answers to common questions - this is not particularly helpful and is likely to be counter-productive.

Step Three: Practice with People

It's essential that you practice with a real person in advance. You need to practice giving succinct yet comprehensive answers as well as creating a strong first impression.

If there's more than one of you at your school who are applying for medicine (or dentistry), it would be worth considering that you could help each other and work together. Share resources, have practice sessions together and give each other constructive criticism. Even if you have only a couple of times a week when you're both free, it can really help to just sit down with someone and discuss an issue such as organ donation – each take a different stance, set a timer and see how you get on. Try not to be intimidated and keep calm. Five minutes might sound like a relatively short period of time, but it should be enough to get the most important points across.

Although many schools will arrange a practice panel or one-to-one interviews for you, very few will offer full MMI practice. If you feel you'd benefit from a full MMI circuit, consider attending a medical interview course which contains a mock MMI circuit (www.uniadmissions.co.uk/medical-school-interview-course).

DON'T ASSUME THAT YOU WON'T GET ASKED TRADITIONAL STYLE INTERVIEW
QUESTIONS IN MMIs. YOU DEFINITELY WILL!

Station 1: Role Plays

You may be asked to role play as a medical student or a junior doctor. This is testing your ability to communicate information in a clear manner and your ability to handle stressful situations. You could be interacting with an actor or the examiner. You may need to talk to either a patient, family member or another doctor.

Examples Scenarios:

Your Role	Actor's Role	Location	Your Task
A Level Student	3rd Year Medical Student	University Open Day	Interact with the actor as you would at an open day
A Level Student	Your neighbour	The front yard	You accidentally run over your neighbour's dog with your car. Break the bad news to them
1st Year Medical Student	FY1 Doctor	On the Ward Round	You notice that the FY1 doctor appears under the influence of ecstasy. What do you do?
1st Year Medical Student	Another 1st Year Student	GP Surgery	Your friend is thinking about leaving medical school as they don't enjoy it. Find out why and offer help
1st Year Medical Student	Patient	GP Surgery	Speak to the patient who has been waiting for over one hour and find out why they have come to the GP
FY1 Doctor	Patient	On Ward	Explain and apologise to the patient about a drug prescribing error that you contributed to
FY1 Doctor	Patient's Relative	On Ward	The relative is very worried about their father. Calm them down and answer their questions

Don't be scared by some of the horror stories you might hear where candidates were asked to break a diagnosis of cancer or tell a patient they were going to die. These are extremely unlikely scenarios that you won't be expected to handle (indeed many junior doctors struggle with these). Even if you do get a particularly difficult scenario, try you remain calm- these stations are never a test of your knowledge. You are not expected to take a comprehensive history or diagnose a patient. **Role-plays are purely a test of communication.**

General Advice:
➢ Before starting the roleplay, ensure that you have read the scenario and understand exactly what is expected of you. Important things to double check are your role (doctor, student, etc.) and your location.
➢ Take a quick look around when you walk into the room. There are sometimes props positioned that you should utilise if appropriate. For example, you should offer a crying patient tissues or a cup of water.
➢ Always introduce yourself and your role unless the brief makes it abundantly clear that you don't need to (e.g. "Speak to your best friend Jane who is…"). A good opening line is: "Good morning, my name is Tom and I'm a first-year medical student. I'd like to speak to you about…"
➢ The actors are sometimes difficult and quiet on purpose in order to put you out of your comfort zone. Don't be thrown off if they appear to be reluctant to engage – that's their job!
➢ Don't be afraid of asking very vague questions to get the conversation started. Whilst questions like "How can I help?" or "How are you doing?" may appear redundant, they are important in opening a dialogue. Remember that going straight to the task can appear very forced, artificial and rude.
➢ Tailor your language depending on who you're speaking with. Be formal with patients and your senior colleagues; more informal with your friends.
➢ If you're uncertain about the direction the conversation is going, feel free to ask the actor: "Is there anything, in particular, you were expecting? Or anything I can do for you?"
➢ The principles of non-verbal communication still apply here. Maintain good eye contact, have an inviting posture and appear engaged in the conversation.

Station 2: Situational Judgment

The Situational Judgement station tests your ability to prioritise competing demands and resolve disputes in a harmonious manner.

If you have taken the UKCAT then you will have already come across SJT style questions. However, unlike the UKCAT, you may not get given multiple options to choose from. This means that you might have to generate the answer yourself rather than using the options as a guide.

In addition, this station may not have an interviewer. Instead, it may be a written station where you are expected to write your answer out in full rather than vocalise it. The scripts will then be marked collectively at the end.

When faced with a situational question, it is helpful to use a basic framework:
1. Identify the basic dilemma
2. Identify your potential courses of action
3. Consider the advantages & disadvantages of each option you're given
4. Consider any alternative solutions, i.e. options outside the ones you are given
5. Think about how the perspectives of colleagues and patients may differ from your own
6. Balance these to pick an action that you can justify with a logical argument

Treat Every Option Independently

The options may seem similar, but don't let the different options confuse you. Read each option as if it is a question of its own. It is important to know that responses should **NOT** be judged as though they are the **ONLY** thing you are to do. An answer should not be judged as inappropriate because it's incomplete, but only if there is some actual inappropriate action taking place.

For example, if a scenario says, "*A patient on the ward complains she is in pain*", the response "ask the patient what is causing the problem" would be very appropriate. Any good response would also include informing the nurses and other doctors about what you had been told.

There might be multiple correct responses for each scenario, so don't feel you have to answer each of them differently. If you are unsure of the answer, mark the question and move on. **Avoid spending more than 90 seconds on any question**, otherwise, you will fall behind and risk not finishing.

Read "Tomorrow's Doctors" and "Good Medical Practice"

These are publications produced by the General Medical Council (GMC) which can be found on their website. The GMC regulate the medical profession to ensure that standards remain high. These publications can be found on their website and it outlines the expectations of the next generation of doctors – the generation of doctors you are aspiring to join. Reading through this will get you into a professional way of thinking that will help you judge these questions accurately.

Step into Character

When doing this section, imagine you are in the scenarios being presented to you. Imagine yourself as a caring and conscientious junior doctor that you soon will be. What would you do? What do you think would be the right thing to do?

Hierarchy

The patient is of **primary importance**. All decisions that affect patient care should be made to benefit the patient. Of **secondary importance** are your work colleagues. So if there is no risk to patients, you should help out your colleagues and avoid doing anything that would undermine them or harm their reputation – but if doing so would bring detriment to any patient, then the patient's priorities come to the top. Finally, of **lowest importance** is yourself. You should avoid working outside hours and strive to further your education, but not at the expense of patients or your colleagues.

There are several core principles that you should attempt to apply to SJT questions that will help your decision making:

Adopt a Patient-Centred Approach to Care

This involves being able to treat patients as an individual and respecting their decisions. You should also respect a patient's right to confidentiality unless there is a significant risk to the general public. The most important principle is to **never compromise patient safety**.

Working Well in a Team

Teamwork is an essential part of any job. You must be a trustworthy and reliable team member and also communicate effectively within the team. You should support your senior and junior colleagues should they require it. It is important to avoid conflict and be able to de-escalate situations without jeopardising professional relationships where possible.

Commitment to Professionalism

You should always act with honesty and integrity as this is expected of anyone entering the profession. This includes apologising for your mistakes and trying to ensure other people apologise for theirs.

Taking Responsibility for your learning

Medicine is a career where you are continuously learning. You are the sole person responsible for it and you will need to prioritise your jobs to ensure you attend scheduled teaching and courses. You should be able to critically reflect upon your experiences.

Example Questions

Example A:

"The ward nurse informs you that one of your FY1 colleagues is taking lots of morphine from the drug cabinet. What do you do?"

This question is not about your knowledge of morphine but about what to do if someone you know is reported to be doing something that is not correct. The obvious trap here is to say, *"I would go speak to the doctor and inform their boss."*

This would be a very serious accusation; remember that the nurse may be wrongly informed, biased or have a grudge against that doctor. Before you do anything, you must show that you will find out the facts and establish whether this is a recurring problem or not and if there are any obvious explainable reasons for it.

Thus, although the question appears very simple- it actually tests multiple skills. It's important to consider the implications of your actions rather than launch into an answer straight away.

"Taking medication from a patient's drug cabinet is something that worries me. Before I do anything, I would try to establish the facts by talking to others who may be in a position to observe such behaviour. This will ensure that it removes any reporter's personal bias or perceptions. If this is true, I would offer to speak to the colleague in private and ask their views. I would offer my support by covering some of their work to ensure that patient safety is not compromised. I would encourage them to get external help and consider involving my seniors if I felt that the situation wasn't resolving."

Example B:

You are just finishing a busy shift on the Acute Assessment Unit (AAU). Your FY1 colleague who is due to replace you for the evening shift leaves a message with the nurse in charge that she will be 15 to 30 minutes late. There is only a 30-minute overlap between your timetables to handover to your colleague. You need to leave on time as you have a social engagement to attend with your partner.

Rank the following actions in response to this situation in ascending order of appropriateness:

A. Make a list of the patients under your care on the AAU, detailing their outstanding issues, leaving this on the doctor's office notice board when your shift ends and then leave at the end of your shift.

B. Quickly go around each of the patients on the AAU, leaving an entry in the notes highlighting the major outstanding issues relating to each patient and then leave at the end of your shift.

C. Make a list of patients and outstanding investigations to give to your colleague as soon as she arrives.

D. Ask your registrar if you can leave a list of your patients and their outstanding issues with him to give to your colleague when she arrives and then leave at the end of your shift.

E. Leave a message for your partner explaining that you will be 30 minutes late.

This question gives you the opportunity to demonstrate a conscientious attitude by prioritising patient care over personal concerns and team working. It would be unfair on your colleague to not give them the opportunity to ask any questions about the handover. The safest option is (E) as it ensures a comprehensive handover and doesn't sacrifice patient safety. The other options all involve a non-verbal handover which risks patient safety.

If you weren't given these options, you could instead talk the interviewer through your reasoning:

"So to summarise, I am faced with the situation where I am finishing my shift and the doctor taking over is running late. If I overstay, I will be late for my social commitment. If I leave, the handover will be inefficient and important information relevant to patient care may not get passed on.

In this situation, I have the option to write all the remaining tasks on paper and either give them to another person that is coming in to pass on to the next person or leave it in an office for the attention of the incoming doctor. Whilst this may be reasonable, it's not the best as there is a risk that the information may not get passed on at all or not in a timely manner which could compromise patient care.

I feel the best option would be for me to call my partner to let them know that I will be running late and wait for the incoming doctor to do a face-to-face handover"

Many students find the Mnemonic *INSIST* helpful when structuring their answers:

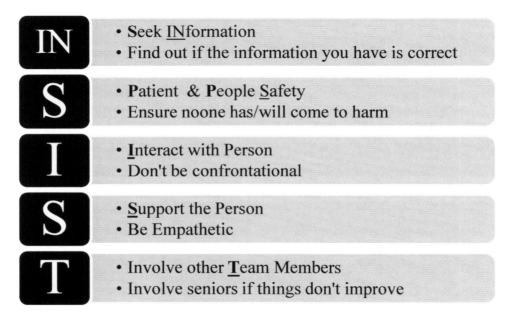

IN
- Seek <u>IN</u>formation
- Find out if the information you have is correct

S
- **P**atient & **P**eople **S**afety
- Ensure noone has/will come to harm

I
- <u>I</u>nteract with Person
- Don't be confrontational

S
- <u>S</u>upport the Person
- Be Empathetic

T
- Involve other <u>T</u>eam Members
- Involve seniors if things don't improve

Station 3: Problem-Solving Questions

You may be sent a problem-solving question a few days before your interview or get given it on the day before your interview is meant to start. These will usually not require detailed knowledge, but rather an ability to use your basic first principles. The important thing is that your argument is clear, logical, and you can give a logical step-by-step rationale for each step you made.

Consider: *A 70 kg man is trapped alive in an air-tight coffin of dimensions 2m x 0.5m x 0.3m. Estimate the amount of time that he has before he runs out of oxygen.*

➤ Clearly you do not have enough information to work this out very accurately, so you are going to have to make some assumptions. First of all, you need to work out the amount of air in the coffin, which requires you to estimate the amount of space being taken up by the man.

➤ If you use the facts that humans are made mainly out of water and that 1 gram of water = $1cm^3$ of water, you can estimate the man's volume as being $70,000$ cm^3 =$0.07m^3$.

➤ This may not be very accurate, but it at least gives you a value to use for the rest of the calculation. If the volume of the coffin is $0.3m^3$, the volume of air in the coffin = $0.3 - 0.07 = 0.23m^3$ = 230 litres of air.

➤ As air is approximately 20% oxygen, you can estimate that there are about **46 litres of oxygen** in the coffin.

➤ If you assume that the man takes in about 0.5 litres of air with every breath, then he breathes in 0.1 litres of oxygen per breath. Now you have to assume the amount of that oxygen that he uses up before exhaling- say about 5%.

➤ So with every breath, he consumes 0.1 x 0.05 = 0.005 litres of oxygen. Therefore, if he can maintain a normal respiratory rate of about 12 breaths per minute, then he will consume 0.005 x 12 = **0.06 litres of oxygen per minute** and so the oxygen will last for $\frac{46}{0.06} = 766\ minutes = 12\ hours + 46\ minutes$.

If you are given a question like this, you will be given a pen and paper to do your working. Try and lay out your working as clearly and methodically as possible to show that you have a clear line of thought. Additionally, write down your assumptions! This will help the interviewer follow your logic and will help you when you are justifying how you got to your answer.

If you are struggling to see how you would go about answering a problem, try looking at the numbers you have been given and think about what is there that is leading you, as you are unlikely to have been given irrelevant data.

If you can only see how to do part of the calculation then make sure you do that part anyway, even if it means estimating a number to use. You will at least get credit for being able to do some of it. However, do think about whether there is an alternative way to do it. If you are stuck, try to see which scientific principles you can apply.

Problem-solving questions can vary hugely. Sometimes, candidates can be handed medical instruments and be asked to use the properties of the instrument to deduce what it could be used for. The important thing to remember is that the interviewer is not expecting you to recognise the instrument right away, but rather wants to see how logical your thought processes are.

Station 4: Data Analysis

Data analysis stations tend to be written stations. There is often no examiner; all the scripts are collected and marked at the end. The format is similar to the UKCAT quantitative reasoning or BMAT Section 1 questions that you may have done. You will be presented with a table or graph and asked to use it to answer a series of questions. A calculator <u>may</u> be provided although don't assume that there will be one.

The best way to improve with these questions is to do lots of practice questions in order to familiarise yourself with the style of questions.

Options First
You will normally be given multiple answer options to choose from. You should look at these first (not the data!) as this will allow you to register what type of calculation you are required to make and what data you might need to look at for this. Remember, Options → Question → Data & Passage.

Working with Numbers
Percentages frequently make an appearance in these types of questions so it's vital that you're able to work comfortably with them. For example, you should be comfortable increasing and decreasing by percentages and working out inverse percentages too. When dealing with complex percentages, break them down into their components. For example, 17.5% = 10% + 5% + 2.5%.

Graphs and Tables
When you're working with graphs and tables, it's important that you take a few seconds to check the following before actually extracting data from it.

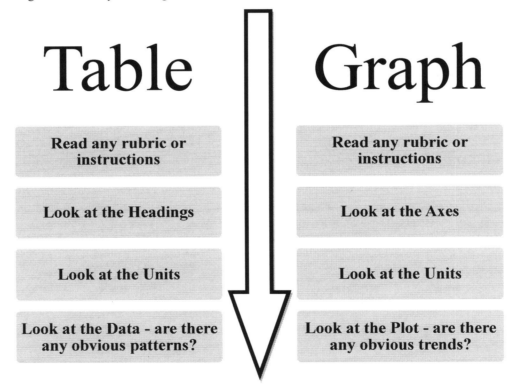

Get into the habit of doing this whenever you are faced with data and you'll find it much easier to approach these questions under time pressure.

Station 5: Video Analysis

In the video analysis station, you will need to watch a short video and then give feedback on it. Normally, the video will be an interaction between a doctor and patient and/or relative.

Common scenarios:
➢ A GP Consultation
➢ Breaking bad news e.g. cancer diagnosis
➢ Explaining medications
➢ Consenting patients for an operation

You may have to give feedback verbally to the interviewer whilst the video runs or at the end of the video. In some cases, there may not be an interviewer in which case you would need to write down your comments. The most important thing is to establish how many times you can watch the video – each viewing should allow you to pick up on more things to comment on. In general, it is better to say too much than too little – it's surprising what marks are awarded for. There are three key areas that you should focus on:

Setting
➢ Seating:
   o Are the chairs arranged appropriately?
   o They should be close together but not so much that they invade the patient's personal space.
   o Is there a desk in the way? Does this act as a physical barrier to communication?
   o Does the doctor offer the patent a seat?
➢ Privacy:
   o Is the location private so that patient confidentiality isn't breached? I.e. Office vs. Cafe
   o Are there interruptions? E.g. phone calls, mobile phones, bleeps, people knocking on door
➢ Surroundings:
   o Does it look comfortable?
   o Is there appropriate equipment necessary? E.g. Tissues and water if breaking bad news

Verbal Communication
➢ Introduction
   o Does the doctor introduce themselves?
   o Do they explain their role?
   o Do they offer a handshake?
➢ Does the doctor check the patient's identity?
➢ Starting the conversation: Does the doctor try to ascertain the patient's purpose for the visit? Look out for phrases like:
   o *"Do you know what has been happening so far?"*
   o *"Do you understand why we are here?"*
   o *"Is there anything, in particular, you were expecting today?"*
➢ Small talk: Does the doctor get straight to the point or use "icebreakers" to put the patient at ease before approaching the main topic?
   o E.g. *"How was your journey?"* or *"Would you like a drink?"*
➢ Does the Doctor avoid medical terminology?
   o Chances are that if you can't understand the terms, then nor can the patient!
➢ Does the doctor ask short and simple questions vs. long and drawn out ones?
➢ Does the doctor try to engage the patient in making it a two-way conversation?
➢ Does the doctor interrupt the patient?
➢ Is there opportunity for the patient to ask questions and how are they answered?
➢ If there are more people in the room, does the doctor only address the patient or all of them?
➢ Is there a clear conclusion and plan from the conversation?
➢ Does the doctor frequently summarise to ensure that the patient understands?

Non-Verbal Communication
➢ Are there signs of active listening and rapport building?
➢ What's the body language like?
➢ Does the doctor pick up on subtle cues by the patient or encourage them to speak?
➢ Does the doctor look stressed or under pressure? E.g. typing rather speaking with the patient or looking at their watch.

Some phrases to look out for:
➢ *"Thank you for coming. I hope my office was easy to find"*
➢ *"What can I do for you?"*
➢ *"I can see the reason..."*
➢ *"Do you understand what is wrong?"*
➢ *"How do you feel things are going so far?"*
➢ *"What would you like me to do"*
➢ *"What can I do to help?"*

Station 6: Calculations

You may sometimes be asked to work your way through a series of mathematical calculations. A calculator may or not be provided. Most questions tend to be based on calculating drug doses although anything is fair game. For more practice, it's worth revisiting UKCAT Quantitative Reasoning questions or BMAT Section 2 questions. Students tend to do poorly in these questions because they're bogged down with the extra unnecessary information that the questions contain or they are unable to convert between units comfortably.

Example Question 1
A 75-year-old woman has severe back pain; she needs a dose 675 mg Tramadol via IV infusion. Her weight is 85kg. The Tramadol IV infusion comes in 20ml vials of 10 mg/mL. How many vials do you need to use?

Solution: The patient's weight isn't needed for this calculation. She needs 675mg and each ml contains 10mg. Thus, she needs: $\frac{675\ mg}{10\frac{mg}{ml}} = 67.5$ ml. Therefore, she needs 4 vials (12.5ml will be left over).

Example Question 2
A 20-month-old, 10kg baby is admitted with severe asthma. He needs urgent Salbutamol 1 mg/kg/hr by IV infusion. Your colleague helps you by diluting Salbutamol 500 mg in glucose 5% 500 mL. What rate should the infusion be given at?

Solution: The child needs 1mg/kg/hr x 10kg = 10mg/hr. The infusion has 500mg in 500ml = 1 mg in 1 ml

Thus, the infusion should be given at: $10\frac{mg}{hr} \div 1\frac{mg}{ml} = 10\frac{ml}{hr}$

Example Question 3
A 65-year-old man is admitted with seizures and needs urgent Phenytoin delivered via IV infusion. The BNF states that the dose should be 10 mg/kg. This should be made up of sodium chloride 0.9% to yield an overall concentration of 25 mg/mL. He weighs 70 kg.

What volume of sodium chloride 0.9% is needed to prepare the IV infusion correctly?

Solution: Dose Required $= 10\ x\ 70\ =\ 700\ mg$
$Recall\ that\ n\ =\ cV$
Thus, $V\ =\ 25\ mg/ml\ =\ \frac{700mg}{25\ mg/ml} = 28\ ml$

Station 7: Writing Tasks

Sometimes, you might be asked to write down your responses to traditionally asked questions e.g. *'Why Medicine?'* instead of vocalising them to an interviewer. This has two important implications:

1) Your answer will need to be more formal than if you were vocalising it. This is because speech is naturally less formal and you can use non-verbal communications to augment your points. Since this isn't available in this task, it's imperative that you treat this as an English language exam as much as an interview.
2) Depending on the allotted time, you should first write out a draft answer on spare paper so that you can avoid ugly crossings out and scribbles. Some medical schools will judge you also on your handwriting.

Station 8: Group Tasks & Discussions

Rarely, there may be a station where you are required to work in a group. These stations require a lot of organisation on the university's part so are generally quite rare. This station's aim is to assess your ability to work in a team and communicate with your colleagues. The exact task you are asked to do can vary dramatically. For example, you might be asked to build a bridge from lego bricks or arrange a medicine-themed musical. Once the task begins, you will normally have to assign a team leader.

The important things to remember are:

➢ Ensure that you participate actively in the discussion and engage with others
➢ Know your place in the group and act appropriately
➢ Your job is not just to generate ideas but to also listen to other people's ideas
➢ If you strongly feel that you're right, then present a logical argument to persuade people
➢ Resolve any potential conflicts politely – getting cross over a minor issue is far worse than accepting a sub-optimal solution
➢ Never interrupt anyone or overpower anyone (even if you're the designated leader)
➢ Don't shoot people down - respect their views; avoid railroading the group down one path by ignoring people's ideas and forcing your views onto them
➢ Ensure you engage everyone in the group
➢ If your group is very quiet, brainstorm by going around the group to get everyone engaged
➢ Sometimes the team leader will end up being quiet as they feel overwhelmed – support them and do everything you can to get them engaged.

Station 9: Rest Stations

Some MMI circuits have inbuilt rest stations. Use this time to calm your nerves and breathe easy. You cannot undo the mistakes you think you may have made in the previous stations and thinking about them can affect your next one. So focus and think about what you're likely to encounter in the stations that you have left – remember that there are unlikely to be two stations examining the same skills or topics.

Feel free to grab a quick drink of water and snacks. Avoid chewing gum and anything that could ruin your clothes. Leave all your snacks at this station – don't take them with you. Five minutes should be plenty to re-energise yourself.

And don't worry if you start at a rest station – lots of research has shown that it makes very little difference to your overall score.

OXBRIDGE INTERVIEWS

Oxbridge medical interviews are more scientifically rigorous and demanding than the traditional style interviews. They are much more likely to focus on the human side of biology (physiology, pathology, pharmacology, etc.) although questions on chemistry and physics are still fair game.

Most applicants will have at least two interviews at Oxbridge - one is likely to be a 'general' one- similar in style to the classical medical interviews (with questions like *how do you deal with stress?* etc.). The second will likely be more science-based. This section focuses more on the latter science-based interviews.

In general, you'll be **tackling a large question with many smaller sub-questions** to guide the answer from the start to a conclusion. The main question may seem difficult, impossible or random at first, but take a deep breath and start discussing different ideas that you have for breaking the question down into manageable pieces.

The questions are designed to be difficult to give you the chance to **show your full intellectual potential**. The interviewers will help guide you to the right idea provided you work with them and offer ideas for them to steer you along with. This is your chance to show your creativity, analytical skills, intellectual flexibility, problem-solving skills, and your go-getter attitude. Don't waste it by letting your nerves overtake or from a fear of messing up or looking stupid.

The purpose of Oxbridge interviews is to gauge your intellectual potential and teachability. Interviewers are trying to identify if you're able to apply basic scientific principles to come up with plausible theories or explanations. You're likely to be asked on topics that you have little prior knowledge; interviewers will be testing to see whether you can logically come to an answer using basic first principles. They will guide you in the process so pick up on their prompts.

Ultimately, the **Oxbridge interview process** is meant to reflect the supervisions that you will reflect at uni. These are led by a senior academic and they're testing what you're like under pressure and whether you can hold intelligent, well-thought-out conversations on topics you won't be totally familiar with. Remember, it's not about the right answer, but your thought process and ideas.

OXBRIDGE INTERVIEWS ARE **NOT** ABOUT YOUR KNOWLEDGE

THEY ARE ABOUT WHAT YOU CAN DO
WITH THE KNOWLEDGE YOU ALREADY POSSES

General Advice

➤ Apply the knowledge you have acquired at A-Level and from your wider reading to unfamiliar scenarios.

➤ **Stand your ground if you are confident in your argument**- even if your interviewers disagree with you. They may deliberately play the devil's advocate to see if you are able to defend your argument.

➤ However, if you are making an argument that is clearly wrong and are being told so by the interviewers - then concede your mistake and revise your viewpoint. Do not stubbornly carry on arguing a point that they are saying is wrong.

➤ Remember, making mistakes is no bad thing. The important point is that you address the mistake head on and adapt the statement with their assistance where necessary.

➤ The **tutors know what subjects you have studied at A-Level** so don't feel pressured to read EVERY aspect of your subject.

How to Communicate Answers

The most important thing to do when communicating your answers is to **think out loud**. This will allow the interviewer to understand your thought processes. They will then be able to help you out if you get stuck. You should never give up on a question to show that you won't be perturbed at the first sign of hardship as a student and to stay positive and **demonstrate your engagement with the material**. Interviewers enjoy teaching and working with students who are as enthusiastic about their subject as they are.

Try to **keep the flow of conversation going** between you and your interviewer so that you can engage with each other throughout the entire interview. The best way to do this is to just keep talking about what you are thinking. It is okay to take a moment when confronted with a difficult question or plan your approach, but ensure you let the interviewer know this by saying, *"I'm going to think about this for a moment"*. Don't take too long- if you are finding the problems difficult, the **interviewers will guide and prompt you** to keep you moving forward. They can only do this if they realise you're stuck!

The questions that you'll be asked are designed to be difficult, so don't panic up when you don't immediately know the answer. Tell the interviewer what you do know, offer some ideas, talk about ways you've worked through a similar problem that might apply here. If you've never heard anything like the question asked before, say that to the interviewer, *"I've never seen anything like this before"* or *"We haven't covered this yet at school"*, but don't use that as an excuse to quit. This is **your chance to show that you are eager to engage with new ideas**, so finish with *"But let's see if I can figure it out!"* or *"But I'm keen to try something new!"*. There are many times at Oxbridge when students are in this situation during tutorials/supervisors and you need to show that you can persevere in the face of difficulty (and stay positive and pleasant to work with while doing so).

Types of Questions:

➢ Observation-based questions ("Tell me about this…")
➢ Practical questions ("How would you determine that…")
➢ Statistical questions ("Given this data…")
➢ Ethical questions ("Are humans obligated to…", "What are the implications of…")
➢ Proximate causes (mechanism; "How does…") and ultimate causes (function; "Why does…") - usually both at once

The questions also have recurring themes because they are important for biological theory and research: Natural and sexual selection, genetics and inheritance, human body systems, global warming and environmental change, and general knowledge of plants, animals, bacteria and pathogens.

The Oxbridge medical courses are all about taking your core science – your anatomy, physiology, pathology – and building on top of them later with clinical experience. By asking the types of questions that you can't just repeatedly practice ("I want to do medicine because…") you are forced to **take a step back, think about what you do know and form a logical argument**. It's not the answer they're looking for, but the way you think it through. That's an excellent indicator of the kind of student you'll be.

Of course, interview preparation for the 'standard' questions is absolutely necessary – your reasons for doing medicine and applying to Oxbridge will roll off the tongue soon enough. But additionally, for those questions where you don't have a pre-packaged answer, keeping calm and realising that you actually know a lot more than you think and relaying this to the interviewers in a relaxed and confident way – whether your answer is right or not – is a very desirable skill.

Final Advice

1) **Don't be put off by what other candidates say** in the waiting room. Focus on yourself – you are all that matters. If you want to be in the zone, then I would recommend taking some headphones and your favourite music.

2) **Don't read up on multiple advanced topics in depth.** Choose one topic and know it well. Focus the rest of your time on your core A-level syllabus. You are not expected to know about the features of Transverse Myelitis, but you will be expected to be able to rattle off a list of 10 cellular organelles.

3) **Don't worry about being asked seemingly irrelevant questions** that you'll often hear in the media. These are taken out of context. Focus on being able to answer the common questions, e.g. "Why this university?" etc.

4) **Don't lose heart** if your interviews appear to have gone poorly. If anything, this can actually be a good sign as it shows that the interviewer pushed you to your limits rather than giving up on you as you clearly weren't Oxbridge material.

5) **Don't give up.** When you're presented with complex scenarios, go back to the absolute basics and try to work things out using first principles. By doing this and thinking out loud, you allow the interviewer to see your logical train of thought so that they can help you when you become stuck.

6) **Practice.** There is no substitute for hard work. Work your way through Oxbridge style problems – there are over 100 available in *The Ultimate Oxbridge Interview Guide* (www.uniadmissions.co.uk/oxbridge-interview-book). Practice questions with other applicants and also consider attending an Oxbridge medicine course for professional practice and advice (www.uniadmissions.co.uk/oxbridge-interview-course).

EXTRA READING

The obvious way to prepare for any Medical School interview is to **read widely**. This is important so that you can mention books and interests in your personal statement. It is also important because it means that you will be able to draw upon a greater number and variety of ideas for your interview.

> ➢ **Make a record** of the book, who wrote it, when they wrote it, and summarise the argument. This means that you have some details about your research in the days before the interview.
> ➢ **Reading is a passive exercise.** To make it genuinely meaningful, you should **engage with the text**. Summarise the argument. Ask yourself questions like how is the writer arguing? Is it a compelling viewpoint?
> ➢ **Quality over Quantity.** This is not a race as to how many books you can read in a short period of time. It is instead a test of your ability to critically analyse and synthesise information from a text – something you'll be doing on a daily basis at Medical School.
> ➢ **Refresh yourself before your interview.** If you've mentioned a book in your personal statement and haven't read it for several months, ensure you flick through it again to refresh yourself.

It's generally a good idea to read at least two books – ideally, one that is science-based and another that explores what it is like to be a doctor. The best students will do much of their reading during the summer and then reference these books in their personal statement. They will also continue reading on a weekly basis throughout the interview process to ensure they keep up-to-date in new healthcare findings, e.g. Student BMJ, New Scientist, etc. If you've mentioned a book in your personal statement or during the interview, you should be prepared to summarise the main points of the books and identify a few areas that you found particularly interesting.

The books given below are not a mandatory reading list but simply a suggestion in case you're not sure what you are looking for. There are literally hundreds of excellent books on medical practice and/or the medical sciences, so take your pick and read something that interests you. As long as you can demonstrate the initiative to do extra reading and interest in what you have read, it really doesn't matter what books you pick.

Medical Practice
1. *Tomorrow's Doctors* by the GMC – especially the 'Outcomes for graduates' section
2. *Complications: A Surgeon's Notes on an Imperfect Science* by Atul Gawande
3. *Trust me I'm a Junior Doctor*: Max Pemberton
4. *Confessions of a GP*: Benjamin Daniels
5. *Sick Notes*: Tony Copperfield
6. *Suburban Shaman*: Cecil Helman

Medical Science
7. *The Selfish Gene*: Richard Dawkins
8. *The Extended Phenotype*: Richard Dawkins
9. *The Single Helix*: Steve Jones
10. *Bully for Brontosaurus*: Stephen Jay Gould
11. *Bad Science:* Ben Goldacre
12. *Bad Pharma:* Ben Goldacre
13. *The Tell-Tale Brain:* V.S. Ramachandran
14. *Nature Via Nurture:* Matt Ridley

UCAS Success
15. *The Ultimate BMAT Guide:* Rohan Agarwal
16. *The Ultimate UKCAT Guide:* David Salt
17. *The Ultimate Medical Personal Statement Guide:* Rohan Agarwal
18. *The Ultimate Oxbridge Interview Guide:* Rohan Agarwal

Organisations

The NHS
The National Health Service (NHS) was established in 1948. Its basic ideology is that treatment is available to all, regardless of socioeconomic status or ability to pay. It remains free (except dental services and nominal prescription charges). Eye tests and prescription glasses are not included on the NHS.

The secretary of health is responsible for the work of the department of health (DoH) which takes overall responsibility for NHS, mental health, social services and public health. The NHS can be broadly split into primary and secondary care. Primary care consists of General Practice surgeries and other community-based services; secondary care is hospital-based and involves specialist doctors.

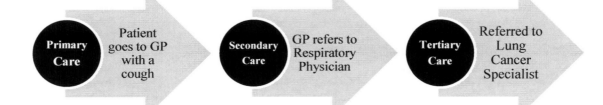

Patients are generally referred to secondary care by their GP or via A&E. Rarely, secondary care specialists may also refer patients onto tertiary care centres in complex cases. As GPs can resolve 90% of patient's problems, this reduces the pressures on secondary care centres. Therefore, it avoids specialist doctors spending time with patients that less specialised doctors could manage with.

The GMC
The General Medical Council (GMC) is the regulating body for doctors in the UK. All doctors must be registered with the GMC in order to practice as a doctor. If a doctor is found to be in breach of the GMC's code of conduct, their licence to practice may be revoked – preventing them from practising medicine in the UK.

NICE
The National Institute of Health and Care Excellence (NICE) provides national guidance and advice on how to improve healthcare. These guidelines are concerned with analysing how effective and affordable healthcare services are.

Clinical Commissioning Groups
Clinical Commissioning Groups (CCGs) are responsible for choosing which services should be offered to people in a local area. They can choose to commission NHS-based services or, in some cases, private ones e.g. Virgin. CCGs basically buy services from hospitals, hospices and other community services.

The EWTD

The European Working Time Directive (EWTD) is an EU law that is designed to prevent employees from working excessively long hours as it would compromise their health and safety. For doctors, this means:

➤ Doctors should work a maximum of 48 hours per week on average
➤ Doctors should get at least 11 hours rest per day (i.e. no shifts longer than 13 hours/day)
➤ Doctors are entitled to a rest break if they work more than six consecutive hours
➤ A minimum of 5.6 weeks of paid annual leave

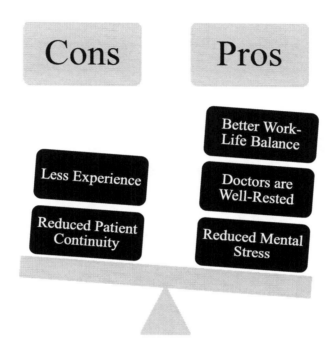

The EWTD helps doctors by ensuring that they are rested and have a good work-life balance. However, it does mean that they get less clinical experience. Furthermore, since doctors get more days off to compensate for periods of long calls (to ensure average hours are <48 per week), it means that there is reduced patient continuity – with different doctors seeing patients on different days.

Doctors can opt-out of the EWTD if they wish to but it must be done without any undue pressure. It remains unclear what the implications of Brexit on the EWTD will be.

Clinical Governance

You don't need to know too much about clinical governance. Essentially, it is a system through which **NHS hospitals and CCGs** (vs. Doctors and other healthcare professionals) are responsible for:

1) Maintaining good standards of care
2) Learning from mistakes
3) Improving the quality of services that patients are provided

Junior Doctors Contract

In September 2015, Jeremy Hunt, the minister for health, proposed a new contract for junior doctors (FY1 to senior registrar). He justified this by saying the NHS needed to be a '7 Day Service' (even though all inpatients were already looked after 24/7). This was based on the apparent observation that patients admitted on weekends had a greater mortality than those admitted on a weekday. This finding was highly disputed with many prominent academics and clinicians accusing the health secretary of misrepresenting data. The major contract changes were:

➤ Removal of overtime rates for work between 07:00 – 22:00 on every day except Sunday
➤ Small increase in Basic Pay of approximately 10%
➤ Reduction of the number of maximum hours per week from 91 to 72

This meant that doctors would be paid the same rate for working Tuesday morning as Saturday evening. This also meant potentially working many more weekends than previously. The British Medical Association (BMA), the doctor's union, declared several days of strikes. These resulted in the cancellation of thousands of operations and clinics. Despite significant opposition, Jeremy Hunt declared in July 2016 that he would unilaterally impose the contract on all junior doctors with it being implemented from October 2016 onwards.

This is a very politically charged issue – it's important you try to remain impartial and apolitical if you're asked questions like, *"Should doctors ever strike?"* or *"Would you strike as a doctor?"*.

Clinical Trials

Clinical trials are experiments done to investigate new treatments. Commonly, clinical trials investigate the safety and effectiveness of new drugs vs. existing drugs. There are three phases:

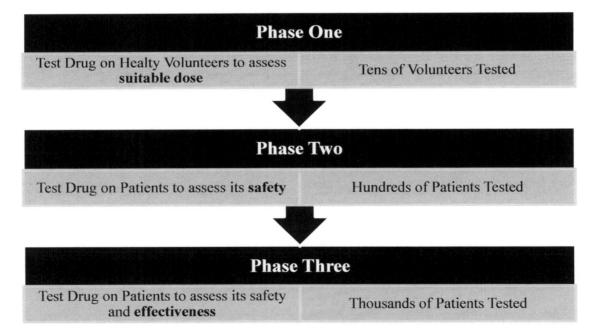

Phase One	
Test Drug on Healty Volunteers to assess **suitable dose**	Tens of Volunteers Tested

Phase Two	
Test Drug on Patients to assess its **safety**	Hundreds of Patients Tested

Phase Three	
Test Drug on Patients to assess its safety and **effectiveness**	Thousands of Patients Tested

Medical Training

After graduating from medical school (5-6 years), every doctor must do 2 years of 'foundation training'. At the end of the first foundation year (FY1), doctors will get full registration with the GMC to practice medicine. After the second year (FY2), they have several choices. They can apply for:

➢ Core Medical Training if they wish to pursue a medical speciality, e.g. cardiology, respiratory, endocrine, gastroenterology, rheumatology, nephrology etc. [2 Years]
➢ Core Surgical Training if they wish to pursue a surgical speciality, e.g. colorectal surgery, upper gastrointestinal surgery, vascular surgery etc. [2 Years]
➢ Other Speciality training if they wish to pursue other specialities like paediatrics, psychiatry, obstetrics/gynaecology, radiology etc. [5 – 9 Years depending on the speciality]
➢ GP training if they wish to become a GP. [3 Years]

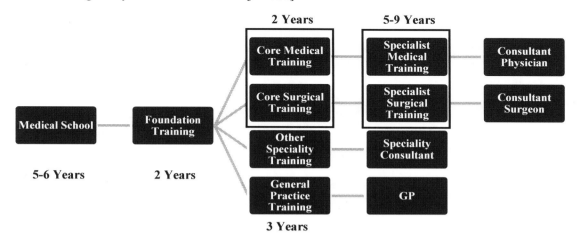

It can take in excess of 10 years to become a consultant in many specialities – more if you include the time that doctors may take to do additional degrees like PhDs and MDs. It may also take longer if the doctor isn't able to pass all their postgraduate examinations in a timely manner, e.g. MRCP and MRCS.

Revalidation

Revalidation is a process that all doctors must undergo in order to prove that they have kept themselves up-to-date with advances in medicine and guideline developments. Revalidation was introduced to restore public faith in doctors following the Harold Shipman Scandal. Doctors must undergo revalidation every five years – they must provide evidence of things like attending conferences, reading research, etc. It is necessary in order for doctors to keep their medical licence and intends to assure patients and employers of the doctor's quality.

The Audit Cycle

An audit is a systematic investigation into a system to see how it is performing when compared to national guidelines. It allows us to identify any potential problems that might be preventing good medical practice. Once these problems are identified, changes are made to try to resolve them. After a period of time, the audit is repeated again – completing the audit cycle. Hopefully, the changes result in an improvement in healthcare.

Doctors are encouraged to do audits as they can lead to valuable improvements in clinical care. Audits can occur at many levels:

➤ Nationally, e.g. National Stroke Audit
➤ Hospital-Based, e.g. ensuring that all patients are reviewed by a consultant daily
➤ On a ward, e.g. ensuring that all thermometers are correctly calibrated

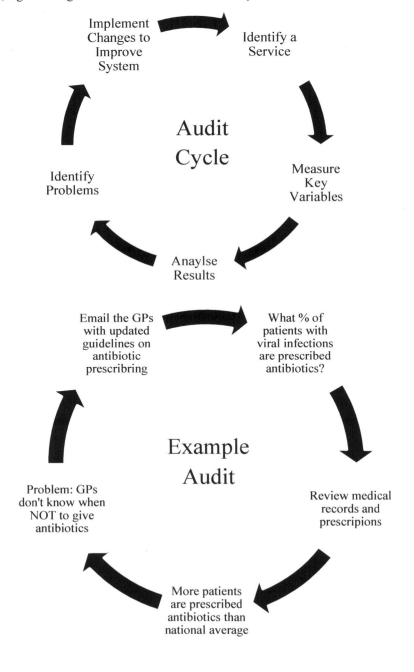

NHS Scandals:

Failings within the NHS can be at several levels; several scandals have rocked the NHS recently. Whilst Harold Shipman is an example of an individual failing their patients, Bristol Heart and Alder Hey are examples of large institutions failing to recognise a problem. The Mid-Staffs scandal was also a failure by the regulatory bodies in addition to the institutions and individuals. Lessons have been learned and changes implemented to make NHS better managed and regulated.

Harold Shipman

Dr Shipman trained as a practising GP. The death rate amongst his elderly patients was unusually high. Further police investigation revealed that he had:

➢ Falsified medical records on his computer
➢ Overprescribed morphine-like drugs to people that needed them
➢ Falsely prescribed morphine-like drugs to those that did not need them
➢ Collected medicine from the homes of recently deceased 'to collect unused medicines for disposal'
➢ Made false calls to 999 in the presence of family but then cancelled the call, stating that the patient had passed away
➢ Forged wills of his patients that then passed away - benefitting him financially

He was investigated and proven guilty of murdering his patients. Further investigations revealed that he may have murdered at least 218 patients. He was sent to prison where he committed suicide. This eventually led to massive changes in the regulation of the medical profession and introduction of several reforms, e.g. revalidation to restore public's faith in the profession.

Bristol Hearts Investigation

At Bristol Royal Infirmary, a newly appointed consultant anaesthetist noticed that cardiac surgery was taking longer and babies were dying at a higher rate than elsewhere. He did an audit which resulted in a formal investigation.

The investigation found that 29 children died and more were left with disabilities as a result of poor standards. Two cardiothoracic surgeons were permanently banned from practising as doctors again. The enquiry found that the poor performance was due to:

➢ Poor management and lack of leadership within the organisation
➢ Poor quality checks on surgical performance
➢ A lack of monitoring led to a delay in identifying the problem
➢ Raising concerns was difficult as senior managers weren't approachable

The enquiry concluded that the key problem was that there weren't enough hospital quality checks to identify failings early on. The enquiry resulted in several big changes:

➢ Hospitals were monitored more closely by regulating bodies
➢ There was a change in mentality to a 'No Blame Culture'
➢ National League tables for hospitals were introduced
➢ A framework for National standards of care was established

Alder Hay Investigation

The Alder Hey organs scandal involved the removal and retention of children's organs without family consent from 1988 to 1995. An enquiry was initiated after a baby died undergoing open-heart surgery at Bristol Royal Infirmary (see Bristol Hearts Investigation). Her mother discovered years later that her heart had been stored by the hospital and generated significant media attention. Hospitals had to pay millions of pounds in compensation to affected families.

An investigation showed that organs were being retained 'routinely' by hospitals across the UK. This resulted in *The Human Tissue Act* that ensured that the removal, storage, use and disposal of human bodies, organs, and tissue was properly regulated and done with appropriate consent. To this day, anonymous organ donation is acceptable but selling organs is illegal.

Mid-Staffs Investigation

In 2008, Stafford Hospital was reported to have abnormally high mortality rates and poor care. This led to an external enquiry which concluded that there were over 1,000 avoidable patient deaths. It also said that patients had received very poor care with many not being cleaned for prolonged periods of time. It said that these were caused by short staffing, poorly trained staff, poor management, and falsification of data to 'balance the books'.

This resulted in:

➢ Introduction of a duty of candour (being open and honest with patients when mistakes occur)
➢ Financial Compensation for affected patients and families
➢ Resignation of several senior managers
➢ Publication of mortality rates for each hospital online

MMR Vaccine Controversy

The Measles, Mumps and Rubella (MMR) vaccine controversy started in 1998 after Andrew Wakefield, a medical researcher, published a fraudulent paper in *The Lancet* that showed an apparent link between the MMR vaccine and autism. The Sunday Times investigated the paper and found that Wakefield had multiple undeclared conflicts of interests, had manipulated data and broken several ethical codes. The GMC found Wakefield guilty of serious professional misconduct and removed him from the medical register. *The Lancet* also fully retracted his paper. Multiple large studies were conducted to investigate the issue – none of them found any link between MMR and autism.

As a result of the paper, vaccination rates in the UK dropped dramatically which resulted in significant increases in measles and mumps resulting in several avoidable children dying. A similar pattern was also observed internationally. There has been a concerted effort to re-immunise children that didn't have the MMR vaccine in recent years to improve healthcare.

Medical Ethics

The GMC is pushing for medical school interviews to become more heavily focussed on assessing the values held by the candidate. Do not get bogged down by excessive amounts of detail. Instead, familiarise yourself with the main principles and points of debate in medical ethics. I recommend reading *Medical Ethics: A Very Short Introduction* by Tony Hope, which gives a brief and accessible overview. When presented with a question on medical ethics, it can be useful to think about how the main principles of medical ethics apply.

You may be asked questions that appear difficult or you may have your own views. You need to demonstrate that you understand the ethical issue and apply your knowledge to come up with a plausible reply. Sometimes, the answer may not be immediately obvious to you. It is normal. Do not get deterred by this. Think it through. Apply the principles of medical ethics and the answer will be clear. The main principles of medical ethics are often said to be:

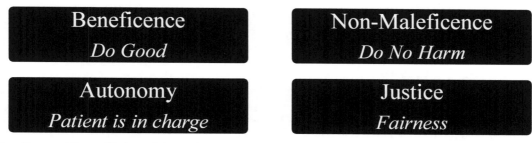

Beneficence: The wellbeing of the patient should be the doctor's first priority. In medicine, this means that one must act in the patient's best interests to ensure the best outcome is achieved for them, i.e. 'Do Good'.
Non-Maleficence: This is the principle of avoiding harm to the patient, keeping with the Hippocratic Oath "First do no harm". There can be a danger that in a willingness to treat, doctors can sometimes cause more harm to the patient than good. This can especially be the case with major interventions, such as chemotherapy or surgery. Where a course of action has both potential harms and potential benefits, non-maleficence must be balanced against beneficence.

Autonomy: The patient has the right to determine their own health care. This, therefore, requires the doctor to be a good communicator so that the patient is sufficiently informed to make their own decisions. 'Informed consent' is thus a vital precursor to any treatment. A doctor must respect a patient's refusal for treatment even if they think it is not the correct choice. Note that patients cannot demand treatment – only refuse it, e.g. an alcoholic patient can refuse rehabilitation but cannot demand a liver transplant.

There are many situations where the application of autonomy can be quite complex, for example:
➢ **Treating children:** Consent is required from the parents, although the autonomy of the child is taken into account increasingly as they get older.
➢ **Treating adults without the <u>capacity</u>** to make important decisions. The first challenge with this is in assessing whether or not a patient has the capacity to make the decisions. Just because a patient has a mental illness does not necessarily mean that they lack the capacity to make decisions about their health care. Where patients do lack capacity, the power to make decisions is transferred to the next of kin (or Legal Power of Attorney, if one has been set up).

Justice: This deals with the fair distribution and allocation of healthcare resources for the population.

Consent: This is an extension of Autonomy- patients must agree to a procedure, treatment or intervention. For consent to be valid, it must be **a voluntary informed consent.** This means that the patient must have sufficient mental capacity to make the decision and must be presented with all the relevant information (benefits, side effects, and the likely complications) in a way they can understand.

Confidentiality: Patients expect that the information they reveal to doctors will be kept private- this is a key component in maintaining the trust between patients and doctors. You must ensure that patient details are kept confidential. Confidentiality can be broken if you suspect that a patient is a risk to themselves or to others, e.g. terrorism, child abuse, informing the DVLA if a patient is at risk of seizures, road accidents, etc.

When answering a question on medical ethics, you need to ensure that you show an appreciation for the fact that there are often two sides of the argument. Where appropriate, you should outline both points of view and how they pertain to the main principles of medical ethics and then come to a reasoned judgement.

It is important to know that sometimes the beneficence and autonomy may be in conflict. For example, a patient is denying treatment that could be lifesaving. It is possible that sometimes the patients make decisions that are not correct or in conflict with beneficence duties of a doctor. When faced with such scenarios, try to understand the reasoning of the patient. Is it because of fear, ignorance or something different, e.g. religious beliefs. If the decisions of the patients are fully informed and the patient has the capacity to make well-informed decisions (patient is not confused due to illness/drugs or mental illness), clinicians should respect the autonomy of the patient.

Mental Capacity Act

The primary purpose of the 2005 act is to govern the decision-making process on behalf of adults who lack the capacity to make decisions for themselves. There are several principles to be aware of:

1. A person must be assumed to have capacity unless proven otherwise.
2. A person is not to be treated as unable to make a decision unless all practicable steps to help them to do so have been taken without success.
3. A person is not to be treated as unable to make a decision merely because they make an unwise decision.
4. An act must be in their best interest.
5. The act must be the least restrictive with regards to the individual's freedoms.

Capacity

Medical capacity arose from the Mental Capacity Act. It's the patient's ability to decide that they can make specific decisions about their care. The capacity is time and 'point' specific, meaning that they may not have the capacity to make complex financial decisions but can take decisions if they would like to have/decline specific treatment. This can change in time so there may be a time when they have capacity but other times when they don't (even within days or hours, depending on their clinical condition). For example, a patient admitted with a severe infection may not have capacity on their first day in hospital but this may change as they improve with treatment.

When assessing capacity, it is important to know that the individual does not have an underlying mental illness or a reason to compromise their decision-making abilities.

Important things to consider are:
- Can the patient understand the information?
- Can the patient retain the information?
- Can they analyse the information correctly?
- Can they communicate their choices clearly?

Any missing steps can lead to the patient having a 'lack of capacity'. It is important to understand this as doctors are often faced with situations where patients may make decisions that are not in keeping with the acceptable norms (e.g. Jehovah's Witness refusing blood products and having serious blood loss). Carrying out procedures or treatment that directly contravenes a patient's wishes who has capacity is a breach of patient's autonomy.

Doctors should consider a formal mental capacity assessment in the following scenarios:
1. Sudden change in mental status
2. Refusal to treatment, e.g. unclear reason or due to irrational biases/beliefs
3. Known psychiatric/neurologic condition
4. People at extreme of ages < 18 years or > 85 years

Medical Law

Understanding the principles of medical law is essential. Here is a brief overview of some key legal cases and principles that you should familiarise yourself with:

Mental Health Act

This act basically governs how heath care professionals interact with people with mental disorders and their rights to force treatment. The original act was passed in 1983, but there has been a significant amendment in 2007. The most significant components for health professionals are the definition of holding powers which allow doctors to detain and treat a patient with a mental illness against their will. Most notably, these are the section 5(2) and 5(4) defining doctors' and nurses' duties respectively. Other orders to be aware off are Section 135 (magistrate order) and section 136 (police order). You should hopefully have covered these during your psychiatry rotations.

Data Protection Act

This act gives the GMC power to control how data is collected, recorded and used. Personal data under the act is defined as identifiable information. It's important that data is:

1)   Processed fairly and lawfully
2)   Gathered for specific purposes.
3)   The data is adequate, relevant, accurate, and kept up to date

This governs how doctors collect patient information and who they can share this information with. Practical examples are doctors being allowed to break confidentiality for acts of suspected terrorism and road traffic accidents.

Gillick Competence

Children under the age of 18 can consent to treatment if they are able to understand, weigh up, and decide they want the treatment. However, they cannot refuse treatment until they are 18 years old. For children under 18 with no parent/guardian who aren't Gillick competent, you are able to act 'in their best interest'.

Bolam Test

The Bolam test is a legal rule that assesses the appropriateness of reasonable care in negligence cases involving a skilled professional. The Bolam test states *"If a doctor reaches the standard of a responsible body of medical opinion, he is not negligent"*. In order for someone to be shown to be negligent, it must be established that:
1)   There was a duty of care
2)   The duty of care was breached
3)   The breach directly led to the patient being harmed

Euthanasia

Euthanasia is a deliberate intervention undertaken with the express intention of ending a life to alleviate pain and suffering. The two main types of euthanasia are:

➤   Active Euthanasia: Doctor causes the patient to die, e.g. by injecting poison
➤   Passive Euthanasia: Doctor lets the patient die, e.g. withdrawing life-sustaining treatment, switch off life-supporting machines

Active Euthanasia is classed as murder in the UK and is illegal. Passive euthanasia is legal. You should know the main arguments for and against active euthanasia (covered in *'Why is euthanasia such a controversial topic?'*).

QUESTION TITLES

Whilst the list of questions provided is not exhaustive, it does cover the vast majority of styles of questions that you are likely to be asked. However, there are no guarantees and you could potentially be asked things that you've never heard of anybody else being asked in interviews.

Nevertheless, don't be afraid of the unknown. Keep in mind the qualities that interviewers are looking for and go for it! Remember, what's more important is your ability to deliver genuine answers that are tailored to you – **don't try to rote learn and recite the example answers given in this book.**

Motivation Questions

Medical Ethics Questions

Knowledge-Based Questions

Communication Skills Questions

Personal Attribute Questions

Voluntary & Work Experience Questions

Miscellaneous Questions

Oxbridge Questions

MOTIVATION

1) Why Medicine? Why do you want to be a doctor?

You are almost guaranteed to be asked this question in every medical school interview you attend. Hence it is essential that you have prepared a flawless answer for it. The best way to approach this question is by being very honest and very detailed in your answer. It can be difficult to know where to start when answering this question. You could look at your personal statement and bullet point the reasons you stated there of why you wanted to do medicine or start a mind-map to help you reflect and drag out the deep-rooted motivation behind your decision to study medicine. This could be the opening of your single long interview or a station in MMI.

Bad Response A:

"I have always been a caring person. I cared greatly for my pets when I was younger and took a great interest whenever my friends or family became ill. Whenever I was taught a new scientific fact about the human body, I would always be the first in school to ask questions and do my own research to find out more. I have always admired doctors and looked up to them as role models in my life. There is no other profession that I respect more. In addition, my mum is a doctor and she'd like me to be a doctor too."

Bad Response B:

"I want to be a doctor because I would like to help people and save lives. I don't think I am made for an office job and medicine offers lots of variety. Doctors play an important role in society which is something I would love to aspire to. The money's not bad either!"

Bad Response Analysis:

This answer shows very poor insight into the intricacies and the unglamorous reality of the medical profession. The candidate's example of their caring nature is distanced from the reality of using specialised medical skills and knowledge to treat patients. This answer is very focused on the past and does not mention how the candidate currently feels about medicine. The candidate does not explain himself or herself in enough depth; they need to reflect more and explain why they respect the medical profession. The opportunity to show your qualities, i.e. hard work, keenness to learn, your empathic nature, is missed in the above response.

Each point has been poorly expanded on and leaves a lot to be desired. The answer is idealistic and does not demonstrate an understanding into what life is actually like as a doctor. Everyone says they want to help people and save lives, so saying it in this way will not help you to stand out from the crowd. Although medicine does offer a lot of variety, the way this answer is phrased makes medicine seem like more of a last resort instead of something you have a burning enthusiasm for!

Doctors are indeed key members of society, but the answer fails to describe how and why this is, and instead, it seemingly focuses on the desire for prestige. It is perhaps best not to mention pay in your answer to this question, even if it is a factor for you!

Good Response A:

"I am very interested in people. I love working as part of a team and forming personal and professional relationships with others. I find it exceptionally rewarding to learn about how other people view the world and believe medicine provides the opportunity to make uniquely trusting relationships between a patient and a doctor. I also have a great passion for science and scientific discovery. I am fascinated by scientific mechanisms and their complexities and I greatly enjoy the process of learning about them. My work experience has also consolidated my belief that a career in the medical profession is right for me. I was confronted with the unglamorous reality of medicine for both the patient and the doctor, but I began to understand how rewarding the job of a doctor can be. I greatly admire the concept of making the care of the patient the doctor's first concern."

Good Response B:
"I found my volunteer work as a care assistant in X Hospice incredibly rewarding and this confirmed for me the decision to choose a career that would allow me to interact with a great variety of people and play a crucial role in their wellbeing."

Good Response C:
"There are many different reasons for why I think being a doctor is the right career path and lifestyle choice for me. First of all, I think medicine as an academic discipline is absolutely fascinating and it is a genuine privilege to be able to even partly understand the way our bodies work. To be able to put this theory into practice in order to change and save lives would be the ultimate achievement. The skills obtained through studying and practicing medicine are lifelong and transferrable throughout all walks of life, however, the ever-evolving nature of medicine ensures that doctors are constantly learning new things and adapting their practices. These attributes of medicine are incredibly important to me and I believe I would thrive under the pressure this would inevitably bring. I also believe I am a good communicator and would love a job that involves lots of interaction with other people: a vital part of being a doctor is interpersonal communication and teamwork, which I feel I excel at."

Good Response Analysis:
There is no one right answer; there should be lots of reasons for why you want to be a doctor! The above answer incorporates lots of different reasons to want to pursue medicine – think about the qualities/attributes you think are important to being a doctor, and which ones reflect you personally.

Some of these mentioned above include: academia and hard work, practical skills, adaptability, communication and teamwork. It may sound cheesy/over-used to say you want to go into medicine to help people, but it is actually true, so find a unique way of expressing this. Despite this answer being relatively short, all of these features are incorporated into it and demonstrate an insight into the life of a doctor. Moreover, I think it is also important to demonstrate an understanding that it is a lifestyle, more than just a job!

These answers are robust and complete. They show that the candidate understands that a wide range of skills are necessary to be a good doctor, that they have made a well-considered application to medicine, and that they are passionate about a range of aspects of medicine. References to a candidate's work experience is especially creditable as it shows an active interest in and a realistic perspective of medicine.

Overall:
You must avoid a generic answer by making your response personal and including fine detail. Your answer to this question should be relatively long; make sure you highlight your passion for medicine and use reflective language. You may find it useful to make some leading comments, which the interview can ask you follow up questions on; this can allow you to take control of the direction of the interview and show off your strengths. Be warned that your answer may be dissected by follow-up questions. For the above example, a potential follow-up question and a good potential answer are outlined below.

A good candidate can use the follow-up questions to give more details about their motivations and demonstrate even more of the qualities that the interviewers are looking for. Equally, if you give an interest in science and using science to help people as your primary motivation for studying medicine, be prepared to explain why you would not rather go straight into a career in research. Similarly, think about what areas of human science have sparked your interest already. You can use what you have included in your personal statement to build your answer. For example, you could say "my project on the genetics of diabetes drew my attention to the rising epidemic of obesity and diabetes". Be prepared to have some discussion about your project, diabetes or obesity or something completely different, e.g. public health issues and clinicians playing a role in disease prevention! It is important to be aware of what you have stated in your personal statement and read around relevant topics

2) Why do you want to be a doctor and not a nurse?

This question does not usually come up by itself; it will often come up after a non-specific response to the question: "why do you want to be a doctor". If your response is along the lines of helping people and nothing else, then be prepared for this question. Both roles have very similar aspects so you should be able to clearly identify the distinguishing features and base your answer on these.

A Bad Response:

"I am very interested in science so I would love to combine my passion for helping people and this thirst for scientific knowledge. A nurse is only able to provide basic primary care for a patient while a doctor must diagnose a patient and then provide the treatment. The medical curriculum for a doctor involves the human anatomy and I would really love to learn about this in a lot of detail. Most nurses are women and I am a guy, I would get picked on if I became a nurse. Furthermore, doctors receive a much better salary which makes a career as a doctor seem more financially appealing."

Response Analysis:

The sentence about nurses being women is completely wrong and will be a grave cause of concern to the interviewers. The statement about money should also never be mentioned in a medical interview. Remember, you are going into medicine because you are passionate about helping people- money is not a factor at all. The third reason is a valid reason that is the standard response to this question, but unfortunately, the candidate has displayed a lack of knowledge on the role of nurses. Senior nurses are able to diagnose patients as well as prescribe certain treatments. Furthermore, nurses must undergo a rigorous education covering most of the same courses that medical students have but often in a lot less depth. It is, therefore, wrong to say you want to be a doctor because of science; you must say that you want to be a doctor because there is more science involved.

A Good Response:

"I am very interested in science so I would love to combine my passion for helping people and this thirst for scientific knowledge. Although a nurse is able to prescribe basic medications and provide some diagnoses, I feel that a medical education would give me a much greater understanding of science. This would allow me to deal with more complicated cases which really interest me. Finally, a career as a doctor has the additional possibility of going into clinical research as well as clinical duties. This is certainly something that I am considering."

Response Analysis:

This response is significantly better- it explains that the main difference between a doctor and a nurse is the level of science that a doctor must understand. They show an understanding of the role that nurses can play which also adds to the response. Additionally, they add a possible career interest after medical school which shows that the candidate has really thought about a career in medicine.

Overall:

Everyone in the healthcare profession must know some level of basic science, but it is the advanced knowledge that a doctor possesses which distinguishes them from other members of the healthcare team.

3) Do you think nurses are important?

This can be the leading question or a follow-on question from *why doctor* or *why medicine*, more so if your response was inadequate or badly structured. The answer to this question is obviously yes (you would be both foolish and disillusioned to answer no), but we must answer it in a way that distinguishes ourselves from other candidates. The best way to do this is to bring in specific examples; these could come from your work experience or perhaps your volunteering placements. The role of the nurses has evolved with time and they are taking on more diverse roles, e.g. educating the patients, researching, and acting as a go-between patients and doctors.

A Bad Response:

"Nurses are very important to the NHS and play an integral role in the day to day running of the health service. Although nurses cannot provide diagnoses or prescribe treatments, I have always found it nice to have the nurses around. All of the patients at my work experience really liked talking to the nurses and although they were not as important as the doctors, they made a real difference to the care of the patient."

Response Analysis:

The first factual error here is that nurses do provide prescriptions or diagnoses. Certain senior nurses are qualified to prescribe certain drugs, and furthermore, certain nurses are available to do initial checks at GP surgeries. Nurses in the UK must undergo a rigorous training program before they qualify followed by further training on the job, so it is wrong to dismiss them in this peripheral manner. The next statement that "it is nice to have the nurses around" further worsens this. It gives the wrong impression that nurses are serving no real purpose and just happen to be around the hospital. Although this may not have been the intention of the candidate, it certainly comes across in this manner and will not impress the interviewer. The final mistake is stating that nurses are not as important as doctors; this is definitely not the case and we will see how to correct this in the good response.

A Good Response:

"Nurses are very important to the NHS and play an integral role in the day to day running of the health service. In GP practices, certain senior nurses are able to examine and prescribe treatment to patients with minor conditions; the patients can be sent to a doctor if the nurse thinks it would be beneficial. This means that they help alleviate the strain of resources on the NHS and play a critical role alongside doctors. Furthermore, in my work experience, patients always found it nice to have the nurses around. The doctors may only visit the patients for a few minutes every day to see if everything is going well, but it is always the nurses who remain with the patients throughout the day; it is the nurses who often help the patients with their daily needs. I remember one nurse who would always cut up a patient's food for her and then feed her. My work experience showed me that nurses play a very important but different role alongside doctors and a crucial role in patient care."

Response Analysis:

This response is much better than the previous one, although note the level of similarity. Firstly, some of the specific roles of nurses is addressed and the factual errors of the previous answer have been corrected. Secondly, the rather loose statement that "it is nice to have nurses around" has been justified with a specific example. The answer also brings in a specific job (cutting up food) performed by a nurse showing that the student has thought about their work experience. Finally, the equal but different roles of doctors and nurses are acknowledged. The response shows that the student is aware of the changing NHS, limited resources, and different strategies that are being used to deliver cost effective services and the use of skill knowledge framework.

Overall:

This is a very standard question that may come up in a lot of medical interviews. There are lots of small traps in the question that are shown by the bad answer, but providing specific examples from work experience/volunteering will help you stand out from the rest.

4)   If you want to save lives why not become a clinical research scientist?

This question tests your motivation to study medicine and become a doctor, but also that you have a greater knowledge of the healthcare and research field in general. It is possible to do both and many clinicians do research alongside their clinical practice, so if you're unsure on whether or not you are interested in research, then explaining that the two are not necessarily mutually exclusive may be impressive to the interviewers. It is also worth considering the nature of the course at that particular institution, for example, if there is an opportunity to take an intercalated science degree or possibility to take time off for further study.

A Bad Response:

"It's true that with clinical research one has the potential to save many more lives overall, however, it lacks the patient contact that I really think I would enjoy in medicine. I haven't done any work experience in a clinical research lab, but following my medical work experience, I really think I've found the profession I want to enter. Furthermore, I believe I would enjoy a medical degree more than a pure science degree simply due to content and what I'm interested in right now."

Response Analysis:

This response is quite negative towards clinical research and doesn't analyse the merits and demerits of either career. It also does not give the impression that you're particularly informed about either job or certainly not how the two can occur together. Where you can, try to keep your answer focused on the question – this response does not talk about 'saving lives' after the first sentence.

A Good Response:

"Medical research is certainly something I might be interested in and during my medical degree, I'm planning to get involved in some local research projects. If I found an area I was particularly interested in, I would consider applying for the academic foundation programme so I could continue to do research during my foundation training. The concept of 'saving lives' is not the driving force behind me wanting to study medicine and become a doctor. A lot more of the workload, from what I have seen and experienced, is centred around quality of life. Whilst this certainly has the potential to be improved by clinical research, I think I would get great satisfaction from being on the front line of delivering that care and that is why I believe studying medicine is the right choice for me."

If the university you are applying to has a big research centre, you can include this in the answer by stating: *"This school is known for the quality research work and if an opportunity came, I would consider involving myself in the clinical research whilst pursuing medicine as a doctor."*

Response Analysis:

This answer breaks down the question and addresses each aspect separately. You sound well informed if you've researched things such as the academic foundation programme. Interviewers will not expect you to have done work experience in every related profession just so you can rule it out, but suggesting you know your own ignorance on the subject and that you'd like to experience it is unlikely to be a bad thing!

Overall:

Try not to fall into the trap of simply explaining why you don't want to do clinical research, but take a step back and think about every part of the question. It's a good idea to be well informed about the opportunities to get involved in clinical research at the institution you are interviewing at and during your training so that you can speak fluently about both the answer to their question and why you'd do well studying medicine at their university.

5) What makes this university and its medical course right for you?

Do not confuse this question with 'Why do you want to go to medical school?'!

In your medicine interview, you need to sell yourself to the interviewers and part of that is explaining why you'd suit the style of course that they offer. Try to research a little about the course before your interview and think about what attracted you to apply to that university and what it is about the course structure you particularly like. Also, try to highlight what you will bring to the course, particularly at universities offering a Problem-Based Learning style course where what the students themselves bring alters the teaching and dynamic considerably.

All universities are different, so it is important to have researched what the university has to offer that would benefit you and why/how you would fit in there. It is essential that the student knows what they are signing up for, and must show that they are the kind of person that would thrive in the sort of environment at that particular university. Thus, the answer to this question should make clear that they understand about the university and are the right sort of person for the challenge. Also, look into the extra-curricular activities and societies you might be interested in joining, e.g. your tennis or roving skills may be handy when applying to the university with an active tennis/roving team. Remember, the aim of the game is to portray how well you would fit into their university, and to demonstrate how you would contribute to university life. Sell yourself!

Having visited the university on an open day and chatted to some of the staff and students can be a good thing to talk about as it demonstrates your interest in the university enough to visit and your volition to seek out peoples' opinions. Obviously, the interviewers will assume you've applied to study medicine at other institutions, but for this question a little ego massaging can go a long way.

Bad Response A:
"I've always wanted to study at Uni-X because it has such great facilities for both medicine and for other aspects of student life. These facilities combined with the excellent teaching you have makes me think that Uni-X offers a course that would work well for me. I looked into the PBL-style course but I much prefer the idea of actually knowing something before starting to see patients, so that's why I've chosen a more traditional course like the one Uni-X offers."

Bad Response B:
"I want to go to this medical school because my interest in physiology and my desire to have a career where I can help people means I want to be a doctor. This medical school is in the top 5 in the league tables, so I think it would be good for my career to study here."

Bad Response Analysis:
This response sounds far too generic and does not give the interviewers the impression that you've visited the university or spoken to any current members. Try to explain why that specific university course is good for you and also why you would be good for that course. This response goes some way to doing that by saying that you would prefer a more traditional course. However, lots of places offer a more traditional course so make sure your answer is specific to that university. A poor candidate will often give an answer that does not properly answer the question, is not very specific to the medical school, and shows no/little consideration of the learning environment in the medical school, prioritising other factors disproportionately.

Good Response A:
"I understand that this university is extremely demanding and challenging, but this sort of pressurised environment is one in which I would thrive. I work well under pressure, and am also sure that the strong support networks that are established here will help me to complete my degree to the best of my ability. I am an active learner, and am always keen to be involved in teaching discussions. Therefore, I think that I would benefit greatly from the supervision system that is unique to this university. I am enthusiastic, sporty and outgoing, thus, would be keen to get involved with so much more that the university has to offer outside of my

degree. I am very much an active person in all aspects of my life, which I think would make me fit in well amongst all the highly motivated students that come here."

Good Response B:
"The structure of the course at this medical school really appeals to me. I think I would get the most out of clinical experiences by already having a good understanding of the basic medical sciences, and so the split between pre-clinical and clinical studies here seems a great way to achieve that. Also, I am particularly interested in anatomy and know that this medical school offers some of the best opportunities for learning anatomy from cadaveric dissection, which seems the best way to learn it to me. Also, I like that there are opportunities for regular small group teaching at this medical school, so I am pushed to demonstrate my understanding of what I have been learning and get the opportunity to ask about anything I am unclear on. When I visited the school on the open day, I was particularly impressed by the choir."

Good Response Analysis:
This response demonstrates that the student is aware of the sort of learning environment that they would be in if they came here, and seems determined that they would do well under that sort of pressure. They also show knowledge of the supervision system that operates at this particular university, which is good because that is unique to this university. Additionally, the student considers life outside of work, which is good because the university is keen to have well- rounded individuals who will make the most of the opportunities there.

A good reply will be specific and will highlight the school's achievements, matching them to the applicant's own interest, linking what is said elsewhere to compliment this, e.g. personal statement, information in school's website or prospectus and own interest etc.

Overall:
Overall, to answer this question well it is essential to show knowledge of the university system and how your own attributes would make you suit that environment. It is important to show that you actually want to come to this university for reasons other than its prestige. The student must demonstrate that they have thoroughly researched the university and really do want to go there more than other universities, for well thought through reasons.

You need to give **specific** reasons for the medical school for which you are being interviewed. Answers like "this is the best school", or "my parents wanted me to attend the best school" may please the interviewer but you need to say something of substance. The medical school's website will usually give details of its course which you should familiarise yourself with and identify how it differs from courses at other medical schools. Show that the teaching style offered is right for your learning style and that the school offers excellent support to its students. A large difference among medical schools is between those that do the integrated course type (where clinical and theory-based teaching are given in parallel) and the split course type (those that give 2-3 years of pre-clinical theory followed by 3 years of clinical teaching). Candidates opting for the former often say it is because they cannot wait to get onto the wards and practice patient interaction throughout their time at medical school. Candidates opting for the latter often say that they want a solid grounding in basic medical science before entering the clinical sphere so that they can better understand their clinical experiences.

You may have visited the school on their open days so you could start your answer by adding something that you found interesting that matches with your style/personality, and if possible, link it with something in your personal statement. Following this, you can highlight the other equally important aspects of student life, e.g. social details of the medical school (societies, sports teams etc.), showing that you have put well-rounded consideration into your choice of medical school. So if the school has a good sports team or runs a drama club, you could link your sport/drama skills. A good candidate will demonstrate specific knowledge about the medical school, be positive about it, and have a matching personality/portfolio for choosing it.

6) What do you know about the course structure here?

Background Analysis:

It is very important that you take the time to research the details of the course structure for each of the medical schools to which you have applied and how they differ from other medical schools. The websites and prospectuses of each medical school will give details of the way their course and teaching are structured. A good early thing to think about is whether pre-clinical science and clinical experience are integrated throughout the course or split into different years. Medical schools also often differ on how much problem-based learning they use, the amount of small group teaching, and whether there is the opportunity to do an intercalated degree year. It is very worth identifying a couple of points that you can talk about that particularly attract you to the course at the medical school you are being interviewed for over other medical schools.

A Bad Response:

"I think that the course here is structured so that for the first few years you study only medical science, and hospital experience is put off until the final few years. This attracts me because it is the scientific side of medicine that really appeals to me so I am looking forward to being immersed in that. As I'm not really that keen on the more clinical side, I am glad I wouldn't have to face that for a few years."

Response Analysis:

Firstly, this candidate gives very little detail about the course structure, suggesting that they have paid only cursory attention to the details of what makes studying at this medical school different. Furthermore, while there is no problem with having a leaning to the more scientific side or to the more clinical side of medicine, be careful that you do not give the impression that there are aspects of the course that you simply do not want to do. This candidate's answer could easily be interpreted, whether rightly or not, to suggest that he is not motivated for clinical studies and that there is a potential risk that medicine is not for him.

A Good Response:

"I know that the course here is split into 3 years of pre-clinical science, including an intercalate degree year, followed by 3 years of clinical studies. I enjoy this structure because I think I would like to have the background understanding of the relevant physiology, pathology, etc. before starting my clinical learning so that I can get the most out of my clinical experiences. I also know that there is a wide variety of subjects that you can pursue for your intercalated year, with the opportunity to get involved in both laboratory and clinical research. I am really attracted by this because I would like to get some research experience while at medical school. Another thing I noticed about the course structure is that you do anatomy in the first year and as part of that, students get to have weekly dissection sessions. I think I would find dissection fascinating and have heard from friends at medical school that it is the most useful way to learn anatomy. I'm also under the impression that this is the most dissection experience available at any medical school in the country, so that aspect of the course here really appeals to me."

Response Analysis:

This answer shows that the candidate has evidently been proactive in researching the course in detail and even discussing elements of it with current medical students. Furthermore, it shows that the candidate has given a fair amount of thought to what they are looking for in the course. The candidate's comparison of the course structure to that of different medical schools and explaining why they think this course structure really is best for them is also a good aspect of the answer.

Overall:

Quite simply, make sure you have looked at the course structure of the medical schools you apply for. Think about what structure and what kind of teaching may fit you best. If you have an idea about what sort of doctor you might want to be, then think about how the course structure at medical school can help you get there. For example, if you aspire to being a surgeon, then maybe think about medical schools which give more rigorous anatomy teaching or are associated with tertiary centres for surgery.

7) *How do you handle emotional issues at work?*

This question is asking you to show that you have the ability to overcome and cope with stressful situations. In answering this question, it is important to identify specific coping strategies you have used and describe how they have enabled you to cope well with stress. You need to provide evidence of self-discipline and conscientiousness. It is important to constructively analyse how you dealt with your emotional issues and describe what you learned from this experience.

A Bad Response:
"When I was working at the checkout of a supermarket I would occasionally encounter rude and disrespectful customers. I would sometimes find myself getting annoyed, aggravated, and angry with these customers. To handle these emotional issues, I focused my attention on my work, where I worked faster and did not interact with customers so much."

Response Analysis:
The emotional issue described here is very valid but the coping strategy is not. The candidate is ignoring the underlying cause of his emotional issue rather than trying to find an active solution to it. The answer can be improved slightly by rephrasing as shown below:

"When I was working at the checkout of a supermarket I would occasionally encounter rude and disrespectful customers. To handle these emotional issues, I tried to understand why the customers could be rude or angry. I started interacting with them and would ask them the reasons of their annoyance. I offered my help to make the checkouts less painful. I learned that understanding their reasons and being able to come up with something to reduce customer's anxiety/stress made them, and myself, feel better."

This response is better than the one given as it shows that you have the maturity to deal with stressful situations and can remain calm under difficult scenarios (something that can often happen with angry patient or relatives in your medical career). This response shows that rather than being angry in retaliation or shying away from the situation, you feel confident and can look for resolutions of the problem.

A Good Response:
"During my work experience, I encountered a number of situations that I had not anticipated. It was very difficult to see patients who were connected to many machines and monitors. It was difficult to see people who looked so frail and so dependent on machines; it felt like the things that made them human had been taken away from them. I felt a sense of hopelessness at seeing these patients, where it seemed to me as though the patients had lost their sense of dignity. I believed that it was necessary to share how I was feeling with the doctor I was shadowing. I raised my concerns and asked the doctor to explain the situation I was observing from his perspective. My informed understanding of the situation taught me that the monitoring and ongoing treatments were necessary to ensure the best quality of care and prognosis for the patient. I learned how all patients must fully consent to the treatment they are being given and how all health care staff make the concerns of the patient their first priority. I also felt it was important to talk to the patients and family members themselves about their experience at the hospital."

Response Analysis:
The response above talks about an 'emotional issue' very much in the context of the sort of emotional 'issues' or 'challenges' that a medical student will experience much of in the future. The coping mechanism here is not particularly structured or formalised but it is clear and fundamental. It highlights how the candidate identifies the perspective of the doctor and patient as being important to understand the situation.

Overall:
It is very important to reflect on what you learned through your experience and the success of your coping strategy. Give a true life example to answer this question and modulate the analysis of your chosen example accordingly. It might be useful to comment on the advantages and disadvantages of the coping strategy you used and what you would do differently next time.

8) Medical school is very intense; how will you manage your time to deal with all of your work?

Part of the interview is not only to judge your suitability as a doctor but also your suitability for university in general, and specifically medical school. In this kind of question, you need to demonstrate a mature approach to the possible challenges that you will face in medical school as well as some of the possible ways that you will overcome them.

A Bad Response:

"I understand that medical school can be challenging but I can assure you that I am a very competent student. I have always found school incredibly easy, often finishing all of my set work very quickly and then leaving. I got 13 A*s at GCSE with a UMS average of 96.73%; I feel that this has set me up for the challenges of medical school and I look forward to learning all about the human body. Furthermore, at school, I participated in many extracurricular activities which took up a lot of my time, I plan on giving all of these up to make even more time."

Response Analysis:

This response is at one end of the spectrum; the applicant completely fails to acknowledge any of the challenges that the life in medical school/university involves and says that they are more than competent enough to time-manage at university. The applicant may be very competent but medical school is challenging for everyone and the interviewers are looking at a realistic understanding of these challenges. The applicant says that they finish their work quickly and leave, almost showing disinterest in their work. Furthermore, the applicant at the end says that they will give up all of their extracurricular to make more time for medical school - this will make the interviewer wonder if the applicant really cares about any of the activities that they do.

A Good Response:

"I completely understand that medical school will be a very challenging experience but I believe I will be able to deal with these challenges. For me personally, I find that a schedule really helps me focus my time. When I moved from secondary school to sixth form, I noticed a large difference with a big increase in the amount of free time and self-directed learning that I needed to do. At first, I wasn't too organised but then I bought a diary and set aside time every day for each subject. This allowed me to structure my learning but it also ensured that I did a little bit of work on each subject every day. This meant that I would not have to cram for my exams at the end. I realise that the transition from sixth form to university will be even bigger but by setting a schedule for myself, I will be able to manage my time effectively. Finally, I take part in a lot of extra-curricular but I realise that, regretfully, I may have to give some of them up. I am very passionate about all of my extracurriculars and I would hate to give any one of them up but if I must, then I will do so. I will see what the best is for me and keep some to pursue and leave some if I have to."

Response Analysis:

This response is significantly better than the previous response as the applicant has a mature approach to the challenges that they could face at university. They outline a previous time they faced time issues and then showed how they learned from that. Self-reflection is key to the realistic approach that interviewers are looking for. Also, notice the difference in approach to extra-curricular activities. Both applicants say that they might give up some activities but there is a genuine sense of regret in the second applicant. This also shows that the applicant has thought ahead about how they might manage time at university.

Overall:

A balance is needed to answer this question; the applicant should be confident that they will be able to overcome the challenges of time management. They should not be too overconfident like the first response but at the same time, they should not be scared or panicking in any sense. The applicant must show that they have thought about this previously and give a measured response.

9) Tell me about an experience that has made you reflect on becoming a doctor.

First, it is important you know the roles and duties of a doctor. Doctors support and are supported by teams. The traditional monopoly that doctors once had is no longer relevant with the contribution made by other health professionals in caring for patients, investigating, prescribing, and treating. Team-working allows delivery of integrated care. However, doctors still act as the team leader in many situations. Continuous learning through practice and the desire to improve the quality of the patient experience is also essential. Other key characteristics include communication skills, perseverance, and ability to stay calm under pressure.

Next, it is important to keep a reflective diary of your work experience. Before the interview, you should go through this and take note of the key examples, reflect on them and come up with clear ways of getting across what you saw and what you learnt. Do not be blindly positive and say that everything you saw seemed brilliant. Make sure you get across that you saw the hard side of being a doctor, that you appreciated it, but that you are still up for the challenge. This will impress interviewers more because it shows that you have a realistic view of medicine. You may have mentioned this in your personal statement and use that here as an example.

A Bad Response:
"I organised work experience at my local GP surgery because primary care is such a fundamental part of the NHS and I was keen to see what healthcare in the community is like. Working there once a week has allowed me to form some close relationships with patients and understand their perspective."

Response Analysis:
This answer simply describes what the candidate has done – there are no case examples or learning points. This means that this student may not have made the most of their time on work experience. It also does not relate to the question well. The candidate has failed to mention any duties of a doctor or comment on anything interesting that made her think during her time there.

A Good Response:
"During my time in cardiology, I witnessed an emergency situation and it amazed me how the whole team came together, under the leadership of the doctor, to stabilise the patient. While on my GP placement, one of the key things that really stood out to me was the underlying importance of communication skills in the doctor-patient relationship. Trust is key to this relationship and thus essential to providing patient care. I am also aware of the daily challenges doctors face. In every setting, whether it was in the GP practice or in the hospitals, the doctors worked very hard with very long days and faced many stressful situations. But speaking to the doctors and seeing them overcome these obstacles really inspired me. I understand that a career in medicine will not be easy, but after my work experience I am even more determined and motivated to pursue a career in this rewarding field."

Response Analysis:
This answer provides specific examples with learning points, e.g. "importance of communication skills", while also mentioning some key characteristics. The interviewers will not think it is overly negative if you mention some of the harder challenges you saw – they will appreciate that you are going into medicine with open eyes. Gaining a patient's trust, maintaining it, and acting in the patient's best interests forms the bedrock of the doctor-patient relationship; understanding this shows that this student is a strong candidate.

Overall:
A good answer will use specific examples from the experience to illustrate what they have learnt. It will also use keywords that describe the characteristics of a doctor.

10) Lots of people go into medicine because of their family background - is that true for you?

It is not uncommon for medicine to run in the family. Many students applying may well have parents that are doctors. This can be both positive and negative, but it should not technically affect whether you are given a place or not. However, if you are from a medical background, then it is even more important to show that you have your own independent reasons for wanting to study medicine, rather than just because your family did the same. Equally, if you are not from a medical background it is still important to have strong and independent reasons for wanting to pursue the career.

A Bad Response:

"Both of my parents are doctors, therefore, I gained an insight into the medical profession from a young age. I was also intrigued by listening to my parents discuss their experiences, and knew from a young age that I wanted to follow in their footsteps. I understand that I am in a privileged position to have doctors as parents, and feel that I have gained valuable knowledge from them which will benefit my future studies."

Response Analysis:

This response is not very good because it suggests that the student has not been independent in choosing to study medicine, and is just following the path of their parents. It would be better if the student could show that they have looked outside of medicine as well, and have come to their decision on their own accord without being blinded by what they have seen through their parents. It does not seem from this response that the student has done much other research into the career other than through their parents.

A Good Response:

"Although my parents are doctors, I would not say that I have decided to go into medicine because of this family background. I am aware that the prejudgment exists that if your parents are doctors and you too decide to follow that career path, then it must be just because either your parents want you to or because that is the only experience you have seen, thus, have not thought of anything else to do. Whilst this may be true for some people, for me, it could not be further from the truth. My parents have always encouraged me to do what I want and pursue whatever path I enjoy. When I was younger, I was in fact slightly reluctant to think about becoming a doctor, thinking that I would be judged for copying my parents.

However, it soon dawned on me that pursuing a medical career would not have to mean copying my parents. I am able to make my own decisions, and have done as much research and work experience as others who don't have doctors as parents. I made sure to do work experience in parts of the hospital where my parents did not work in order to avoid them having any influence over my experiences there. In this way, I was able to realise for myself that medicine is a career that I am dedicated to pursuing, as I thoroughly enjoy all aspects of the job, as well as the interesting and challenging scientific knowledge and understanding that I will gain during my studies. Therefore, overall I may have gained an initial insight into the medical profession through my parents, but it is because of my own reasons that I want to follow this path."

Response Analysis:

This response is much better as it convinces me that the student has decided to study medicine for independent reasons, more than just because their parents are doctors. The student was obviously concerned that it may appear as though they were just taking the easy option if they decided to follow the same path as their parents. However, through independent research and experience of their own, they have overcome this worry to realise that medicine is truly the career that they wish to pursue, regardless of what their parents do.

Overall:

Having parents that are doctors may carry with it some prejudice for the student applying to medicine. If an interviewer asks you about this, it is obviously better to tell the truth but you may need to back up your reasons for choosing this career path perhaps more than some others. It is important to ensure that you have independently come to the decision to study medicine, rather than doing it just because your parents do. However, this does not mean that if you are not from a medical background then this question is easy you for as you will still have to have equally strong reasons and motivations for pursuing medicine. Therefore, to answer this question well, all candidates will need to show that they are truly motivated to study medicine for well thought out and researched reasons.

Interviewers need to assess if you are keen to take medicine as a career and it is not something that you are doing due to family or social reasons. This question could be the leading question or a follow-up question from a previous one; more so if your response lacked structure or requires further clarification. For example, your interviewer could start with "why medicine" to "why doctor" and finally ask the above question. Your response may have included experiences drawn from your work/voluntary experience. You don't need to be repetitive but you should try to use examples to develop your answer by adding substance and the knowledge you gained.

Make sure your response is structured and conveys your motivation, showing that the decision to choose medicine is yours and is not influenced by external factors. You should also express an understanding for the challenges that life as a medical student and doctor means.

11) Is there anyone in your family who is already a doctor?

This question may look similar to the previous one but it is slightly different. The previous question is exploring your motivation whilst this one is testing to see if you feel different because you do/don't belong to a family of doctors. Some people may feel they are at a disadvantage if they are the first in their family to pursue a career in medicine, however, many students whose parents are doctors may feel like they have even more to prove. Whatever your family situation, use it to your advantage! Use your experiences to demonstrate that applying to medicine was your independent decision and you are fully committed to it.

A Bad Response:

1) *"Yes, my (family member) is a doctor. I'm very lucky to have always been immersed in the world of medicine, to have met many doctors, and to have gained an understanding into what life as a doctor is like. My (family member) has very kindly helped me with work experience and other necessary elements to my medicine application."*

2) *"No one in my family has ever been a doctor before. I believe this has been an advantage to me as no one has helped me with my application to medicine."*

Response Analysis:

The first response does not explore the answer deeply enough. The answer does not demonstrate that their application to medicine was their own decision and that they have really taken the opportunity to understand life as a doctor. The second response does not use the opportunity to demonstrate why this has been an advantage. The answer could also be perceived as though the student is putting other students down to their own advantage.

A Good Response:

"Yes, my (family member) is a GP. I have been incredibly lucky to grow up in a family who not only support my decision to pursue medicine fully, but who have also given me an insight into the realities of what life is like as a doctor. I have seen the dedication it requires, the hard work, and the sacrifice. I have also seen how joyful it can be to make a difference to patient's lives; I have seen how a doctor can be such an important part of so many families; I've seen how the dedication, hard work, and sacrifice can pay off. What my family has taught me has really confirmed my decision to study medicine."

"No, I am the first in my family to try and pursue a career in medicine. In some ways, this has been a challenge as it has been my responsibility to discover what life could be like as a doctor. I've put myself out of my comfort zone contacting people I don't know to arrange work experience, voluntary work, or simply to ask questions about their jobs. The experience has been new for my whole family, and I am lucky that they are all incredibly supportive. I've really enjoyed learning as much as I can and I believe it has confirmed my decision to apply to medicine."

Response Analysis:

This first response is for those who do have doctors in the family. The answer demonstrates the student has really learnt from those around them and is not naïve about what life is like as a doctor – the positives and the negatives. The answer still demonstrates that the student is sure that they want to apply to medicine. Sometimes interviewers may twist the question to suggest the student has it easier than others if their parents are doctors, but this is not the case. This answer shows that the student knows they are lucky but that applying to medicine is still their own decision.

The second option is for those who are the first in their family to apply for medicine. The answer is an opportunity to demonstrate commitment by actively trying to find out about life as a doctor, especially if it is a challenge.

Overall:

Whether the answer is yes or no, use your answer as an opportunity to demonstrate commitment to your application to medicine.

12) What do you think is the most important quality for a doctor to have?

There are many essential qualities that describe a doctor. It is best to pick one and argue your case.

Open and honest: A good doctor should listen to what a patient says and respond carefully. It is not simply a matter of making an accurate diagnosis, but letting the patient know that the doctor has listened to their concerns and is offering a response that is most appropriate for their unique situation.

Empathy: Empathy is an attempt to understand how a patient feels and how their condition is affecting their everyday life. Empathy is a very powerful thing and is an essential part of any doctor's bedside manner; it can vastly improve the patient experience.

Curiosity: The medicine industry is changing all the time and it's important to keep up to date with new findings, innovative research, and emerging theories at all times. Even after graduation, you shouldn't stop learning. It is important to be analytical about everything you read; this is the cornerstone of evidence-based practice. It is essential that you are able to understand the impact of mistakes or bad judgement and keep your knowledge up to date.

Communication skills: Communication is key for any physician, which includes both listening to the patient and providing information in a way that it can clearly be understood. This will help doctors understand unhealthy patterns the patient may be experiencing and intercept them to ensure that treatments will be effective.

A Bad Response:
"The most important quality a doctor should have is teamwork because they need to work with others every day."

Response Analysis:
The response itself is correct and contains all true information but it is lacking in detail. It does not explain why they believe this quality is the most important. It also does not mention any key medical terms such as "multidisciplinary team" which suggests a lack of understanding on the candidate's part. Such a response may not be very damaging if the interviewer asks a follow-up question to clarify your response, but they may not and thus you have missed an opportunity to sell yourself.

A Good Response:
"I can think of several qualities that the doctors must possess, e.g. hard work, dedication, and knowledge, but I believe teamwork is an essential quality in a doctor. They form part of a multidisciplinary team which is responsible for patient care. Working effectively as part of a team is necessary to achieve optimum care for the patient. However, leadership is also very important in this role; doctors often have to make key decisions and ensure their decisions are carried out. A doctor will have to swap between the dual roles of team member and team leader to ensure great patient care."

Response Analysis:
This answer clearly explains why the candidate feels that teamwork is an essential quality but it also goes on to compare it to another quality. By showing knowledge of other important qualities, it shows that the candidate can present a balanced view.

Overall:
A good answer will add detail and explain the reasons behind their choice, using key medical terms. It will also offer a balanced view and may detail other great qualities. You can choose any but give reasons for why you have chosen that one. Choosing one does not mean that others are less important and you may have a different view than others. As long as it is something that is relevant to your role, it is acceptable. For example, being a good sales agent is a good quality for a supermarket but not for doctors, so make it relevant.

13) What are the worst and most difficult aspects of being a doctor?

This might seem like a surprising question; you have just spent months developing your passion for this amazing job and forming a perfect answer as to why this job interests you; now they suddenly ask you to give some negative aspects of the job. This, in fact, is a very serious question designed to see if you have really thought about a career in medicine. Being a doctor just like any other job will have its advantages and disadvantages; you must show that you have thought about both of these aspects.

Like other professions, doctors face many challenges that have the potential to permeate through to their personal lives. However, the nature of these challenges is quite unique. The aim of this question is to get you to identify these difficulties and discuss how they may impact the life of a doctor.

A Bad Response:
"By far one of the worst and most difficult things about a medical job is the screaming patients. I myself have a very short temper and do not really know how I am going to deal with them. However, I have thought about this greatly and decided that I will go into radiology to avoid all contact with patients and spend most of my time looking at X-Rays. The second drawback of medicine is the long hours; I have calculated the pay rate per hour of a junior doctor and it will be significantly less than most of my other friends at that point in their lives. The vast amount of paperwork will be incredibly irritating. But I have decided to be a doctor as I like it."

Response Analysis:
This is an exaggerated response but each of the drawbacks highlights a key issue. The first issue is the student seems to lack any kind of empathy and patience; they view "screaming patients" as something to be avoided and they suggest that the best method to do this would be a career in radiology. There will always be difficult patients but it is your job as a doctor to be understanding and provide the best possible care (also note that radiologists will have to interact with patients). The second complaint on pay rates is factually correct but suggests that the student is only going into the career for the money. Finally, the complaint about paperwork maybe true but it is not specific to medicine and does not display the maturity required.

A Good Response:
"I think there are a lot of difficult aspects of being a doctor, however, the most difficult part would be the personal sacrifices they have to make on a daily basis. Most people do not realise that being a doctor isn't just a job but a lifestyle. It requires a lot of dedication and time, often to the detriment of their own personal and family lives. It can be a toll that is often hard to bear and its impact should never be underestimated as the daily stressors one faces as a doctor are unique. Doctors face complicated choices in patient care which can involve life and death decisions. This can have a heavy psychological impact. Although they face many difficulties, I believe the upsides of patient satisfaction go a long way to helping doctors overcome some of the inherent challenges that come with the profession. Moreover, I think it is vital to focus on maintaining a healthy work-life balance and taking care of yourself as much as you can within the demands of the profession. There are, of course, many wonderful things about being a doctor, but it is important to be realistic about the challenges."

Response Analysis:
This response aptly identifies some difficult circumstances doctors find themselves in and the impact it can have on the health care professional. Because it is not such a generic answer that any member of the public would be able to come up with, it shows that the student has done their research and understands the reality and the challenges of being a doctor.

Overall:
While considering your answer, make sure you expand on the points you make by explaining the reasons behind your beliefs and provide examples when you can. Examples show that you have thought thoroughly about not only the benefits of becoming a doctor but also the hardships. You need to show that you are prepared for the challenges a doctor faces and that you are prepared for the task.

14) Which 3 skills are most important for a doctor to possess?

This is a very common interview question and it is important to have some idea as to how to approach this question prior to the interview. This will ensure that you deliver a clear and logical answer. This interview question attempts to evaluate your understanding of what makes a good doctor whilst also assessing your ability to prioritise the 3 main skills, as the list can be quite lengthy. Candidates who list 4,5 or 6 skills will be marked down for not following the brief. The key to answering this question is, therefore, to clearly state the 3 skills which you feel are important and expand on why you think they are important. Adding personal experiences/scenarios can help in supporting your answers.

A Bad Response:

"Doctors should possess a number of skills which include good communication skills, empathy, and the ability to listen to patients. This is key to ensure good patient care and also patient satisfaction. They will often face having to give patients what is complex information in simple terms. In that way, doctors need to be able to avoid jargon. Patients may also present with pain or anger about what happened to them and, therefore, doctors need to be empathetic towards them and try to stand in the patient's shoes. This will improve patient care as doctors will better understand how their patients feel and tailor what they say and do to reassure anxious and angry patients. Finally, it is important to listen to patients attentively. This will enable doctors to understand the patient perspective and ensure that no important information that the patient has said during the consultation has been missed."

Response Analysis:

Whilst the candidate has identified 3 important skills, the answer could have been better structured. In fact, the ability to listen to patients will likely fall under the communication skills category. Nonetheless, these 3 skills were well-discussed as the candidate highlighted why they were important. However, talking at length about communication skills may begin to sound repetitive and show that you have not considered the whole spectrum of skills that doctors should possess.

A Good Response:

"There is no single characteristic that makes a good doctor. The 3 most important skills, in my opinion, include good clinical knowledge, good communication skills, and good patient care skills. The skills that doctors learn during anatomy, physiology, pharmacology lectures are core to understanding disease and its treatments. Good clinical knowledge is key to ensuring patients are treated safely and with the best medical care possible. Good communication is important and can be achieved by actively listening to the patient. This ensures that clinical data has been gathered correctly during history taking and it also achieves a therapeutic effect as patients can express their feelings. Furthermore, doctors should deliver information in an appropriate manner to patients as it benefits both patients and doctors; studies have shown that good communication improves patient-doctor relationships, improves patient compliance with treatment, and also improves the job satisfaction of the doctor. Furthermore, patient skills are perhaps the most important for patients themselves; patients want their doctors to be empathetic, caring and patient. This will further enhance the doctor-patient relationship and patient satisfaction."

Response Analysis:

This answer is clearly demonstrating a good understanding of the necessary skills required to be a good doctor. It opens nicely with a statement acknowledging that a doctor requires a number of varied skills but is able to pinpoint 3 skills. It cleverly groups the 3 skills into 3 broad groups; e.g. communication skills rather than good listener which enables the candidate to cover most skills that doctors require whilst also further expanding on the answer. Lastly, the candidate understands the importance of each skill in clinical practice.

Overall:

It is important to have thought about what you think doctors should possess as skills and try and group them into broad categories if you can.

15) What are the biggest challenges facing doctors today?

You can choose what you feel comfortable and knowledgeable in to give a satisfactory answer about your chosen challenge. It could be something like financial pressures on the NHS, resources, shortage of doctors and nurses, chronic diseases or issues that affect training, e.g. European working time directive (EWTD). A good candidate will offer justifications for their answer, including why the problem is so severe and why it will affect most doctors. A recent good example could be the new doctors' contract and its impact on the NHS. You could use an article from recent press as an opportunity to show your keenness to continue to learn and to keep updated on issues that affect patient care. Read around them to prepare a good argument. Some examples to choose from might include: smoking ban in public areas or the obesity epidemic.

A Bad Response:

"Obesity is the biggest problem facing doctors because it can make people ill in so many different ways."

Bad Response Analysis:

The student has identified an important issue but hasn't developed their point sufficiently. This is a fantastic opportunity to showcase your knowledge of modern medicine and demonstrate that you have a good understanding of the difficulties of being a doctor currently. This answer would be better if the student expanded on the extended implications of obesity, e.g. the financial & socio-economic costs of the additional disease burden due to diabetes.

A Good Response:

"I would say the current obesity epidemic is perhaps the greatest challenge facing UK doctors today. This is because it is affecting a huge proportion of our population and impairs so many aspects of a person's health and healthcare management. Obesity often causes hormonal problems, such as Type II diabetes as well as cardiovascular problems, joint problems and many more. Therefore, obese patients often have to be seen by many doctors as they often have multiple co-morbidities, which complicate their treatment. Also, surgery in obese patients is much riskier than on slim patients. Indeed, the growing number of instances where patients have been too obese to fit on normal operating tables shows the sheer logistical difficulties for doctors treating an obese population."

Good Response Analysis:

This is a much better response that identifies multiple facets of obesity that cause problems and then expands on each of them. The student makes good use of their extra knowledge, e.g. the link between obesity and diabetes. It acknowledges the broader implications of obesity on a population basis and its contribution to morbidity.

Overall:

You can also draw on your work experience and reading when answering. In terms of challenges facing doctors in the UK, some good things to think about are the problems from the growing obesity epidemic and the difficulties of having an ageing population. If you're thinking of problems facing doctors on a more global scale, some big problems that are worth thinking about may include the dangers of multi-drug resistant bacteria and the limits they put on the use of antibiotics.

16) What are the disadvantages of a career in medicine and how would you convince someone not to pursue a career in the field?

The difficulty of this question is in striking a balance between demonstrating that you have a realistic understanding of the challenges of a career in medicine while not undermining your assertion that you are fully committed to medicine. Remember, by discussing what you perceive as the disadvantages of a career in medicine, you are giving a reflection on what it is that motivates you. I.e. it shows that you're aware of the challenges modern doctors face.

In this question, there is the opportunity to show that you have thought about how you personally would deal with these disadvantages and what approaches you might employ to cope with them. A good response should probably give at least two disadvantages.

A good way to convince someone not to pursue a career in medicine may be to recognise that different people have different strengths, values, and priorities. Thus, whilst medicine is right for you, it may not be right for someone else. You could tie this into the disadvantages of the field already discussed.

A Bad Response:

"I read in the news that the government is planning to change the contract for junior doctors so that they are actually going to earn less money than before. This is definitely a disadvantage, but I still reckon the doctors earn quite a lot so still think it is worth it."

Response Analysis:

There are several reasons why this is a bad response. Firstly, even though it may not actually be the case, the interviewers could easily infer from the answer that the candidate is mainly motivated by money in their application for medicine. This is partially because the candidate failed to either clarify what they meant or offer other disadvantages which are more important to them. Seemingly being motivated mainly by money can be frowned upon by interviewers, who may suspect that those motivated by money may be more likely to drop out of medicine later to earn more in other careers.

Secondly, while it is certainly good to demonstrate awareness of current developments in medicine, the controversy to which the candidate is referring has other elements that are more important – such as changes that are claimed to risk patient safety. Finally, this answer has shown no appreciation for any other challenges of a career medicine, nor any evidence that the candidate has thought about how they would handle these challenges. This would not be a good way to convince someone that medicine is not the field for them, other career paths have similar issues.

A Good Response:

"I saw on my work experience how a career in medicine can expose you to experiences that can be distressing. When shadowing a FY2 doctor, I saw how he struggled somewhat to not be distressed while comforting a very upset patient who was suffering greatly and had a terminal diagnosis. This made me think about how doctors are always going to be exposed to these kinds of situation and how that could potentially be very emotionally draining. While that is definitely a disadvantage, I think I am quite a resilient person and could find ways to handle this to an extent, such as focussing on the reward of when you actually can help people. Another disadvantage could be the impact that being a doctor has on your personal life.

The duty for doctors to be conscientious means they must prioritise the welfare of patients over other aspects of their own lives. This can often mean that doctors and medical students have to make personal sacrifices, such as missing social events because they need to work late or pitching out of bed to go back into hospital in the middle of the night when they are on call.

While this is a disadvantage you often wouldn't get in other jobs, I feel that it is an inevitable result of the special level of responsibility you get in a career in medicine and reflects how medicine is a profession and not just a job. I remember very clearly from my work experience a doctor telling me how important a feeling of vocation is to motivate you when medicine sometimes seems impossibly stressful or demanding. This resonated a lot with me and made me think in depth about what motivates me to pursue a career in medicine and whether I feel like I have a vocation. I would encourage this 'someone' to do the same and really analyse whether their motivations would really make them feel like it was all worthwhile during the most difficult moments of a career in medicine. If they do not think so, then hopefully this would show them that medicine is not the right career for them."

Response Analysis:

This response is by no means perfect, but it demonstrates some good features. Firstly, it shows a realistic understanding of some of the disadvantages of a career in medicine and that the candidate has thought about these challenges and how they could handle them. It also shows an appreciation of some values that are important in medical practice such as conscientiousness, diligence, and empathy. It also gives the interviewer and opportunity to ask more about work experience. This candidate should be ready to justify their claim that they are a resilient person, as this is something the interviewers might pick up on.

A vocation is defined as a feeling of summons or calling to a particular state, course of action or career, and is often considered important for thriving in, and enjoying, a career in medicine. This candidate does well to show that he learnt from his work experience and has reflected on the challenges of medicine and his own motivations. The challenges of a career in medicine could potentially have been explained in more detail.

Overall:

You can see how a question like this can be used to give the interviewer more information about your understanding of the nature of a career in medicine, your motivations, your values, your work experience and much more. It can be worth taking a second to pause before answering and think about exactly what you are going to say so that you give a clear and well-structured answer that can incorporate some of these elements. Go further than simply listing the potential disadvantages of a career in medicine to show that you have given thought to what motivates people (and yourself) to medicine and whether this is based on a realistic understanding of medicine.

This question is a double-edged sword. A badly phrased response can convey that you are choosing medicine due to influences from someone and it is not an independent decision. Alternatively, if you are not open and honest about the obvious factors (i.e. hard work, long hours, and the ongoing need to make work-life balance), this means you have not really given the career enough thought and don't understand the challenges of being a doctor.

17) Why do doctors leave the NHS?

This question tests your understanding of your future employer, and being well read can show your dedication and motivation to study medicine. There are clearly many reasons for why doctors would leave the NHS and your answer could speak generally about them or focus in on one specific reason. Either way, you need to acknowledge the complexity of the situation. The best people to find this sort of information from are doctors themselves who have or know people who have left the NHS. Thinking broadly about the destinations of people who leave is a good starting point – generally, people leave to continue medicine elsewhere (abroad or private practice) or to pursue a different career (in pretty much anything!).

A Bad Response:

"One reason some doctors choose to leave the NHS is to work for private practices. This throws up some ethical questions over private practice and whether those that can afford it should be able to jump waiting lists and see specialists that would not be available to the general public. To me, it doesn't seem right that the government and NHS help to fund the training of doctors that then leave the organisation to work in direct competition but for a select group of the population."

Response Analysis:

This response does well in considering doctors that leave the NHS to work in private practice, but more elaboration is needed about other areas that the NHS loses its doctors to. It's worth mentioning the breadth of the issue and reasons people leave, even if only to frame your answer to focus on one aspect as that will show your appreciation of the bigger picture.

A Good Response:

"There are a whole host of reasons for why doctors may leave the NHS – to continue medicine elsewhere, to have a different career, to take time out to do research, or even to have a family. During my work experience, I had a discussion with one of the junior doctors about a friend of theirs who had left the NHS to work in management consultancy in the city after his F2 year. This is a good example of the quality of doctor and training that medics receive with the NHS – that this person had the transferable skills to be able to enter a completely different work environment. However, I feel uneasy about the idea that the NHS and government subsidises medical education if people then leave the NHS so early.

Another currently topical reason that the NHS may lose doctors is to work abroad due to the issues surrounding the junior doctors' contracts. We have yet to see whether the high numbers (I read 7 out of 10!) quoted in the media that suggest they may leave to work elsewhere actually do. However, this would start a very new era for the NHS and medicine more internationally if doctors were less compelled to stay to work in the country they train in."

Response Analysis:

Starting your response by showing your knowledge of how varied the reasons doctors may have for leaving the NHS are will show the interviewers your understanding of this complicated situation. Doctors themselves are probably the best people to comment so having an example from your discussions with doctors is likely to be a good idea. Also, notice how much you can respond before you have to justify any of your own opinions about the topics. Topical news stories relating to the issue would definitely be a good thing to bring up (assuming you know enough about them in case they ask you follow-on questions) as it shows you are interested and aware.

Overall:

This is a pretty tricky question so try to highlight what you know about the NHS and as part of suggesting reasons why doctors may want to leave. Where possible, including topical issues is a good idea but make sure you know enough about the issue so that if the interviewers ask you questions about it, you can offer intelligent answers. Any experience or opinions of doctors you know or have met would also be good to include. This is one of those questions where a little prior thought and structuring will stand you in good stead if you are asked this question at interview.

18) How does a medical student's life differ from that of other students?

Studying medicine comes with an expectation to work harder on average than most other students. There are more contact hours than other subjects with practicals and lectures taking up a great deal of time. Work is not limited to contact hours: lecture notes need to be read, essays have to be written, and practicals should be prepared for. Keeping on top of it all can be a challenge. There is also pressure to pass exams. In other subjects, the aim is to achieve the best grade possible. In medicine, you will need to pass the 2nd MB exams in order to become a doctor. These exams certify that you are competent enough to continue towards a professional medical career. Passing these exams can often require cramming in a great deal of knowledge in a small space of time which can be stressful.

Studying at university is a real contrast to being a student at school and organising your work and activities can be a challenge. Tutorials and practicals may clash with performances or sports matches. It is essential to have a system, e.g. a diary or a calendar.

Being a medical student is also a great opportunity to be brought very close to the forefront of scientific knowledge, often ahead of what you will find in textbooks. It is important to find this interesting as you will be studying it for many years. Studying medicine is a marathon. You are studying almost all year round.

There is also a certain standard of behaviour expected for a medical student. As a doctor, you have agreed to a certain level of professionalism and this extends down to medical students. We are monitored by the General Medical Council; medical students are often placed before the Fitness to Practice disciplinary board for actions that would not have warranted any action if committed by other students.

A Bad Response:
"Medical students have a lot of work to do. They will have less time to have fun than other students."

Response Analysis:
The response itself is correct – medical students do have a lot of work. However, this answer is negative in tone and focuses on the perceived lack of fun that medical students experience. Medical students are known for their ability to balance a social life with work; indeed, this is an essential skill for doctors to ensure a proper work-life balance.

A Good Response:
"I am aware that medical students work harder than their peers. There is an expectation for continuous learning and they will be studying for much longer than their friends. However, they still have time to enjoy themselves and ensure they are well-rounded individuals; this will require excellent organisation skills. There is also an added responsibility associated with medical students. They must show a certain level of professionalism so they are forced to mature earlier than others."

Response Analysis:

The answer highlights this candidate as competitive and a very reflective thinker. It acknowledges the increased level of work and how this is reflected in the career of a doctor. They are also aware of the need for doctors to be balanced people and how organisation plays a role in this. "Certain level of professionalism" shows that the candidate is aware of the expectations placed on them as doctors and medical students. The need for maturity is also an important point mentioned. Doctors have an added responsibility to be role models and this responsibility is often passed to medical students.

Overall:
A good answer will relate features in a medical student to how it will impact their role as a doctor. It is important to use buzzwords, such as "organisation" and "continuous learning".

19) Would you choose a party over a patient? What if they weren't your patient? What if you weren't on call?

This kind of question is very common in medical interviews - it is a hard question to answer as you want to show commitment to your patients, but at the same time, your answer needs to be realistic- there are going to be times in your professional life where you will have to decide between a professional and personal commitment.

A Bad Response:

"I would always choose the patient first. My first commitment is always to my patient; the Hippocratic Oath states that as doctors we must all look after our patients. I myself do not go to any parties and spend most of my spare time reading Gray's anatomy (the larger version because I finished the student's version last year). It doesn't matter if the patient is my patient or someone else's patient; I am making a lifelong commitment to the betterment of everyone in the human race."

Response Analysis:

This person might at first seem like the perfect doctor; they spend all of their time reading anatomy books and would drop everything to treat a patient. The first problem with this is that the response is not realistic. No person would actually spend all of their time reading anatomy textbooks, and if they did, they would quickly burn out. Even if you do not go to many parties, you should always try to answer the essence of the question; would you stop a leisure activity to go to help a patient?

Remember that medicine is a stressful career and it's important that you have some time off so that you can de-stress. Spending all your free time on reading medical textbooks or sacrificing your personal time to look after patients is likely to lead to burn-out which is not a good idea!

A Good Response:

"This all very much depends if I am on call and if I have something else planned at the time. I understand that it is very irresponsible to plan on going to a party when I am on call and I would never do this. Even if the patient was not my patient but I was on call, I would choose the patient. My duty as a doctor does not just extend to my patients but anyone who requires my help. However, if I was not on call, I would be less likely to go because doctors must balance their social life and work life. Some downtime is required for doctors to recuperate and this will allow a better performance on the job. Obviously, if there is an emergency and the on call doctor was suddenly unreachable I would feel compelled to go out of basic human compassion."

Response Analysis:

This response is significantly better as it demonstrates the responsibilities that a doctor must have; being a doctor does not just end at the hospital, it is a profession that you must carry with you wherever you go. The answer clearly delineates some circumstances in which they would/wouldn't go to work and provides justification for these.

Overall:

For this question, you must not be afraid to say that there are some circumstances in which you would choose your social life. If you do end up saying that you would always drop anything you are doing to go to see any patient, then a particularly cynical doctor might ask if you believe doctors should have any free time at all!

20) What else do doctors do apart from treating patients?

This question is assessing your knowledge of the working life of a doctor. When answering, you have the opportunity to discuss the work that doctors must do to treat the patient indirectly including administrative work, and any other work-related activities that doctors might take part, in e.g. teaching. You will gain extra credit if you show awareness that the role of a doctor changes as you progress from FY1 to consultant level.

A Bad Response:

"Although the primary role of a doctor is to treat patients, it takes several years of training before you are allowed to treat patients without supervision. As a result, most doctors start their careers by doing administrative tasks like clerking patients, writing notes, ordering tests, writing discharge summaries, etc."

Response Analysis:

This is a poor answer that is very brief, misses a lot of information, and makes incomplete claims. Foundation doctors do undertake a lot of the administrative work on the wards but they are also heavily involved in the implementation of patient care. The important point to understand is that they are not as involved in the planning of treatment. You should note that consultants and other senior doctors spend significant parts of their time on work that is not directly treating patients. No effort is made to draw a distinction between work that is directly involved in treating a patient and that which is indirectly involved. There has been a missed opportunity here to show off understanding of the scope of a doctor's job. Many of the missed points are described below.

A Good Response:

"Whilst the primary role of a doctor is to treat patients, there are lots of other aspects of a doctor's job which are essential in order to allow a doctor to treat their patients. Some of these tasks are those which are indirectly involved in treating a patient. For example, examining a patient and clerking them into hospital are the first steps that must be taken before a patient can be treated and are essential in this process. Similarly, there are administrative tasks that must be performed in this process such as writing up notes, ordering tests, etc. It is usually the foundation doctors who do these tasks on the wards and they are also involved in the implementation of care to patients on the wards.

As doctors progress through their training, they are more likely to be involved in the planning of treatment for their patients while the juniors implement this care. As you become more senior, you are also likely to be involved with the emotional side of treating patients, for example, breaking bad news and dealing with patients' relatives. The emotional side is something that people might not consider when thinking about treating patients but it is as important as the medical care. In cases of patients with terminal illnesses, doctors might not be able to treat their illness but they will be involved in developing palliative care plans. Doctors can also take on separate activities like teaching, research, and hospital management but it could be said that these roles all ultimately lead to improved treatment and care of patients."

Response Analysis:

This is a great answer which shows a broad understanding of the work undertaken by doctors. It clearly demonstrates knowledge of the process involved in treating patients and is able to make distinctions between directly treating a patient and the tasks which facilitate this. It also acknowledges important differences in the work undertaken by junior and senior doctors. The mention of the emotional side of illness shows that the candidate has thought compassionately about treating patients and not just about treating a disease. The final point about other roles doctors can perform again shows a broad understanding of the work that doctors can get involved in and makes an astute point that virtually all of a doctor's work does impact patient treatment in some way.

Overall:

Organising some work experience is a great way to see for yourself all of the different tasks that doctors do. This question might seem like a trick at first, but having done some shadowing you will see all of the other work that doctors must do in order to be able to treat their patients.

21) What are your long term plans in life?

This question is somewhat complex as it does not really have a set answer. It really depends on what exactly you see yourself doing in the future. There are however a few things that can come across as a little one-dimensional and should be avoided.

A Bad Response:

"In the future, I see myself making working in a large university hospital making life-saving decisions, whilst also having a good personal life where I am able to travel the world and devote to leisure activities like golf. I am hoping to own a house in London and send my children to private schools for them to receive the best possible education money can buy. I also hope to specialise quickly in an interesting speciality that will allow me to reach these goals."

Response Analysis:

This is a rather poor answer as it is solely focused on money. It does not give any indication of other goals and completely ignores some of the key points that characterise the medical profession such as helping others and providing good care. Whilst financial safety and gain are a valid goal, it reflects rather poorly to fully ignore aspects such as patient care in this type of answer. Also, the days where medicine was essentially a money printing profession are long over.

A Good Response:

"For the future, I am hoping to achieve a variety of goals both on a professional and private level. On a professional level, I am hoping to reach excellence in my chosen field of practice enabling me to deliver the best care I can to my patients. I am hoping to positively influence their lives by caring for them. On a personal level, my goals include caring for my family and providing for them. I also hope to be able to spend time with them to see my children grow up and become responsible adults. In my free time, I would like to pursue my other interests, e.g. music and photography."

Response Analysis:

This answer is better than the previous one because it draws a clear distinction between professional and private goals. Your professional goal should always be to provide the best care for your patients that you are capable of. On a private level, you can pretty much have any goals you want. Just make sure that they are reasonable and don't conflict with what people generally see as good moral conduct.

Overall:

This question is tricky as you have a lot of freedom in answering it. The best way to deal with this question is to answer honestly about what you want to get out of life. Spending a few minutes thinking about this question prior to the interview will make answering it a lot easier. It is also acceptable to say that you haven't really planned that far ahead, but then make sure you can argue why.

22) Where do you see yourself in 5/10/20 years' time?

This question can be asked for a number of reasons – simply to get to know you a little better and stimulate further questions, to assess your ambitions in medicine, or to assess your understanding of the medical training system. You don't need to know which area of medicine you want to specialise in, but if you do have some idea, then don't be afraid to suggest it provided you have done the research and know a bit about the speciality training.

They are probably unlikely to ask you where you see yourself in 5 years given that you'll still be studying medicine.

A Bad Response:
"In twenty years, I hope to have moved to New York and be the chief paediatric heart surgeon at Mount Sinai hospital. I also hope to be a tenured professor at New York medical school after developing a technique that allows us to engineer heart tissue from pluripotent stem cells- earning a large amount of money as a result. By this time, I will have found a husband and will have settled down with three children. Finally, having established myself at the top of my field, I will begin looking at the political office- I eventually hope to join the US senate."

Response Analysis:
This is obviously an exaggerated response but there are a few key lessons. Never say in an interview that you are planning to move abroad and leave the NHS, even if this is your intention. The NHS provides significant funding to your medical course and they see this as an investment; they need you to stay with them in the future. By committing to medical school, you are making a commitment to the NHS (even if this is something you intend to go back on at a later date).

The second overwhelming mistake with this answer is that everything is too definite. You have no idea what you will be doing in a few years' time let alone the next 5/10/20 years. Whilst such a detailed answer can show that you're ambitious, it also shows a lack of realism. Finally, never mention money in a medical interview (if this is the primary reason you have chosen this career- think again!) - it will make the interviewers doubt why you really want to go into the field.

Good Response A:
"In 10 years' time, I hope to be a speciality trainee doctor, potentially in paediatrics. It's not an area I've had a lot of experience in but it is something which interests me now, although I'm very open to having my mind changed as I train! In fact, from speaking to junior doctors during my work experience, it seems that a lot of doctors don't actually end up in the speciality they thought they might do. Medical school takes 5/6 years then there's the 2-year foundation programme and applying to speciality training. I read in the Student BMJ about broad-based training which is 2 years, so if I did that then it's possible I could just be starting speciality training in 10 years' time.

If I do focus my career in paediatrics, then in 20 years' time I would hope to be a consultant following 8 years of speciality training after the foundation programme."

Good Response B:
"Hopefully I'll get into a medical school this year, so then in 10 years' time it will be 4 years after I'll have graduated. And if all goes to plan, I'll have completed FY1 (and so have fully registered as a doctor with the GMC), FY2, and have started my core training years. I think I might like to be a surgeon, so I currently see myself being a core surgery trainee, but I know that this might well change by the time I get to that stage. Until then, I just want to experience as many different parts of medicine as possible so that in 10 years I'll have a more informed idea of what I want to do"

Good Response Analysis:

This response clearly demonstrates that you know about the training programme and have researched what you can expect. The comment about broad-based training also shows dedication and ambition as you are clued up and seriously considering the shape of your future career. If you were interested in taking an intercalated degree or a year abroad to work once qualified, then you may also want to mention that here.

Overall:

Use this question to demonstrate your understanding of the career you are applying to study for. Chatting to doctors during work experience is a great way to find out about the training programmes and career timelines you can expect. Also, being openly flexible for things like intercalated degrees, years working or studying abroad and starting a family, etc. will show that you have a realistic grasp of the future and the demands of a career in medicine.

It may appear daunting to think about the future, but it is not that difficult to predict where one might be as the duration of medical school and path after that is very well defined. One may not be able to predict if they see themselves as a hospital doctor or in general practice or what speciality (surgical, medical etc.) they would opt for, so it is absolutely fine to say that you do not know exactly what type of doctor you want to be. Indeed, it shows maturity to appreciate that what interests you and the priorities you are looking for in your job may change somewhat through the long process of medical training. You can use a question like this to demonstrate your knowledge of how training works after medical school and an appreciation that in such a demanding and competitive career you cannot always expect to stick to a rigid career plan.

23) Do you think problem-based learning would be suitable for you?

You should be aware that different medical schools each have a different format of delivering their programme. Some will deliver lectures and be classed as having the more 'traditional' approach, whilst many schools are now offering a problem-based learning (PBL) course where you will be given regular cases for you and your group to prepare. You will then be met with a facilitator to discuss the answer. With an increasing number of schools offering PBL style learning, this question is worth perfecting. Try and approach this by firstly demonstrating a good understanding of what PBL is. Then discuss situations where you have already done some PBL and why it suited you. Finally, conclude that it is therefore suitable for your future studies.

A Bad Response:

"PBL would be good for me because I cannot imagine myself sitting in lectures all day. I don't think I would be able to concentrate for that long. I would rather be given a case and then go home and think about it and talk through the answers with my peers. We get given far too much information in lectures these days. I would rather spend my time on only the core knowledge which will likely come up in my exam and is useful in clinical practice."

Response Analysis

Whilst the candidate has highlighted reasons why he/she would prefer PBL to a more traditional method of learning, in that they would prefer to work out the answers to the problems themselves and would like to participate in discussions, it may not be a good idea to suggest that he/she only wants to learn the minimum to pass the exam, but to demonstrate to the examiner that the PBL will provide you with the foundation of the topic, and that your responsibility is then to do some further reading and research.

A Good Response:

"I think that PBL would suit me as I have always found that I learn and remember information best when I have been given cases and topics to research at school- perhaps because it forces me to read a length about the topic rather than being given information in a lecture. I also really enjoy undertaking group work, and therefore, I think I would thoroughly enjoy participating in group discussions. Furthermore, I believe I can learn a lot from my colleagues as each person has their own way of thinking when it comes to their approach to problem-solving. Lastly, PBL gives you the ethos and skills to teach yourself and continually update your knowledge, which is invaluable, as doctors must continually learn and teach."

Response Analysis:

The candidate is able to apply his/her current positive experience of PBL to demonstrate its suitability to his/her learning style. Interviewers also really like to hear that learning in medicine is lifelong and that PBL gives you the skills to teach yourself.

Overall:

With many schools offering PBL, it is important to know exactly how it benefits its students. If you want to go one step further, you may want to show that you have read up on its effectiveness by quoting a few studies- look up things like GenScope, or even Google PBL in the British Medical Journal. This will definitely impress the interviewers!

24) We have much better applicants than you – why should we take you?

The aim from the interviewers is to play 'bad cop' and try and stir you up a little. Do not be fazed by this- it is their job and they do not mean to make you feel bad! They are simply assessing your ability to deal with criticism, which you will be inevitably faced with at some point in your career. The simple answer is that you are actually the correct person for this course -don't be afraid to say so! This, of course, needs to be backed up by evidence of what specifically sets you apart from the hundreds of other applicants.

Bad Response A:

"I guess you probably do have much better applicants than me. I just wanted to try to get a place into medical school but I guess, like you have highlighted, I am probably not good enough. There are perhaps a lot of applicants with better grades than me, but I have wanted to be a doctor ever since I could remember- I think that is a good enough reason."

Bad Response B:

"I'm confident that I'm the best candidate for this course. I got 10 A stars at GCSE, and have excellent predicted grades and a very high BMAT & UKCAT score. I would be crushed if I didn't get in."

Response Analysis:

The first candidate shows a concerning lack of confidence in themselves. A confident answer accompanied by confident body language (good eye contact, sit up straight) will go a long way. Contrastingly, the second candidate is on the opposite extreme and comes across as arrogant. A lack of personal insight and willingness to take feedback on board is equally as bad in an interview setting.

Do not accept that there are other applicants that are better than you- you will find things that differentiate you from others. Even if your grades are a little lower, you may excel at other things such as music, art, or sport and thus become an asset to the university in that way. Make sure to highlight this during your interview.

A Good Response:

"I have all the foundations necessary to make a great doctor and the ability to build on those during my time here at medical school. I am excited at the prospect of learning so much here. Furthermore, I bring with me great academic skills- I have shown that I have a great scientific aptitude by securing good grades during my schooling years and also scoring a bronze in the science Olympiad. I believe this will stand me in good stead for my further academic studies. Furthermore, I am an avid football player, playing not only for my school but also for my local club. I believe that I could actively contribute to the football clubs of this university."

Response Analysis:

This answer demonstrates confidence and enthusiasm. The candidate is able to utilise his/her achievements as a selling point and shows the interviewer what he/she can bring to the university. Remember that you are an investment for them and they love to hear what you aim to bring to them during your time at university.

Overall:

The aim of the interviewer is to try to shake you up a little. If you know that and are expecting that from the beginning, it won't be such as shock and you will be prepared for tough questions like these. Remember to highlight your achievements to date, and try to sell yourself to the interviewer by showing them how much you plan to contribute to their university.

25) What do you expect to get out of this degree?

Ultimately, a medical degree leads you to a career in medicine. However, there is so much more available to be gained from the degree, and the effort that you put in correlates with what you will get out of it. Therefore, it is important to show in this response that you are passionate and enthusiastic about the degree, thus will get as much out of it as possible. It is also important to recognise that this means more than just the academic side of things, as there is much more to being a doctor than just knowledge.

A Bad Response:

"I expect to finish this degree with the knowledge, understanding, and competency to become a doctor. I expect to be taught all of the necessary information which will help me to be a good doctor, and also to learn some skills which I can use in practice. I expect to make some good friends who will hopefully stay friends for life. I also hope to make some good contacts in the medical profession."

Response Analysis:

Although none of this response is technically incorrect, it only shows the bare minimum that you could get out of a medical degree. It is possible to get so much more out of the degree than just the basics, but this candidate has not demonstrated that they are aware of this, or perhaps they are just not enthusiastic enough to put in the extra effort. This suggests that the student may not be as much of an asset to the university community as others may be, as they are not willing to reap the many other benefits that both the degree and university has to offer.

A Good Response:

"Of course, the main thing that I want to get out of this degree is how to be a good doctor. However, I am aware that this incorporates many more aspects than just the academia. Certainly, I am keen to gain all of the knowledge and understanding of the academic aspects which I will need for my future career. However, I am eager to go above and beyond that, and I am excited by the fact that the learning opportunities at this university are seemingly endless, for example, opportunities to get involved in the debating club.

Therefore, I will be able to extend my knowledge and understanding of medicine above and beyond what is required to just pass the exams. As well as academia, I expect to gain important skills that will be necessary for embarking into the medical profession. These will include both clinical skills and other important life skills which all form part of the job. Furthermore, I am sure that during this degree I will meet so many amazing people and form friendships which will last a lifetime, thus making up an important part of this degree, and it is important to have people around you to support you on the way and make the most out of my time at university. I also hope to get involved in sports and societies so I can make achievements outside of the degree."

Response Analysis:

This response is thorough and shows that the student is genuinely passionate about the degree and will gain a lot out of it. Students are able to get through the degree by putting in minimal effort (although this is still quite a lot), but the university will be impressed that this student wants to get out a lot more than just the bare minimum. It is true, as in most things, that the more effort you put in, the more you will get out of it. This response demonstrates that the student is keen to make the most out of all of the fantastic opportunities that are available at this university and will fully benefit from a place on the course.

Overall:

Overall, a good response to this question will demonstrate that the student is passionate about the degree so will gain a lot more out of it than someone much less enthusiastic. Candidates should recognise that there are many other aspects to be gained other than knowledge, such as life skills and lifelong friendships. This is a good time to mention any university societies that you've come across during the open days or from reading prospectuses. It is also important to show that you are keen to learn more than just what you are taught directly in lectures as the university will be looking for people who are self-motivated to learn more outside of the provided material.

26) Why is it important for medical professionals to be empathetic towards their patients?

This is a really important question because it tests whether a candidate truly understands and appreciates what being a doctor is about. It would be useful to have a good think about what empathy means (in particular how it differs from sympathy), and why this might be important in the doctor-patient relationship. This question is based on the idea that a patient's ideas, concerns, and expectations must be addressed with as much diligence as their clinical symptoms or disease, and is an important message to convey when answering this question.

A Bad Response:

Medical professionals have to show empathy to depressed patients to try and cheer them up. Patients need support when they are in hospital and empathising with them will help them to get better quickly. Empathy makes patients think you are a nice doctor, which is an important requirement as a medical professional. It also gives you a good feedback rating as a doctor, which would help you to progress through your career faster, and make patients like you more than your colleagues.

Response Analysis:

This response states all of the wrong reasons for the importance of empathy; additionally, it confuses the term empathy with sympathy. It fails to address any of the reasons that empathy is actually important.

A Good Response:

To me, empathy means putting oneself in the patient's shoes and imagining how things must seem from their perspective, which I believe is really important as a doctor. Firstly, empathy is essential because a patient's ideas, concerns, and expectations are just as important as their clinical symptoms, and must be addressed with compassion. If you imagine what the patient is going through from their point of view, you might think of new ways in which you can improve their care that may not have seemed obvious at first glance. Additionally, if someone is caring and shows that they understand how the patient is feeling, the patient is more likely to feel at ease and be open about discussing their ideas and worries, which would ultimately help to deliver better care. Overall, I think empathy helps to break down the doctor-patient barrier, making patients feel more comfortable in an otherwise seemingly daunting and unfamiliar environment.

Response Analysis:

This is a good response because it explains briefly what empathy means to the applicant (and demonstrates that the term hasn't been confused with sympathy) and then goes on to back up this idea with examples of how it is important. It mentions a variety of reasons for the importance of empathy, and uses keywords and phrases such as "ideas, concerns, and expectations," and "compassion" which are things that interviewers are likely to be looking out for to show that candidates understand the crux of doctor-patient interactions, and have thought beyond simply solving the patient's clinical problem.

Overall:

This is a really important subject for candidates to appreciate and is likely to come up in some form at the interview. Knowing what empathy is, and 3-4 reasons that it is important will be helpful, not only for the interview but also for future careers. Easy pitfalls with this question are confusing empathy with sympathy, thinking that empathy is something that is only used when patients are upset to cheer them up, and believing that empathy is useful for personal gains and career advancement, which should never be mentioned in an interview as a reason!

27) What would you do if you didn't get into medicine this year? What if you didn't get in after a gap year or after 3 years of applying?

The reason interviewers may ask you this question is to assess how determined you are to studying medicine. The most important thing to remember in your response to this question is to demonstrate self-improvement. It is crucial to accept that the reason you may not be successful could be due to the quality of your application, but demonstrate that you are willing to improve during your gap year.

A Bad Response:
I am very passionate about studying medicine so if I didn't get in this year I would apply again next year. During my gap year, I would go travelling. If I didn't get in after my gap year, I would keep re-applying so as to maximise my chances of getting in as my mind is set on studying medicine.

Response Analysis:
This response is very passive and bland. Remember that the question demands a response that demonstrates that you actually want to improve your application and not just take a gap year. A good response would express that you have a clear plan if your first option (getting into medicine) should fail, demonstrating organisation and foresight. The answer is also very vague and gives no specific description as to why a gap year would help you and how you are making the most of the undesirable situation. Although you are showing determination by stating that you would keep re-applying, it's unrealistic to apply for 4 or 5 years in a row and you would need to have insight into your own shortcomings.

A Good Response:
First of all, if I didn't get into medicine this year I would be very disappointed. However, I would receive as much feedback as possible regarding my personal statement and my application as a whole and see where I could improve before reapplying next year. If it means retaking some subjects to achieve better grades, then I would do so. I would make the most of the situation and try and take part in as many enriching experiences as possible – I have always been particularly interested in travelling and would organise a volunteering project in South America.

If I didn't get in after my first gap year, I would reapply again after one further gap year. After 3 years, as much as I would like to say that I would apply yet again, I would need to have a realistic expectation of my abilities. I would need to realise that studying medicine might not be possible and instead try and study a subject allied to medicine, like biomedical sciences. This may lead me to going into medical research or perhaps applying for graduate entry medicine afterwards.

Response Analysis:
This response is far better. Not getting into medicine would leave you disappointed, and stating this shows that you definitely *don't* want to be in this situation. 'Receive as much feedback as possible' demonstrates that you are not only going to improve your application but are willing to listen to criticism and critiquing before self-improvement, an important attribute to have during medical school and as a doctor. Show a clear plan for the gap year - this doesn't have to be travelling, it can be anything you're interested in like music or languages, but remember to demonstrate how it would help you. This answer, unlike the last, shows that you understand your personal limitations after years and that other options are also available although not ideal. It's preferable to state an alternative as close as possible to medicine, like biomedical sciences, as stating something totally unrelated undermines your initial attraction to medical sciences.

Overall
This question will usually be asked at the end of the interview just to see whether you have a backup plan. Stating that you have planned a gap year does not mean that you don't want to get in this year, but rather you understand the challenges of the application process, and with improvements, you are confident that you can get in next time.

28) *When you have time off, what do you like to do to relax?*

This is a common opening question at interviews, especially at Oxbridge universities. Whilst this question is supposed to help the candidate to calm down by thinking about their favourite past times, it can elicit a knee-jerk response in over-prepared candidates! Use this question to focus on portraying yourself as an interesting and well-rounded person. Talking about an interest or hobby should be fairly straightforward if you enjoy it enough, so take the opportunity to get on top of any nervous energy.

Obviously, this question should reflect on you as a person – any made-up answer will come across as unconvincing, or worse, that you don't particularly enjoy your hobby. The important thing is to show that you have a multifaceted personality, are prepared to work hard, and you are not just a book worm. Extracurricular interests offer respite from work and an opportunity to meet people outside of medicine. Regardless, ensure you only tell the truth. There is no point saying that you do scuba diving but not know about altimeters! Your interviewer may have the same interest as you and it will become very obvious and look bad if you have been less than honest.

A Bad Response:
When I finish a long day of studying hard, I like to read the latest BMJ before I go to bed. I also like to watch TED talks about medical topics for a bit of light relaxation.

Response Analysis:
This is exactly the response the interviewers do not want to hear. An example of this attitude is a candidate who had in fact brought with her every issue of the BMJ since 2000 in case the interviewer quizzed her on an article! They, of course, did no such thing and her extreme preparation was completely in vain. Interviewers don't expect much in-depth knowledge – they are looking for the right attitudes and qualities that will make a good medical student with the resilience and character to succeed.

A Good Response:
I really enjoy painting. I'm currently in the middle of a large commission of landscapes, but I mostly enjoy doing my own art, especially painting people- I'm really fascinated with people's stories. I also use painting and art as a way to process challenging situations and circumstances in my life.

Response Analysis:
This kind of response is often warmly received. If the interviewer is intrigued, they may ask more questions which can put the candidate at ease since they are talking about a topic they (presumably!) know a lot about. In terms of choosing a hobby to talk about, most medical students are musical to some degree, so standing out from the crowd may be difficult unless you play an unusual instrument or have achieved a lot. Conversely, choosing a hobby that is too niche may confuse the interviewer and set the interview off to an awkward start, unless you can show real passion and enthusiasm which may intrigue the interviewer to find out more. In addition, mentioning enjoying pseudoscience hobbies such as homeopathy is not advised due to the obvious conflict between medicine and alternative therapies.

Within any hobby you mention, figure out how you can apply the skills involved in that hobby to medicine. For example, in this response, the candidate shows that they enjoy a dextrous skill (useful for surgery!), that they are good at it (talking about gaining a large commission), and far more importantly, that it's a useful emotional outlet for the stresses of life. This question is essentially making sure that the candidate is not all about medicine and that they have a way of dealing with the distressing and challenging situations they will find themselves in and can healthily process their emotions. This answer also has the bonus of implying one of the candidate's main motivations for medicine – their love of people – which they may be able to link back to later in the interview. For this reason, being genuine (rather than reciting a prepared answer) for this kind of question is essential.

Overall:

A medical student with a healthy way of processing the stresses of medicine will be far more successful than one who lives and breathes revision notes – remember that medicine is more than scientific facts and figures, and in fact, the most challenging aspects are often dealing with patients and bad situations. Knowing that you can cope with the stresses makes the interviewer more likely to invest in you as a candidate.

Medical schools are looking for well-rounded individuals. Pursuits that require a lot of practice (sport, music, and drama for example) are a good way of demonstrating diligence. Furthermore, life as a doctor can be hugely physically draining (from hours and hours of running up and down wards, standing in an operating theatre, etc.) and so playing some sport helps show that you have the fitness to handle this. However, you don't have to stick rigidly to interests like these. Any hobbies outside of medicine can be important in helping to deal with the stresses of a medical career. A question like this is an opportunity to let some of your individuality and character shine through.

MEDICAL ETHICS

29) What are the main principles of medical ethics? Which one is most important?

There are a few principles which are generally accepted as the core of medical ethics. It can be useful to read a little about them to make sure you have a good grasp on what they mean. See the Medical Ethics section for more details.

In answering this question, good answers will not just state what the main principles of medical ethics are, but why they are so important. You don't need to go into too much detail, just show that you know what the principles mean. In choosing which principle is most important, it is good to show balanced reasoning in your answer, i.e. that you recognise that any single one of the principles could be argued to be the most important but for specific reasons you have picked this one.

A Bad Response:
"It is really important for doctors to empathise with their patients, so empathy is probably the main principle. If doctors empathise with their patients, this means they will do what is in the patients' best interests, so it is the most important principle in medical ethics."

Response Analysis:
Empathy is obviously an important component of the doctor-patient relationship and the ability to empathise is crucial for all medical professionals, but it is in itself not a principle of medical ethics. The candidate seems to be getting at the idea of beneficence but does not really explain what they mean or why it is so important. If you are asked to make a judgement on which medical principle is most important, it is a good idea to have mentioned other medical principles earlier in your answer to compare it to. Thus the main way in which this answer falls down is in having shown no real appreciation for so many of the medical principles mentioned above.

A Good Response:
"The main principles of medical ethics are usually said to be beneficence, non-maleficence, autonomy and justice. It is very difficult to say which is most important as, by definition, they are each crucial in medicine and they are all very linked with each other. For example, if a patient wants a treatment that a resource-limited health system, like the NHS, can't offer without compromising the healthcare to someone else then this is a conflict between autonomy and justice. If I had to pick, I would say that beneficence is probably the most important principle as if it is applied to all your patients then it should imply justice and if a patient is properly respected, then it should also take into account the importance of autonomy."

Response Analysis:
This candidate showed knowledge in both the main principles and understanding of what they mean and how they could be applied practically. Notice how this candidate showed their understanding without actually defining each principle, though there wouldn't necessarily have been anything wrong with doing so. This candidate recognised the difficulty in picking a 'most important' principle, in so doing showing balance and humility. Their insight into the conflict between different principles further shows a good understanding and suggests they have given medical ethics a good degree of thought.

Overall:
This question can be a really easy one if you familiarise yourself with the main principles of medical ethics so that you know you can define them and recognise how they might apply in a clinical setting. The question of which is 'most important' has no single right answer – it can be good to say this and then make sure you have a reasonable justification for whichever principle you pick.

30) Should doctors ever go on strike?

This question offers the candidate an opportunity to show an awareness of contemporary issues in medical governance and an appreciation of some dilemmas faced by doctors who try and balance a duty of care with a right to strike.

A Bad Response:

"Doctors should always feel able to strike. It is their right to demonstrate their disgruntlement at any perceived unfairness in their working conditions. Why should they put up with poor pay just because the government is trying to save money? Doctors have spent years training and have an extremely stressful job and should be remunerated proportionally to this. Cutting pay is outrageous!"

Response Analysis:

The candidate has failed on a number of fronts. Firstly, the candidate focuses purely upon the idea that a strike is due to poor pay. Though this could be the case, it is certainly not the major issue that junior doctors took with Jeremy Hunt's proposed reforms. Indeed, it was more to do with concerns regarding patient safety in relation to new working hours for junior doctors. Secondly, the candidate takes a very uni-dimensional approach and completely ignores the idea that the conditions of doctors striking should perhaps be different from other professions given that their strikes may well have a direct effect on the health of a large number of the population. Thirdly, the candidate has trivialised the aims of the government to the extent that it seems they do not really understand what the government are trying to get out of this situation (or at least have an appreciation for what the government's true position is).

A Good Response:

"I think it is important to balance the right of doctors to strike when they perceive unfairness and concern with patient safety. Doctors are in a unique and difficult position in that their striking will undoubtedly have an impact upon the health of those patients that they commit their lives to helping. This is a very difficult situation but we must also remember that doctors deserve to be provided with safe and fair working conditions. Therefore, as long as an adequate emergency cover is provided, I believe that the right to strike is a key means for doctors to alert the government to issues in the way that some of the country's most vital healthcare staff are being treated."

Response Analysis:

This response shows a deeper appreciation for the difficulty of the question of doctors going on strike. The candidate balances the two sides of the coin well and then comes to their own conclusion. This demonstrates that the candidate has thought about this and they present their opinion clearly and concisely in a way that invites healthy debate between the candidate and examiner.

Overall:

It is important to always present a balanced view, demonstrating consideration for both sides of the argument. It is fine to eventually present your opinion on the matter (indeed this is what's encouraged by the question!), however, it must be educated and balanced. Do not be too much like a bulldozer in your approach and not consider the other side of the argument (even if you do think it's a rubbish one!).

31) What do you understand by "confidentiality"?

Confidentiality is a legal obligation and an ethical obligation (required by professional codes of conduct). It means not sharing information about patients without their consent and ensuring that written and electronic information cannot be accessed or read by people not involved in the patient's care. Informed consent and patient capacity are considered essential in maintaining the privacy of the patient. Confidential data is any information that could be used to identify the patient; this includes name, address, etc.

Confidentiality is important for several reasons. One of the most important elements of confidentiality is that it helps to build and develop trust. Patients may not trust a healthcare worker who does not keep information confidential and we know that trust is key to a doctor-patient relationship. A client's safety may be put at risk of discrimination and stigma if details of their health are shared publicly, e.g. a HIV diagnosis.

Discussions about the patient should take place in the workplace and not be overheard to general public. To ensure confidentiality, information should only be disclosed to third parties (such as another government agency or a family member/carer) where a patient has consented to the release of the information. Further workers need to ensure that any information that is collected is securely stored and disposed of.

There are few exceptions to the general rule of confidentiality and they all have legal bases. These include: if a serious crime has been committed; if the client is a child and is being abused/at risk of abuse; or if you are concerned that the client might harm someone else. When legal obligations override a client's right to confidentiality, there is a responsibility to inform the patient and explain the limits of confidentiality.

A Bad Response:
"Confidentiality is what prevents us from sharing patient information with others. It means that we cannot talk about patients in open places in case others overhear."

Response Analysis:
The response itself is correct and contains all true information but it is lacking in detail. Using the word "cannot" implies that the candidate does not understand the ethical obligation; it would be better to use "should not". This answer does not discuss the importance of confidentiality and how it gives patients the confidence to disclose. It also doesn't address the limitations of confidentiality and scenarios when it can be breached.

A Good Response:
"Confidentiality is the legal right of the patient to not have their information disclosed to outside parties. Patients entrust us with sensitive information relating to their health and other matters when they seek treatment so we also have an ethical obligation to keep confidentiality. Patients share in confidence and help build the patient-doctor relationship. There are also some circumstances where confidentiality may be breached. These can include notifiable diseases and cooperation with social services or when a crime is involved."

Response Analysis:
This answer has a clear definition of confidentiality and mentions the ethical obligation healthcare workers have to keep confidentiality. This candidate clearly understands the importance of patient trust and how it affects the patient-doctor relationship. They also discuss the conditions in which we can breach confidentiality which shows that the candidate has a great understanding of the issue.

Overall:
A good answer will clearly define confidentiality and discuss its importance with "patient trust" as a buzzword. It will also discuss the conditions in which confidentiality may be broken.

32) When can doctors break confidentiality?

As doctors, we have an ethical & legal obligation to protect patient information. This improves patient-doctor trust. However, there are circumstances under which doctors are allowed to break patient confidentiality like:

➢ The patient is very likely to cause harm to others, e.g. mental health disorder
➢ Patient doesn't have the capacity, e.g. infants
➢ Social Service input is required, e.g. child abuse
➢ At request of police, e.g. if a patient is suspected of terrorism
➢ Inability to safely operate a motor vehicle, e.g. epilepsy

A Bad Response:

"Doctors can break confidentiality when they believe that it will benefit the patient. Confidentiality is an important aspect of medical care because it protects patients from having information that is private to them being disclosed to the public. Confidentiality can also immediately be broken if a patient who has been advised not to drive is found to be driving as it causes a risk to the public if the driver is involved in an accident."

Response Analysis:

The first sentence in this response is a little vague; ideally, the candidate would expand on how exactly breaking confidentiality would benefit the patient. For example, is it because the patient in question is in grave danger from abuse, threatened by a weapon or details about them need to be disclosed in order to catch the criminal? The question does, however, appreciate the importance of maintaining confidentiality. To state that confidentiality can be broken immediately without first consulting the patient (as in the driving scenario) and advising them of disclosing information themselves is technically inaccurate.

A Good Response:

"Patients have a right to expect their doctors to maintain confidentiality and doing so is very important to maintain a good patient-doctor relationship as well as maintain the public's trust in the profession. However, there are a number of circumstances under which doctors may break confidentiality. As stated in the GMC guidance, it may be broken if it is required by the law, if it is in the public's best interest due to a communicable disease such as HIV or a serious crime needing to be reported such as a gunshot wound. It is always important to ask patients first if their information can be disclosed and to encourage them to disclose things themselves. For example, if a person with uncontrolled epilepsy is driving, you have a duty to report it to the DVLA but you must give the patient every chance to tell the DVLA about their condition themselves. In this case, you can only break confidentiality if the patient refuses to inform the DVLA so that you can protect them and the general public."

Response Analysis:

The response identifies the importance of maintaining confidentiality. The candidate nicely references an appropriate source for doctors such as the GMC to state instances in which confidentiality is broken. This shows that the candidate has read guidance that medical students and doctors are expected to know and is able to apply her knowledge to answer this question. The examples are accurate.

Overall:

It is important to be familiar with key 'hot topics' in medicine such as consent and confidentiality and to carry out a little background reading on these prior to attending a medical interview in order to provide them with accurate examples. Examiners will indeed be impressed if you understand these core concepts and their importance to medical practice. The GMC website's 'good medical practice' is a very good site to visit in order to obtain further information on these topics and others that are likely to be assessed in your interviews.

33) Do you think pharmaceutical companies should be able to advertise on merchandise?

This question is asking whether it is right for drug companies to advertise their drugs for the treatment of various diseases directly to patients and doctors. This is an interesting question that could allow good candidates to shine if they can present a well-thought-through argument. The major considerations here are whether it is fair for advertisers.

A Bad Response:
"Yes, they should be able to advertise because patients will then be aware of the additional drugs available to them to treat their disease. In addition, doctors will be more informed about drugs and know what drugs to use in specific conditions."

Response Analysis:
Though the candidate touches on the important point of making sure patients are fully informed of all treatment options, he fails to address the significant other issues associated with this problem. For instance, what if the evidence base for the use of this drug is poor? Will the drug company ensure that the merchandise they advertise on is widely disseminated around the country to people of every social demographic (ensuring equality of healthcare opportunity)? The candidate has taken a rather simplistic and blinkered approach to this complex question that requires far greater thought and balance in the answer.

A Good Response:
"On one hand, it seems fair that patients should be made aware of all the potential drugs that may help their disease even if they are not currently licensed by NICE. This allows patients to make a fully informed decision and not providing all available options encroaches upon their autonomy. On the other hand, suggesting to patients that a potentially very expensive new drug that is the key to their survival will put patients' families under pressure to potentially self-finance the drugs and/or put their doctor under massive pressure to prescribe the drug. In the circumstance that the cost-benefit of the drug is not deemed acceptable by NICE, then this raises the issue of having patients who can afford these new drugs receiving different treatment from those who cannot. This directly contravenes the principles of this country's national healthcare system. Furthermore, advertising to doctors raises the issue of influencing them to prescribe the drug. It can be argued that the product being advertised will lead to a bias in the prescribing habits regardless of the proven efficacy or cost benefits."

Response Analysis:
This answer provides several different dimensions that demonstrate careful consideration by the candidate. Impressively, the candidate manages to slip in references to NICE, ethical principles, and topical issues such as healthcare being stratified based on patients' wealth. This shows a deep appreciation for topical healthcare issues as well as providing a balanced view. To improve, the candidate could have presented their own opinion and conclusion.

Overall:
This is an opportunity to shine as the question provides a wide scope for dropping in lots of your "extra" reading (see the "good" answer). Other points may be that there would need to be legislation in place to ensure that the drug companies follow firm evidence when advertising these drugs (e.g. regarding drug superiority over another). Candidates should be aware that this sort of starting question might then lead onto a wider discussion regarding the application of the free market to healthcare and all that entails. Therefore, in preparing for these sorts of questions, candidates should read more widely than just that directly relevant to these questions. There's no point being polished and efficient for a precise sort of question given that it's likely a variant of the question that will be asked come interview time anyhow!

34) You are a junior doctor and on your way back from work after a busy night shift. At the car park, you find someone who has collapsed and requires CPR. You remember that you aren't insured to do CPR outside the hospital – what do you do?

This is a potentially tricky question and some background reading into the laws that govern the application of healthcare in the UK would, of course, be desirable. However, most interviewers will not expect you to be familiar with the intricacies of the law and so will simply be looking for good reasoning ability. You should approach this question systematically. An example of such a systematic approach is the following: Firstly, does the junior doctor have a duty of care to this member of the public? Secondly, what standard of care is expected of them? Thirdly, can they be held to account for increasing the harm to the member of the public?

A Bad Response:

"No, because if something goes wrong then the person's family may sue the junior doctor. Additionally, the collapsed person isn't the doctor's patient and so they have no responsibility for them."

Response Analysis:

Several issues arise with this answer. Firstly, the law states that they will only be liable for damages if their action leaves the recipient in a worse position than if no action at all had been taken. Given that the person would have almost certainly died without CPR, it seems that the junior doctor would be justified in administering CPR without fear of liability. Secondly, the candidate states that the doctor has no duty of care because the person is not their patient. This may be true; however, the interviewers would begin to severely question this individual's morality if they were to not apply their potentially lifesaving skills in this situation simply because they did not have a formal duty of care. Remember that even as a member of public, it is crucial to raise an alarm, seek assistance to ensure that the patient gets the treatment.

A Good Response:

"I'm not entirely sure of the finer points of the law, however, I believe that a doctor should give CPR in this scenario. This is mainly from a moral point of view due to the doctor having the knowledge to save this person's life. I seem to remember that doctors can administer treatments without consent if the individual is unable to give consent and it is in the patient's best interests. Both these conditions seem to apply here. As long as the doctor feels they are able to provide CPR to the level expected of a junior doctor (they are not drunk for example), then I feel they should administer the CPR. Even if they are not able to provide CPR, they should raise alarm to get help by calling 999."

Response Analysis:

The candidate does well to present a good, logical argument with a nice conclusion at the end. Importantly, they admit to the interviewer that they are not an expert on the law but show how the small bits they do know (when treatment without explicit consent is appropriate) may be applied to this situation. The candidate even touches upon counter-arguments, e.g. what if the doctor is incapacitated for some reason (the candidate suggests a situation whereby the off-duty doctor may be drunk on a night out).

Overall:

This is a typical question where the interviewer is unlikely to expect you to know what the law is, however, wants to see how you think your way through tricky problems. They may well drip-feed you pieces of information to see how you think on your feet and how you can adapt your argument as new information comes to light. Plenty of practice in thinking about these sorts of dilemmas will make you more comfortable with these questions. An extended question to think about relating to this would be: Has the patient clearly denoted a Do Not Resuscitate wish?

35) *Do you think people injured doing extreme sports should be treated by the NHS?*

The crux of this question comes from the implication that those who do extreme sports, such as skydiving, are people who voluntarily take risks with their health and should not expect taxpayers to pay for their medical care if they are injured. This is reflected in a private healthcare where people who take risks would have to pay a higher fee. Patients often argue that they have the right to healthcare since they themselves are taxpayers and by paying to support others they also have the right to seek treatment.

We can analyse this question with the principle of justice because healthcare systems, such as the NHS, have limited resources so we must place restrictions on how funds are spent. It would release funds that could be spent on others who have not purposefully put themselves in harm's way. However, the principle of autonomy also plays a role; a person's autonomy has to be respected. They have a right to decide how to live their life and participate in extreme sports if they wish. Looking at a third principle, beneficence, it is important to be non-judgemental and act in the best interests of the patient, which means treating injuries. Most medical professionals will prioritise the principles of autonomy and beneficence over justice.

We can draw a parallel between the situation proposed and denying treatment to those who are ill due to lifestyle choices. These conditions are often seen as "self-inflicted" and include smoking- or obesity-related diseases. If we begin excluding those who participate in extreme sports, it is a slippery slope before we exclude lifestyle diseases from public funded treatment.

A Bad Response:
"People who do extreme sports put themselves at risk; their injuries can be avoided by simply following a different lifestyle. This is not fair to others who are leading normal lives. However, people who do extreme sports also pay taxes which contributes to the running of the NHS so they are entitled to use it."

Response Analysis:
The response is good because it shows a balanced view. However, it misses the opportunity to get into detail. For example, they did not discuss patient autonomy and the patient's right to lead their life as they see fit. Doctors can give advice but should not penalise them for not following it. Another ethical principle that was not fully discussed is justice. The NHS has limited resources so should we redistribute our funds to only people who cannot avoid their injuries? Another fault with this answer is that it misses the key connection between the question and the treatment of alcoholics and smokers with a self-inflicted disease.

A Good Response:
"The NHS is a publicly funded institution and for the general public. We should not limit anyone's access to it. This goes against the principle of non-maleficence. Others may argue that people doing extreme sports are causing themselves avoidable harm and their injuries are self-inflicted so the NHS funds could be better spent elsewhere – thus following the principle of justice. However, this is analogous to the treatment of alcoholics and smokers. We treat such people within the NHS because the service is for the promotion of better health (beneficence) so it is not ethical to withhold treatment."

Response Analysis:
This answer starts with a strong opinion and gets straight to the point – this will catch the interviewer's attention. This is then followed by a balanced argument showing the candidate is able to consider opposing opinions. Drawing a parallel between the question and the treatment of other lifestyle diseases is essential in an excellent answer. Being able to refer to current topics or issues in the NHS is the sign of an excellent candidate. This answer also discusses all the ethical principles apart from autonomy – the answer would be improved if autonomy was also used.

Overall:
When answering an ethical question, use the ethical principles (autonomy, beneficence, non-maleficence and justice) to structure your answer. Giving a balanced view also shows you understand both sides of the argument and makes you stand out as a strong candidate.

36) Should the NHS fund IVF? What about injuries that arise from extreme sports such as mountain climbing?

This question essentially addresses two different subjects, both relating to a similar basic issue: shortness of funds. Since we're in the UK and are arguing on the background of the tax-funded NHS, the basic question is how far society can be held responsible for covering the costs of treatment resulting from the actions of individuals.

A Bad Response:

"The NHS should fund neither IVF nor health care for extreme sports injuries. IVF is a service that is hugely expensive and has a fairly low success rate. Funding cycle after cycle of IVF is just not sustainable and at some point, the patient has to accept that they just cannot get pregnant – especially if the difficulties are simply due to the mother putting her career first and now being too old to conceive. There are plenty of children looking to be adopted. The same applies for injuries resulting from extreme sports. It is unacceptable for society to pay the bill for when somebody's hobby goes wrong. If individuals believe that they need to go mountain climbing and get hurt in the process, it is up to them to cover the bill, not society. The NHS just does not have the funds for this."

Response Analysis:

This response is judgemental and shows very little understanding of what the NHS is about and, more importantly, what it means to be a doctor. The idea of the NHS is to provide healthcare for everybody – indiscriminate of their income and social class and that includes support with conception. In addition, there are tight regulations in place when it comes to cyclic treatments such as IVF, where 2 cycles are covered by the NHS and all further cycles have to be covered by the patient. In regards to the extreme sports, this answer shows great ignorance with regards to a doctor's duty of care. Whilst it can be argued that extreme sports-associated injuries are the individual's fault, what about diseases associated with smoking and alcohol, poor diet or even simple activities such as driving? These can just as easily be attributed to individuals and cost the NHS much more money than extreme sports.

A Good Response:

"This is a very complex question. It addresses the question of what treatments are affordable and logical in times of shortening funds. Instead of focussing on these two very specific examples, this question should be approached on a more general level. In principle, the NHS is based on the idea that everybody living in the UK should have access to healthcare. This includes treatments for infertility as well as for injuries associated with extreme sports. The most fundamental idea of the NHS is to not differentiate between diseases themselves but to ensure that everybody gets treatment. Unfortunately, during times of shortening funds, there need to be limits to this as some modern treatments are very expensive. It is for that reason that in IVF, for example, only a limited number of cycles is NHS-funded. On a more doctor-centred level, being non-judgmental is of central importance. It is our duty to treat everybody, irrespective of race, creed, gender or the cause of their injury or disease."

Response Analysis:

This is a good response as it acknowledges the complexity of the issue whilst relating it back to the specific question. It is non-judgemental in that it does not assign blame and tries to address the root cause of the problem. For a good response, it is important to provide a differentiated and logical answer that does not fall victim to personal opinions or rash impulses.

Overall:

Medical Ethics is rarely ever black or white, there are always grey areas. The main challenge of this question is to avoid rash and sweeping statements and to answer in an undifferentiated manner. The IVF part of the question is a particularly difficult subject, mostly because it is very difficult to assign responsibility for the inability to conceive. The mountain climbing part is somewhat less challenging as blame is assigned more easily. Be careful, though, as it is very easy to fall into the blame trap.

37) Why is euthanasia such a controversial topic?

Euthanasia is a topic that comes up a lot in many ethical discussions in medicine. It is a very controversial topic as the definition of euthanasia itself is a complicated one and it also stands in fundamental conflict with what it means to be a doctor: to preserve life.

A Bad Response:

"Euthanasia describes the medical killing of people. It can be seen as controversial as the bottom line is that it is murder to end a life. In euthanasia, a doctor kills his patient because the patient's life is considered not worth living and he (the patient) would be better off being dead. In that sense, it represents the most merciful step to take."

Response Analysis:

This is a bad response as it is too undifferentiated for an issue as complex as euthanasia. The question asks about the controversy surrounding it and this is in part due to the very nature of euthanasia. Whilst the above answer superficially touches on these issues, it does not explore the issue sufficiently to be an appropriate answer. Be aware of how complex the matter is and do not trivialise it.

A Good Response:

"Euthanasia is a controversial topic for a multitude of reasons that come from a variety of different backgrounds. One of the reasons for controversy lies in the very definition of euthanasia. Euthanasia is defined as the ending of life to alleviate suffering. This almost makes it sound like a form of treatment. The controversy arises when one considers the very meaning of being a doctor. It is the doctor's duty to safeguard and protect life, not to end it. On the other hand, the idea of duty of care and patient well-being is the very thing that may justify the ending of life to alleviate suffering. In essence, the controversy on an ethical level arises in part from the conflict between safeguarding life and ending it to reduce suffering.

Other causes for controversy lie in issues such as communication where the question is asked how, for example, a comatose or paralysed patient can communicate their wish to live or die. A further point to take into consideration is the idea of life not worth living. Once we accept that there is a life that can be declared as not worth living, where does that lead us? Some fear that it will lead to a slippery slope where definitions of unworthy life become increasingly arbitrary.

The GMC code of good medical practice and UK law currently don't permit euthanasia."

Response Analysis:

This is a good answer as it directly addresses the complexity of the issue and then attempts to provide explanations and examples for the different issues. The answer also attempts to demonstrate the controversy in that it provides the point of view of the two main camps involved in the discussion. This is important as only with opposing opinions can there be controversy.

Overall:

This question is a challenging one as it is easy to get lost in one's own opinion. It is important to have a correct definition of euthanasia as it is very easy to answer this type of question wrong if the definition is incorrect. Whilst one has to be careful with one's own opinion, it provides a good starting point as it will allow for examples and arguments of both sides.

38) What is the difference between euthanasia and physician-assisted suicide?

Background Analysis:

Euthanasia is the act of deliberately ending a person's life to relieve suffering. Assisted suicide is the act of deliberately assisting or encouraging another person to kill themselves. In a practical example, a doctor administering a patient with a lethal injection to stop their suffering would be euthanasia. If the doctor handed the lethal injection to the patient so they injected it themselves, this would be physician-assisted suicide. The best answers to this question will go beyond knowing the different definitions to being able to interpret what implications these definitions have on the differences between euthanasia and physician-assisted suicide legally and ethically.

A Bad Response:

"Aren't they basically the same thing? It means when a doctor helps someone who is seriously ill to die so that they are not in any more pain. I know it is illegal and I think maybe that when it is counted as murder, then it is euthanasia and when it's counted as manslaughter then it is called physician-assisted suicide."

Response Analysis:

This is clearly wrong. In an answer like this, it is better to simply admit it if you don't know what the definitions of these terms are, instead of trying to guess them.

A Good Response:

"The difference between euthanasia and physician-assisted dying is that in the former, the doctor is actually doing the act that kills the patient, whereas, in the latter, the doctor is merely assisting the patient to kill themselves. There are several important differences between the two. For example, in physician-assisted suicide, the patient's desire to die is, by definition, a requirement. This is not necessarily the case for euthanasia, which can be voluntary, non-voluntary or involuntary. It is because of this that some people argue that physician-assisted suicide is more morally acceptable because it is in accordance with patient autonomy whereas euthanasia is not necessarily. However, it is sometimes argued that this discriminates against those who are too disabled to commit suicide, even with physician-assistance, and that in these cases, active voluntary euthanasia should be allowed as ultimately the intention is the same. Legally, there is also a big difference – active euthanasia is regarded as murder or manslaughter whereas physician-assisted dying is not, though it is still illegal."

Response Analysis:

This answer shows good knowledge of the definitions of euthanasia and physician-assisted suicide, as well as the different types of euthanasia. It shows an appreciation for the ethical distinction between the two and some of the controversy that surrounds the issue. It is always a good idea to include ethical principles like autonomy in your answer. The candidate could perhaps do more to explain whether they think there is an ethical difference between physician-assisted suicide and active voluntary euthanasia.

Overall:

These distinctions are of huge importance in medicine and are the source of much debate and controversy, so it is worth familiarising yourself with them now. The best answers will demonstrate not only knowledge of these concepts but also an understanding of what they mean and how ethical arguments tie into them.

39) Do you think it's ethical that drugs are trialled in third world countries but once they're developed, they can't be used by most of the country's population because of their cost?

It is important in answering this question to address both sides of the argument and reflect on the benefits and disadvantages of both. Here, the interviewer wants to see that you are able to consider different perspectives other than your own. That you are able to argue your point clearly and logically and that you have a valid and credible understanding of medical ethics. It is essential that you develop a good awareness of medical ethical issues in preparation for the interview. It is very important that you are able to make a good ethical assessment of a given situation and make ethically-informed arguments.

A Bad Response:
"It is very cruel that drugs should not be given to the people of the countries in which they were trialled. These people are so close to drugs that have the potential to cure them or their family. These people suffer disproportionally to those in other countries because third world countries lack the functional resources. We need to help third world countries and not withhold resources from them to disadvantage them further."

Response Analysis:
The candidate is focused on a very narrow-minded view of the situation. This impairs the candidates' ethical analysis of the situation, preventing a balanced viewpoint being expressed as well as a lack of logical reasoning given to support the viewpoint expressed.

A Good Response:
"Many third world countries are not able to afford drugs independently from other sources of financial support. Consequently, the third world country is being exploited for financial gain by other countries and organisations; its resources are being used but the country receives very little - if any - benefit. As a result, third world countries are likely to fall further into poverty, increase inequalities within the global community, and inequalities within the population of that third world country. However, many research studies can only be afforded if they are undertaken in third world countries. Therefore, we need to ask ourselves if we would rather not run the drug trials and not have these lifesaving drugs available for anyone, or run the drug trials in countries that will not benefit from them in the foreseeable future. It could be argued, from a utilitarian perspective, that developing the drugs is always worthwhile as the drug will ultimately be able to save lives somewhere in the world. The most ethical response would be to use some of the profits from the production of the drug to support the third world country."

Response Analysis:
This response goes through a step-by-step logical approach to addressing all the different factual and ethical issues involved. It tries to explain why both sides of the argument are justified as a result of the contextual limitations of the situation. It identifies the key ethical question at the centre of the discussion and ends on that. The responses go further as to suggest a solution, demonstrating a good grasp of the ethics involved. The response is detailed. It does not reach a fixed conclusion which suggests that the candidate has explored each side of the argument and has found both arguments similarly convincing.

Overall:
Answering ethical questions requires a different technique to answering most other interview questions. The basis of answering these questions relies on a good understanding the basic theories of medical ethics and requires practise. You should listen to and engage in ethical discussions with peers, teachers or anyone who is interested and try to gain a balanced view of medical ethical situations.

40) Parents who withhold vaccines from their children commit a form of child abuse. Do you agree?

Parents have to make decisions in the child's best interests, making sure they are safe; thus acting as the child's advocate. Previously, the law viewed children as property that parents could control as they saw fit; we now recognise that parental authority arises from parental responsibility. Parents need to intervene when children's immaturity could lead them into danger. They also need the power to make medical choices because most children do not have the capacity to do so.

However, it is essential to take into account the large scale of harm posed by infectious diseases. The primary risk of this parental decision is borne by the child. The danger is very real; a parental choice not to vaccinate can directly harm other children and increase the risk of outbreaks. If vaccination rates are high enough, the concept of herd immunity offers additional protection to everyone – both vaccinated and unvaccinated.

On the other hand, vaccination is not risk-free. They can carry side effects of fever, joint and muscle pain, and swelling. However, in comparison to the much greater risks of not receiving vaccination – many of these diseases kill – vaccination remains the best option.

A Bad Response:
"I believe these parents are guilty of child abuse. A vaccination is highly important to prevent disease in a child. By knowingly preventing a child from receiving a vaccination, they are allowing the child to be susceptible to a host of dangerous diseases. Thus, putting the child at risk."

Response Analysis:
This response conveys a very strong opinion. In interviews, it is always best to give a measured response that shows both sides before coming to a conclusion. This opinion is also contrary to current law – parents can refuse vaccinations and the law does not prosecute for child abuse – so this answer seems poorly researched. However, the answer does contain correct information, it has just not been presented well.

A Good Response:
"I think it is important to explore the reasons that parents may refuse a vaccination for their children. Some refuse based on religious grounds and it is important to respect that. However, some may be refusing due to misinformation; we are still recovering from the Andrew Wakefield scandal that linked autism to the MMR vaccine. In these cases, it is important to give information and educate parents.

Parents have a duty of care to their children and often want the best for them; they could believe that the best is refusing a vaccine which is where education comes in. A vaccination also provides a protective effect to the community to herd immunity so it is not just their child at risk, and it is important to explain this as well. There are also risks and side effects associated with vaccines so parents could believe they are protecting their child based on this. I believe it would be misguided to label all parents who refuse vaccinations for their children as child abusers. It is important we address the underlying issues."

Response Analysis:
This is a very comprehensive answer. It provides ideas for both sides of the answer and gives a measured response. Always avoid condemning patients and instead promote education – doctors need to educate the public as well as treat them. All the information provided is correct and used as evidence to their argument. The candidate also demonstrates empathy by placing themselves in the parents' position.

Overall:
A good answer will demonstrate knowledge of current procedures and will try and view the issue from the patient's perspective. Avoid condemning patients or their actions but instead give a more neutral opinion.

41) Should doctors be banned from smoking?

This question revolves around the idea of how far doctors not only act to improve patient's health but are also responsible to provide an example of healthy living. The question is if it is legitimate to demand of doctors to live a healthy lifestyle since they will be advising their patients to improve their lifestyle by, for example, quitting smoking.

Bad Response A:
"Doctors should not be banned from smoking because they have a right to do what they want to their bodies, as long as it does not harm anyone else."

Bad Response B:
"Doctors have an important position in the public eyes as they act to improve public health and demand of their patients to do their best to improve their health as well. It is common knowledge that a healthy lifestyle is central to maintaining good health, which includes smoking cessation. Having your doctor tell you that you are supposed to stop smoking as it is bad for you, but then he is smoking himself will make the patients lose trust in the healthcare system. It is the health professional's duty to provide a good example to his/her patients by living a healthy lifestyle. This includes smoking. Therefore, I believe that doctors should be banned from smoking."

Response Analysis:
The first response is very superficial and doesn't explore any of the key ethical issues. The second response lacks insight into the complexity of the question. It fully ignores the ethical component of the question. Whilst it can be argued that as a medical professional, one should provide a good example to one's patients and not smoke, the same principle of autonomy and self-determination that applies to the patient also applies to the doctor. One's choice of career does not limit these freedoms. This is important to recognise.

Good Response A:
"This is a challenging question as doctors hold a special place in society. On one hand, they are mere individuals like everybody else with the same rights and responsibilities as every other citizen, which includes everyday choices such as smoking. On the other hand, they hold a special position in the public eye by providing an instance of moral direction giving. This is where the question of the smoking ban for doctors comes into play. Doctors will advise their patients to improve their lifestyle in order to improve their health and in many instances, this includes smoking cessation. If now the advising doctor himself is a smoker, this advice can be seen as losing a significant degree of strength as he does not act on his own advice. It is, however, important to realise that besides the professional side of the doctor, he or she also has a private side to which they are entitled to make whatever decision they want, provided it is legal, and this includes smoking. Therefore, whilst it would be preferable for doctors not to smoke simply because it would be preferable for anybody not to smoke, it is wrong to ban doctors from smoking merely because they are doctors."

Good Response B:

"As I see it, the main arguments for a ban on doctors smoking are that it may indirectly have a negative effect on the health of patients. By setting a bad example, it could be said that doctors who smoke are failing to discourage their patients from doing the same. If a patient knows that their doctor smokes, they are perhaps less likely to take the advice from that doctor to quit smoking as seriously, as they know it is hypocritical. On the other hand, it could be said that banning doctors from smoking starts a slippery slope of interfering in doctors' private lives: why not ban them from drinking alcohol and give them target BMIs as well? These clearly start to impede on the doctor's autonomy. In balance, I think that doctors have a right to smoke if they want to, as long as they ensure it is not having a negative impact on their patients. This could mean banning doctors from smoking on hospital premises, for example."

Response Analysis:

This answer is better as it acknowledges the complexity of the issue and also tries to explain the background to why such a question arises in the first place. It attempts to describe the role doctors play in society and how this is related to the judgement of their choices and decisions when it comes to their private life. This is important as it considers the ethical idea of autonomy and self-determination that is a central part of this question.

Overall:

Generally speaking, this question ties in with the idea of leading by example. Similar questions include obesity or alcoholism in doctors. When answering any of these questions, it is essential to realise that doctors, just like everybody else, also have a private life in which they are separated from their profession and are just as entitled to making decisions out of their own free will as anybody else, especially when it comes to their own bodies and health. They are doctors and humans. Sometimes the role and responsibility may be at conflict and one must find a way. Doctors, as humans, have the autonomy but also have a responsibility in preventing disease. Passive smoking can be dangerous and a doctor that smokes may not be a good role model for his patients. Candidates should be exploring this in their reply when putting up arguments for both and summarise with what they think would be a better option.

42) What are the ethical implications of an obese doctor?

Obesity is an escalating global epidemic in many parts of the world. Obesity affects virtually all age and socioeconomic groups. It is no longer limited to developed countries but has spread to developing countries as well. The UK has the highest level of obesity in Western Europe. Obesity levels in the UK have more than trebled in the last 30 years and, on current estimates, more than half the population could be obese by 2050.

Obesity poses a major risk for serious diet-related non-communicable diseases, including diabetes mellitus, cardiovascular disease, hypertension and stroke, and certain forms of cancer. Its health consequences range from increased risk of premature death to serious chronic conditions that reduce the overall quality of life. Care of obese people will require the doctor to expend more time and medical resources. Thus, obese patients often place an increased burden on the healthcare system and have regular interaction with the healthcare system to receive advice from doctors. It important that doctors can act as health advocates. Obese doctors may be seen as hypocrites as they try and advise patients on weight loss. It is also important that doctors remain fit – they often have to stand for long periods of time and will have to at times, run in medical emergencies. An obese doctor may have difficulties with this task which will impair their ability to fulfil their role.

The media has created the perception that obese patients are "lazy, noncompliant, undisciplined, and lacking in willpower". Such negative attitudes place the patient–physician relationship at risk if patients agree with this belief; it can damage the trust and confidence patients must place into their doctors to receive optimum care. Obesity in doctors can be another barrier to good patient care as they may be reluctant to discuss weight loss strategies with their patients. Physicians should work to avoid bias in health advice regardless of their own BMI status.

A Bad Response:
"Obese doctors pose an ethical dilemma. They are supposed to offer health advice and patients who see doctors who are overweight, they are unlikely to follow their advice. This can impact patient care."

Response Analysis:
This answer merely touches on a few of the issues and does not use key phrases, such as "trust" or "patient-doctor relationship". The positive aspects of this answer include acknowledgement of the ethical dilemma associated with the situation and its possible impact on patient care. A better answer would discuss the health conditions associated with obesity and why it is important for doctors to counsel patients on this, as well as the possible consequences of an obese doctor giving this advice.

A Good Response:
"The concept of an obese doctor may appear as paradoxical to many patients. Many patients are aware of the health implications in obesity so they can start to question the doctor's ability to act as a health advocate. These doubts can adversely affect the patient-doctor relationship. However, doctors face great stresses at work and whilst it's a good idea in principle to have thin doctors, it is difficult in practice, e.g. comfort eating. Finally, being obese could help some doctors empathise with their patients to get them more engaged in discussions about lifestyle advice."

Response Analysis:
This answer provides specific buzzwords, e.g. 'patient safety', 'empathy', and 'health advocate'. These words always add to an answer and present the candidate as a knowledgeable and competitive applicant. It also highlights the potential consequences related to the patient-doctor relationship and offers a realistic viewpoint on the current paradigm.

Overall:
A good answer will employ topical phrases, such as "patient safety", and "patient-doctor relationship". It is important to always discuss any concept brought up in more detail and develop it more. This gives a more interesting answer and shows interviewers that you are a reflective thinker.

43) Are disabled lives worth saving?

When asked ethical questions, there are rarely right and wrong answers. However, with this question, the answer is clearly yes. As a doctor, it is not your position to decide that someone with a disability is living with a quality of life that is not worth sustaining. It is worth discussing cases in which patients decide their lives are no longer worth living but it is not a doctor's decision to make.

A Bad Response:

"If an individual with a disability requires lifesaving treatment or an individual requires treatment that may leave them with a disability then I do not think that the treatment should be given. Individuals with disabilities have a much lower quality of life and it is not fair to subject someone to this kind of life."

Response Analysis:

A response like this would raise a lot of concerns about the candidate giving the answer. The first issue to address is that individuals with disabilities are often able to live with good quality of life, there are lots of ways that individuals can learn to cope with their disabilities. The second is that doctors cannot make decisions about treatment based on quality of life judgements. Doctors must make decisions based on their medical knowledge and the likelihood of success of the treatment. It is not a doctor's place to suggest that life is not worth living if you have a disability.

A Good Response:

"The answer to this question is definitely yes. Whilst disabled people might face difficulties in life that others are fortunate enough not to face, this does not mean that disabled people do not have a good quality of life. However, quality of life is a subjective thing. The idea that disabled lives might not be worth saving suggests that disabled people would be better off dead than living with a disability. There are a lot of disabled people who be offended by this judgement and would tell you that their lives may be sometimes difficult but that they find ways to cope with their struggles in order that they can enjoy life.

There are some cases in which individuals with a disability may make a decision that they do not want their life saved. For example, an individual with locked-in syndrome whose only remaining form of communication was his ability to blink, said that once he was no longer able to blink, he wanted doctors to turn off his life support. The doctors respected this patient's wishes but it would have been wrong for doctors to make this judgement on behalf of the patient. Disabled lives should be saved if the individual with the disability wants to have their life saved."

Response Analysis:

This is a good answer which makes a clear distinction between a doctor's decision that a life isn't worth saving and a patient's decision that their life isn't worth saving. Importantly, the answer is very positive about the lives of disabled people and understands that individuals can still enjoy a good quality of life. As a doctor, it is important to support patients with disabilities and to ensure they can have as high a quality of life as possible.

Overall:

As a potential doctor, I hope you agree that disabled lives are very much worth saving. Remain positive when answering questions like this. If possible, I would recommend trying to get some experience working with disabled people or at least try to speak to someone with a disability. These individuals often have remarkable stories of their resilience and fight and they will tell you that their struggles are worth it to be able to still enjoy life.

44) Discuss the ethical dilemma of Huntingdon's disease when one family member knows they have it and don't want anyone else to know.

Huntington's disease is a devastating neurodegenerative disease with no cure; it affects the coordination of movement and leads to mental decline. The diagnosis is usually confirmed by genetic testing and affected individuals show disease progression in a predictable way. The genetic testing can even predict when symptoms will begin to affect the individual. In the latter stages of the disease, sufferers require full-time care which often affects life for the surrounding family. The disease is inherited in an autosomal dominant fashion which means offspring have a 50% chance of developing the disease, however, it should be noted that individuals suffering from the disease often choose not to have children because of this risk. There is a wide range of ethical issues which arise from the diagnosis of Huntington's disease and they will be explored in more detail in the answers below. When approaching ethical questions like this, the key thing is to explain your reasoning for your thought and to discuss both sides of the argument. Ensure you answer the question too, explain why this is a 'dilemma'.

A Bad Response:

"Huntington's disease is a devastating neurodegenerative disease which develops predictably and sufferers require full-time care in the latter stages of the disease. This is likely to put significant pressure on close family and friends. Importantly, the disease is inherited in an autosomal dominant pattern which means that any offspring have a 50% chance of suffering from the disease. For both of these reasons, it would be wrong for a sufferer of the disease to keep it a secret from their family and partner. Family deserve to know that their relative is certain to require care later in life and details about the potential effect on offspring should not be kept from a partner. It is, therefore, the GP's duty to inform the family and partner in a situation where the individual with the disease does not wish to share their diagnosis."

Response Analysis:

This answer raises two of the important ethical dilemmas surrounding a diagnosis of Huntington's. The progress of the disease is devastating and sufferers will come to require full-time care. This is something that families understandably would like to prepare for however many sufferers do not want this sense of impending doom hanging over their family's heads and would rather break the news later. Similarly, when it comes to reproduction some couples would like to undertake IVF and use pre-implantation genetic testing to ensure an embryo with HD will not be used for reproduction but there are individuals who feel this is morally wrong and so may prefer to keep their diagnosis a secret from their partner. Whilst the answer raises these two points, it doesn't discuss why an individual may not want to share their diagnosis. The question asks about the ethical dilemma so both sides of the argument should be offered. The answer also incorrectly states that it is the GP's duty to inform the family and partner. This would be a breach of confidentiality; the GP can only encourage the patient to share this information with their family.

A Good Response:

"Huntington's disease is a devastating neurodegenerative disease which develops predictably and sufferers require full-time care in the latter stages of the disease. Genetic testing can predict when symptoms will begin to appear which can be very stressful for sufferers. An individual diagnosed with HD may not wish to share this information with their family for a number of reasons. The disease is inherited in an autosomal dominant pattern which means each of the sufferer's siblings has a 50% chance of being a sufferer and also that at least one of the sufferer's parents will also suffer. Since this disease does not have a cure, some say it is unethical to inform people that they will develop this disease long before they ever develop symptoms.

However, others argue that knowledge that the disease will progress allows patients to plan their lives. Other important factors to consider are the ages of family members, some members may be too young to be tested because they may not be deemed mature enough to deal with news of a diagnosis. Individuals may also hide this information from family for financial reasons. If family members are aware of the diagnosis and get tested themselves to discover they too have HD, they will be required to pay much higher costs for medical insurance.

Whilst you may argue that individuals can access free healthcare on the NHS, often the provision of care for individuals with debilitating chronic conditions is not good enough and health insurance is an important safety net. Despite these concerns, if I was the GP for a patient in this situation I would encourage them to tell their family members. Obviously, I would be unable to inform the family myself due to confidentiality but I would stress that it is important that everyone in the family should have the opportunity to think about their long-term plans should they have HD or if they will end up caring for someone with HD."

Response Analysis:

This is an excellent response which really explains why this is a dilemma for a patient. It gives both insightful reasons why a patient may want to keep the diagnosis a secret but also offers the conflicting thoughts that a patient may have in weighing up a decision to tell someone. Finishing the answer by stating what the candidate would do as the patient's GP helps this answer to really stand out and shows that the candidate is thinking about these issues from a perspective of a potential doctor.

Overall:

In any ethical question, ensure you provide a balanced argument but try to come to a conclusion if you can. You will get extra credit if you can understand how doctors fit into these situations and can demonstrate knowledge of legal issues limiting doctors' actions e.g. confidentiality.

45) You are treating a dictator who is responsible for the murder of thousands of people in his country. You are alone with him and realise killing him could save millions of lives. Assuming that you wouldn't get caught, would you do it?

Background Analysis:

As with any ethics question, the first thing to do is to recognise that there are **two sides to the argument** and to think about what these are. Ultimately, it matters less which side you choose than it does your ability to ethically justify your decision and the personal values you show in your argument. This is an opportunity to demonstrate a good understanding of relevant ethical principles and your ability to apply them practically. If there are potential flaws in your argument, it is much better to recognise them overtly than to try and gloss over them. Arguments of both sides should be given and then a reasoned decision on which is more powerful should be made.

A Bad Response:

"I would never kill someone, so I would definitely not kill the dictator. But maybe I just wouldn't treat him as well as I could and so hope that the disease kills him."

Response Analysis:

This candidate has failed to demonstrate the ability to use ethical reasoning to justify their decision or to show an understanding of any of the main tenants of medical ethics. He also has not recognised that there could be another perspective on this problem and that arguments exist for killing the dictator. Finally, the suggestion of compromising care to the dictator certainly requires more justification. While it is true that there is an ethical difference between acts (killing the dictator) and omissions (failing to treat the dictator properly, in the hope he will die), this candidate does not really explain what they mean by this.

A Good Response:

"The arguments for killing the dictator seem reasonably clear – if doing so will save millions of lives then a utilitarian argument could state that this would achieve the best for the most people and so is the right decision, though there are a few problems with this. Firstly, you can't be sure of the assumption that killing the dictator will save lives – how do you know an equally bad dictator will not come through the ranks to take his place? Secondly, a murder by a medical professional completely breaks the implicit trust in universal beneficence to individuals and political impartiality that medical professionals rely upon to practice, especially organisations in conflict regions like MSF. If regimes stop trusting these organisations and allowing them to practice, it could be that more people are harmed than saved. Another strong argument against murdering the dictator is that it would be a clear violation of several cornerstones of medical ethics: respect for the sanctity of human life, non-maleficence and beneficence - the priority of the wellbeing of the patient in front of you, whoever they are. It is a slippery slope as soon as doctors start to judge whether or not the patients in front of them are worth helping. Ultimately, murder is fundamentally wrong in any situation. It is for these reasons and because you cannot even be sure of the utilitarian argument for killing the dictator that, on balance, I would not do so."

Response Analysis:

Although this response is quite long, such a difficult moral problem warrants a suitably thorough answer. This candidate clearly outlines ethical arguments for and against killing the dictator and then comes to a reasoned judgement. The candidate also shows a clear understanding of the concept of utilitarianism and knowledge of the principles of beneficence and non-maleficence, giving the interviewer the opportunity to ask more on those if they want.

Overall:

Notice that both the bad answer and the good answer came to the same conclusion: neither would kill the dictator. It was not the ultimate decision that was the difference between them, but rather their ability to reasonably justify their opinions with ethical argument and explain what they meant.

46) You're given £1 Million to spend on either an MRI machine or on 50 liver transplants for patients with alcoholic liver disease (cirrhosis). Which one would you choose?

Background Analysis:
Decisions about resource allocation are hugely important in a system like the NHS where resources are so limited and those making the decisions must be able to justify them to the public. Analysis of the cost-effectiveness of treatments is done by NICE, which assesses how money can be best spent to achieve the best for the most people. This uses measures such as QALYs (Quality Adjusted Life Years). The other ethical decision here is whether patients should be treated for arguably self-inflicted conditions.

A Bad Response:
"I would pay for the MRI machine. This is because for the patients with alcoholic cirrhosis, their condition is self-inflicted and so they should be given less priority than patients whose diseases are not self-inflicted, like many of those who would be helped by the new MRI machine."

Response Analysis:
This alludes to a common ethical debate about whether, in a resource-limited public health system like the NHS, those with conditions which could be considered self-inflicted should be given less priority than other patients or perhaps be asked to pay for their healthcare. The arguments put forward for this include the idea that this would discourage people from unhealthy or risky lifestyle choices and so remove some of the burdens that these patients present to the NHS, while also benefitting the patients themselves. In contrast, arguments against this state that in many cases the causes of a disease can be multi-factorial, including lifestyle risk factors but also genetic predisposition for the disease, so it cannot be said with complete surety that a person's lifestyle choices are responsible for the disease. Furthermore, such a move would represent a slippery slope towards doctors making dangerous judgements about which patients are worth treating and which are not. What makes this answer bad is that the candidate has failed to support their decision with an ethical argument or to recognise that their valid counter-arguments to his position. Furthermore, the candidate hasn't shown any awareness about how these resource allocation decisions are really made.

A Good Response:
"I suppose my decision would have to depend on a number of factors. To start, I would want to know if there has been any analysis from NICE regarding which of these options has the potential to contribute to the most QALYs. While liver transplants make a relatively quantifiable improvement to the recipients' lives, it is difficult to quantify the amount of benefit from using an MRI machine – use of the machine does not generate QALYs in itself, but the earlier and more accurate diagnosis that it can offer certainly has the potential to do so. Another factor would, of course, have to be the relative need for MRI machines vs. liver transplants. For example, giving a hospital a second MRI machine will be of substantially more benefit than giving it its sixth MRI machine. Ultimately, I think this approach would probably lead me to opt for the MRI machine. This is because, although the liver transplants are of very obvious and substantial benefit to the 50 people who get the transplant, the MRI machine has the potential to last for decades and so help thousands of patients so that its cumulative contribution to wellbeing is perhaps greater."

Response Analysis:
This answer shows that the candidate has an idea about the process behind resource allocation decisions in the NHS and the role of NICE. It is also a thoughtful approach to the problems of working out how to fairly compare very different types of expenses, such as diagnostic tool versus a treatment. It is good that the candidate ultimately picks one of the options as the question explicitly asks for this and their choice is supported by the caveats that it would require deeper analysis and rely on an evidence-base.

Overall:
What matters more is not whether you pick the MRI machine or the liver transplants but your ability to give a balanced and rational ethical argument to support your answer, to demonstrate relevant knowledge and consider the practicalities of applying this in the real world.

47) The UK has one of the lowest numbers of hospital beds in relation to population in the entire EU. Do you think this is a problem?

This question addresses the overall supply situation of the NHS. The number of beds in relation to the population is a good indicator of the overall health care provision to the population in question. The higher the number of beds, the more people can be accommodated in hospitals without increasing waiting times for admissions. In light of ever increasing waiting times for surgery as well as A&E, it is important to consider questions of health care provision. This is particularly the case as an increasing amount of hospitals is driving to reduce hospital bed numbers even further in order to adhere to governmental saving prescriptions.

A Bad Response:
There are several issues with this statement. Firstly, the comparison with Europe. The UK has the best health care system in the world and that is independent of the amount of hospital beds per population. The second issue arising from the question is the overstatement of the relevance of hospital beds as an indicator of quality. The amount of hospital beds per population does not provide much information as they are a poor indicator of the quality of care delivered. Similarly, there is no relationship between the net number of hospital beds and factors such as waiting times.

Response Analysis:
This is a bad response as it demonstrates a large degree of ignorance to the issues surrounding the provision of hospital resources to meet the needs of the population. The number of hospital beds provides a good indication of a health care system's ability to provide the necessary care to a population in question. Rash answers always look bad and being rash in answering questions such as this one will reflect poorly on the applicant's abilities.

A Good Response:
There are always issues with comparisons like this. They mainly lie in their briefness. It is difficult to comment on their relevance and on their specific meaning without further details. Looking at the question itself, however, this statistic paints a somewhat grim picture. Assuming that most European countries have similar interests in the provision of health care to their population, the fact that the UK is so low on the list is disheartening. It in part explains the issues surrounding long waiting times for surgery and it drums home the importance of supporting the appropriate discharge of medically fit patients. It furthermore makes the continuous reductions in hospital bed numbers graver due to the overall worsening of the situation. All in all, the low number of beds is a problem as it provides insight into the overall situation of care provision in the UK.

Response Analysis:
This response attempts to encompass all relevant aspects of the question. The student also demonstrates an understanding of scientific practice by raising issues with the question itself. By doing so, he/she demonstrates that he/she is aware of problems associated with this type of question. The student then goes on to highlight the implications of the question itself, attempting to give as much of a complex insight as possible.

Overall:
A challenging question that is important to be aware of in the times of ever-changing NHS budget provisions, especially with the continuous reduction of the amounts of beds. It is very important to have a good grasp and understanding of healthcare politics and of how healthcare provision could be improved with regards to issues such as bed number.

48) Do doctors hold a special position in society?

Doctors carry a big responsibility in society. They ultimately are responsible for maintaining and restoring the health of the population. In that capacity, they have an obviously very important role. In addition, due to the high degree of training and education involved in becoming a doctor, the profession historically holds a position of intelligence and moral relevance in the population. Historically, doctors, the clergy and lawyers provided the educated and elite classes in many societies. This has changed somewhat but the socially special role of doctors still persists. Doctors consistently score highly in tables related to the public's trust.

A Bad Response:
"Doctors represent the elite of the educated class in our society. They are highly skilled and highly educated and, therefore, by default very intelligent. It is for this reason that doctors hold a special position in society. Being entrusted with the population's health is a very challenging and complex matter that makes the medical profession a highly noble and respect-worthy one. Due to the morality associated with delivering the right treatment, doctors probably represent one of the very few parts of society that can still be trusted to be honest and truthful."

Response Analysis:
This is a bad response as it has little to do with reality. Whilst it is true that doctors hold a somewhat special place in society, this has little to do with the inherent intelligence of doctors nor with the nobility of the medical profession. The student's opinion regarding doctors' morality is simply wrong. Doctors are just as much able of immoral and criminal acts as any other population group. Nonetheless, the student is highlighting an important aspect of what it means to be a doctor. To a certain extent, the public has precisely this perception of doctors as a bastion of morality and character, especially with decreasing relevance of the church. This makes it that much more important to be aware and concise with the understanding of the roles of doctors, even when being a medical student. The public is very much aware that today's medical students are tomorrow's doctors and, therefore, it will expect us to behave accordingly.

A Good Response:
"Due to the nature of medicine and the interaction between doctors and their patients, doctors historically hold a special place in society. There are few people that are privy to such a high degree of very private information about patients than doctors. It is not rare that doctors know more about their individual patients than the patient's close relatives. This necessarily produces a special moral and ethical position for doctors. The public is more likely to trust doctors, simply due to the necessity of doing so. In addition, the educational pathway of doctors sets them apart from many other professions due to its complexity and challenging nature. In addition, doctors represent the guardians of health, arguably one of the most valuable possessions anybody can have."

Response Analysis:

This is a good response as it attempts to address the question in its entirety and also addresses the historical background. The answer furthermore attempts to rationalise the reasons for the trust placed in doctors, attempting to use this to explain the role of doctors in society.

Overall:
A complex question, but one that every medical student should be aware of as it has direct implications on what is expected of them once they qualify and as a matter of fact whilst they undergo training. Being aware of the public's expectations and opinions regarding the medical profession is very important. This special position in the eye of society has many direct implications on individuals in the medical profession, including the way they can for example act in employment disputes such as the recent junior doctor row. When for example taking industrial action, it is always about more than just the doctors as patient care is influenced as well.

49) A Jehovah's Witness is brought in by an ambulance to A&E after being in a road traffic accident and suffered massive blood loss. They need an urgent blood transfusion but the patient is refusing it. What do you do?

This is a classic ethical dilemma and variants on this frequently get asked. It's very important that you're aware of the law surrounding capacity and consent (see medical law section). The key here is to explore the patient's refusal for transfusion rather than falling into the trap of assuming that they don't want it as they are a Jehovah's Witness.

A Bad Response:

"I would give the blood transfusion anyway because the first duty of the doctor is to do what is right for the patient. Therefore, if a blood transfusion is needed to save her life or prevents serious harm, then that would be best. This patient may not know what is best for them right now, but could be thankful after we give her the blood transfusion if it then saves their life"

Response Analysis:

This response fails to consider the finer ethical and legal implications of transfusing someone against their wishes. There is no mention of patient autonomy or capacity. Nor does the response explore the reason for why the patient is refusing the transfusion.

A Good Response:

"Initially, I would try to establish why the patient is refusing a blood transfusion – is it because they lack capacity? Or is it because of a phobia of blood products/needles? Or based on religious beliefs? There is a conflict in this situation between wanting to do what we, the healthcare professionals, perceive is in the patient's best interests, which is giving the blood transfusion and respecting the patient's autonomy. To balance these, I would first make sure that the patient understood the potential consequences of what could happen if they refuse the blood transfusion – including potential death. Also, I would check that they still have the mental capacity to make this decision, including asking about whether they have made a prior declaration about what they would want in this situation, and assessing whether they suffered a head injury in the RTA or could be delirious due to blood loss.

It would also be important to check that the patient is not under undue influence from any friends or family who are with them. If the patient seems to have full mental capacity, understand the consequences of their decision, and not appear to be under the influence of anyone else, then I would respect their wish not to have a blood transfusion while consulting with colleagues so that they can check my assessment of the situation. In addition, I would also explore alternatives to blood transfusion".

Response Analysis:

A fantastic response that gives a structured step-by-step guide as to what the student would do. They clearly have a sound grasp of the medico-legal implications and also avoid the trap of assuming the refusal is due to religious purposes.

Overall:

You might get asked follow-on questions of this theme, e.g. "Another unconscious patient is admitted following a car accident. They are believed to be a Jehovah's Witness. Would you transfuse?"

In this case, as the patient is unconscious you are able to act in their best interest assuming there is no advance directive or family member preventing you from doing so (in which case, you should seek urgent legal advice). A Jehovah's Witness with full capacity can refuse blood transfusion but in this situation, it is possible he may have changed his mind or became a Jehovah's Witness unwillingly.

KNOWLEDGE BASED

50) Do you agree with the privatisation of the NHS?

This is a highly charged question. The interviewee must be able to give a balanced argument whilst still demonstrating a clear point of view. The interviewer wants to ensure your understanding of the healthcare system you are applying to be a part of, and how politics permeates the day-to-day function of the NHS. It is also a chance to demonstrate keen debating skills.

A Bad Response:

"I don't believe in the privatisation of the NHS. I believe the average UK citizen would end up worse-off both financially and in terms of their health if privatisation were to be taken further. It is financially viable for the NHS to remain free at the point of use. This is simply a way of attempting to turn healthcare into a competitive, profitable market, which I believe to be immoral."

Response Analysis:

Although the content may be true, this answer is too unequivocal and does not provide a balanced view of the topic. This answer is also perhaps too emotional and could be perceived as more of a rant than as part of a lively debate.

A Good Response:

"Before you can answer that question, you need to understand what privatisation of the NHS actually entails. The concept of privatisation can be viewed as a spectrum with an entirely publically funded NHS at one end of the scale, and America's private system with commercial insurance at the other. Commencing privatisation of the NHS involves private companies bidding to provide particular services currently already covered by the NHS, which is already happening. Those who are pro-privatisation believe that this increased competition provides patient choice and may actually stimulate improvements in the standard of care.

However, I believe that in the UK we are incredibly lucky to have access to a unique and world-class health care service, and it can be accessed free at the point of use by all. Privatisation directly erodes these fundamental socialist principals the NHS was founded on and could deepen existing inequalities, thereby worsening the general health of the UK population. Since it's conception, the NHS was never set up to be a profitable franchise and privatisation seems to involve prioritising profit over health – something which I don't feel represents the moral values of the NHS. Having different providers for every service also further breaks up an already fragmented system, resulting in less transparency. Overall I believe that privatisation of the NHS is detrimental to patient care."

Response Analysis:

This comprehensive answer incorporates the pros and cons of the question whilst clearly articulating a strong point of view. It is a good idea at the beginning to demonstrate knowledge about what privatisation of the NHS actually involves in practice. Whatever your personal opinions, it is important to acknowledge that we are very lucky in the UK to access free, world-class care and that privatisation represents a threat to this.

Overall:

Take time to explore the meaning of the question and consider your argument. It is important to be balanced and convey both the advantages and disadvantages before arguing your conclusions. It is also important not to be afraid of expressing your opinions, as long as you can back this up – this is not the platform for a political stance.

51) What differentiates the NHS from all other healthcare systems in the world?

This question is obviously aimed at the funding structure of the NHS as well as the question of eligibility. The founding idea of the NHS is to provide medical care for everybody living in the UK, irrespective of their income or social situation, i.e. 'free for all' at the point of entry. The funding model of the NHS is to assign a certain proportion of the general tax income to healthcare. The exact amount is dictated by a judgement of need of funding. Other healthcare systems use different funding models. For example, in the US, all healthcare is privately funded by the individual and in Germany, for example, healthcare is insurance-based.

A Bad Response:

"The NHS is superior in all aspects to other systems of healthcare provision as it is free for everybody and you can get all the treatments without having to pay anything. This ensures that everybody can get all the treatment they want without having to worry about how to pay for it. Having access to the most modern and effective treatments free of charge is essential for the maintenance of good population health, making the NHS the best healthcare system in the world."

Response Analysis:

This is a poor response because it is too one-dimensional. First of all, the question does not ask to make a judgement on which system is better but merely asks for the differences. Secondly, the answers show a principle misunderstanding of the resource allocation within the NHS. The NHS provides only NICE approved treatments and part of the approval process is a cost-efficiency calculation, which is particularly important in the context of modern cancer drugs that are highly effective but also very expensive. Some of these modern drugs do not satisfy the NICE cost-benefit calculation and are not available on the NHS, despite their affectivity.

A Good Response:

"The main points differentiating the NHS from other healthcare systems is the funding structure. Some countries like the USA rely on exclusively private funding for healthcare where every individual is responsible for covering the cost of their own treatment. Other countries like, for example, Switzerland rely on an insurance-based reimbursing scheme where medical costs are paid back by the insurance. In comparison to that, the NHS is funded by tax income. This means that a certain proportion of the overall income is allocated to healthcare in order to cover the anticipated needs of the system during the fiscal year."

Response Analysis:

This response is significantly better. It answers the question and provides examples from other countries, demonstrating good knowledge of healthcare overall. It avoids judgement and provides a good clear answer to the question. It also shows insight into the funding structure of the NHS.

Overall:

In this question, it is important to avoid judgement and being too rash with the decision-making. The question does not ask about superiority, but about differences. Other than the obvious difference in the funding structure, other differences include bodies such as NICE that evaluate treatments for cost-effectiveness and also provide guidelines for appropriate care delivery, as well as the organisation of care delivery with GPs almost functioning as triage points responsible for the distribution of patients.

52) Why do we worry so much about Hospital-acquired infections?

Hospital-acquired infections are a big issue. This is due to several different factors. Firstly, there is the issue of antibiotic resistance which is greater in hospital-acquired infections. Hospital bugs become resistant to commonly used antibiotics due to the selection pressures exerted by the antimicrobial environment. Secondly, many patients in hospital have a dampened immune response as they are ill. This reduces their ability to fight off infections- making them more susceptible to severe and prolonged infections. Lastly, hospital-acquired infections have an important financial impact as well, as they increase the time spent in the hospital. A patient may be cured of their original disease, but then acquires an infection in the hospital prolonging hospital stay.

A Bad Response:

"Hospital-acquired infections play a little role in a hospital setting as patients coming to the hospital are already ill anyway and treatment for an additional illness does not make much difference. Due to the availability of highly effective antimicrobial treatments, even the most persistent infections can be successfully treated. Whilst antibiotic resistance is a big issue in the community, it is less of an issue in the hospital as there are strong intravenous antibiotics available. In addition, hospital-acquired infections are relatively rare due to the strict cleaning procedures in place that prevent the spread of disease."

Response Analysis:

This answer is factually wrong. Hospital-acquired infections are of great worry. Whilst it is true that there are strict cleaning procedures in place to reduce the incidence of infection, they do not prevent all of them from occurring. In addition to that, hospital-acquired infections affect approximately 8% of all hospital admissions which represents quite a significant proportion of the patients. Also, whilst it is true that there are some antibiotics that can be used for some of the more resilient bugs, these pretty much represent the last resort and have quite significant side-effects for the patients.

A Good Response:

"Hospital-acquired infections have to be taken seriously. They are an issue for multiple reasons. The most significant reason is the increased resistance to available treatments. Many of the bacteria responsible for hospital-acquired infections have developed a multitude of antibiotic resistance traits that allow them to evade many of the mainstay treatments. In addition to the resistance, many of the resistant organisms are more virulent, causing more severe disease. This may also be due to the general status of poor health that the patients in the hospital are in. Being sick reduces the immune system activity, not only making the patients more susceptible in general but also giving the disease a more acute and severe course. There are other reasons why hospital-acquired infections represent an issue. They include the financial strain of prolonged hospital stays as well as the associated worsening of the hospital infrastructure as more beds are being occupied for longer, making it more difficult to find room for new admissions."

Response Analysis:

This is a good answer as it provides good insight into the issue surrounding the question. It also shows insight into the complexity of hospital care and what role hospital-acquired infections play in that context.

Overall:

This question deals with an important issue and with antibiotic resistance becoming an increasingly big problem, it is important to recognise the role of hospital-acquired infections in that context as well. Without research into new antibiotics proving increasingly challenging, this is a very important issue that needs to be addressed in order to ensure the future effectiveness of available treatments. With the high prevalence of hospital-acquired infections (8% of all admissions), it definitely is an important factor to recognise.

53) If you were in charge of the NHS what would you do?

Whilst this seems like a slightly rogue and tricky question, your response can demonstrate your understanding of the structure of the NHS and some of the problems currently faced by the organisation. The interviewers may be asking this question to see how much you know already about an organisation you will be working for one day, or they may be asking it simply as stimulation for debate and discussion to see how you think through a problem. Being in charge of large national organisations is something you're unlikely to have experience of and that's absolutely fine! But do expect to have your ideas challenged and to defend your opinions.

Since this is a very broad question, you may want to narrow down your answer right from the start and say that you will focus your answer on a specific bit. For example, say you focus on a particular problem you witnessed during your work experience or have personal experience of.

A Bad Response:
"If I were in charge of the NHS, I would want to reduce waiting lists so that patients get quicker access to the right health professionals. The waiting times for some clinics and operations can be very long and this is not conducive to an efficient system or happy patients. In order to achieve this, I would channel funds into employing extra staff in one area at a time until the waiting times in that area are reduced and then hopefully with the backlog cleared, the future waiting times will stay reduced."

Response Analysis:
This response does well in highlighting a specific subject to tackle, however, it comes across as overly confident and unfortunately with an unfeasible idea. The response also lacks an example or explaining where this idea has come from; either of which would help the interviewers to frame what they hear and ask more productive questions in return.

A Good Response:
"Right now, I must admit that I know far too little about most of the NHS to make any sensible suggestions as to how I would change it. So, with that in mind, if I were in charge I would invite employees of all skills and levels to offer their experiences and ideas as to how to make specific systems more efficient and a better experience for both staff and patients. I think it's the staff on the ground that can offer the best ideas as to how their jobs could be improved. I think it would be easier for people to accept changes if they were proposed by colleagues rather than seen as imposed on them by management.

For example, when I was doing work experience with a vascular surgeon, I attended an outpatient clinic and was interested to find the high number of patients who did not attend their appointments. If I were in charge of the NHS, this could be an example of something I would investigate using staff feedback – is it that the no-shows are actually needed to keep the clinic running to time or is time being wasted?"

Response Analysis:
This response uses your own lack of knowledge about the subject and spins it into a positive, focusing on the people on the ground doing the work and experiencing the system every day having the most informed opinions about it. The use of an example helps to illustrate the argument and reminds the interviewers of how much you absorbed during your work experience.

Overall:
There are infinite things one could do if one were to take over charge of the NHS, so narrowing down your discussion points will really help you here. Current issues seen in the media would also be a reasonable springboard for your response to this question. If the interviewers start to debate with you, then try to explain the rationale behind your ideas but don't feel you have to continue to defend ideas if it quickly becomes apparent they are not feasible! The interviewers are almost certainly interested in seeing how you think through the problem rather than what you actually come up with – no-one is expecting you to have a management degree.

54) How would you approach the problem of low NHS funding?

Resource allocation is a very important point of ethical debate in the NHS. Discussing it gives you an opportunity to show good reasoning abilities, an appreciation for the importance of justice as a principle in healthcare, and a strong moral compass. It also shows that you recognise that it can be challenging for doctors when treatments are available for patients that they are unable to offer due to limited funding. Explaining this to patients can be very difficult and potentially upsetting.

A Bad Response:
I think the NHS funding should be increased by the government. However, I understand that this could be difficult in which case, the money should go towards treating those who need it most.

Response Analysis:
A pragmatic albeit simplistic view on resource allocation. There is little insight into how treatments and procedures are funded by the NHS nor is there any mention of how the applicant would increase funding. Finally, there is no explanation as to what is defined as patients 'who need it most' and who would decide this.

A Good Response:
A good policy for distributing limited funding is prioritisation so that the money is used in a way that produces the greatest possible overall benefit. A good way to quantify this is in Quality Adjusted Life Years (QUALYs) / £K spending. NICE analyses the average QUALY/£K for different treatments and produces guidelines on which treatments produce the most benefit. These guidelines are probably the best way of deciding how to spend NHS money. In the future, it could be necessary to suspend the free provision of non-vital treatments such as IVF. It is also important to ensure that the money is spent as efficiently as possible, e.g.by treating patients in the community instead of a hospital.

Response Analysis:
A much more comprehensive response that analyses the process by which treatments and procedures get approved and allocated. There is a good level of discussion regarding the multiple organisations that contribute to this and a valid plan of stopping non-vital treatments. The use of IVF as an example is well done.

Overall:
This question is also about understanding the interaction between beneficence, autonomy and justice, **and** rationalising treatment that is equitable. Whilst a treatment/intervention/procedure may be good for the patient (beneficence), it may be costly and, hence, limit its use in a large population. This would lead to finding means to restrict treatments to some and that will not do justice and fair to all. Governing bodies like NICE offer guidelines to ensure treatments remain equitable and fair to all.

All patients in a similar situation should be treated similarly. Clinicians should ensure that the treatment options are cost effective and use resources correctly.

55) *What is a clinical trial?*

Clinical trials are an important part of the licensing process of a new drug. There are several stages of clinical trials; all designed to assess safety and effectiveness of a drug. The clinical trial stage follows a series of other trials preceding it in order to provide an idea of safety for human testing. Before entering the clinical trial stage, a drug needs to be deemed safe for human use. To further ensure safety, reduced doses of the drug are usually used for early stage trials. Despite these steps, sometimes things go wrong in clinical trials and participants get hurt. Various institutions tightly regulate clinical trials.

A Bad Response:

"In a clinical trial, volunteers are given an experimental drug to determine its effectiveness in the treatment of a certain disease as well as its safety for use in humans. Human trials are superior to animal trials as they allow a judgement of the effectiveness of a drug in humans. After a drug has passed clinical trials, it is available to the general public in form of treatment. Through this process, we can progress quickly from drug formulation to use."

Response Analysis:

This answer is too short and shows little understanding of how medical licensing works. Whilst the general concept of clinical trials is correct, there are some errors regarding timescale as well as associated procedures and risks. Firstly, it takes about 10 years from the formulation of a drug to it entering the trial phase and even then, only a fraction of all drugs designed even enter the human trial phase. Secondly, there are several levels of clinical trials before a drug can be licensed for safe human use and even then, more time will go by on additional licensing procedures before it is available for use in treatments.

A Good Response:

"Clinical trials represent an important milestone in the licensing process of new medications. They usually are preceded by extensive testing on cells, computer models, and animals to provide an idea of effectiveness and safety in mammals. Human clinical trials themselves are organised in different stages, depending on how close a drug is to licensing. Phases 1 – 3 happen before a drug is licensed and involve increasing sample sizes as well as different parameters of research. Phase 1 trials, for example, involve the determination of safe doses, Phase 2 trials the determination of general effectiveness, and Phase 3 trials aim at comparing established treatments with new treatments to provide a judgement on superiority. It is important to note that not all drugs that enter Phase 1 trials will progress to Phase 3 and to licensing. Phase 4 happens after licensing and usually aims at determining long-term risks and benefits etc. Due to the nature of human testing, clinical trials of all phases are tightly regulated by governing bodies and the declaration of Helsinki as well as the Nuremberg Code."

Response Analysis:

This answer is a good one as it reflects a good knowledge of the process of clinical trials and also gives the examiners a quick summary of how precisely clinical trials work in the different phases. Showing insight into this is important as the term "clinical trial" is often misunderstood. It further demonstrates a good understanding of the challenges of human testing and the responsibilities arising from using human test subjects.

Overall:

Due to the use of human test subjects, clinical trials are an important ethical issue. As they play a central role in the development of drugs and the very real prospect of doctors treating patients that either are part of a trial or have an interest in participating in trials, it is essential for doctors to understand how clinical trials work and what differentiates the distinctive stages. Remember that all new drugs go through the same rigorous process before becoming available to the public.

56) What are the new junior doctor contracts about?

The new contract is supposed to lay the foundation for a 7-day NHS service that ensures good hospital care for all 7 days of the week. There are 3 main areas of change. The first involves safeguards that prevent doctors from being overworked by financially penalising institutions that do not allow for the contractually prescribed rest and break periods. The second set of changes involves the progress in salary. At the moment, the doctor's salary raises each year to reflect the increase in expertise due to increased experience. The new contract wants to bind pay raises to the reaching of new stages of qualification. The third area of change is aimed at core working hours. At the moment, these run from 7am to 7pm on Monday to Friday. This is supposed to change from 7am to 10pm from Monday to Saturday. This has a great impact on the work-life balance of doctors.

A Bad Response:

"The main change to the junior doctor contracts lies in the payment structure. Doctors are expected to work more for less money. This is unacceptable as doctors in this country are already being paid relatively poorly in comparison to other countries such as the US. It is immoral to expect such a highly qualified profession such as doctors to work for such little money. Doctors maintain the health of society and as such should be appropriately compensated for their services."

Response Analysis:

This is a bad response as it falls short of the complexity of the contract changes. Whilst it is true that the changes will result in a decrease in pay, this is only part of the problem with the new contracts. Bigger issues lie in the poor work-life balance as well as in the removal of working time safeguards that protect doctors from being overworked in order to protect patients. Tired doctors make mistakes, which will endanger patient's health. It also fails to explore the impact of this contract on the NHS in the long-term, e.g. junior doctor's exodus to other countries.

A Good Response:

"The new contract entails several changes that will have a great impact on the junior doctor's life, both professionally as well as privately. Changes to working time protection will remove safeguards in place that currently aim to prevent the overworking of doctors. This is essential to prevent mistakes that happen when doctors are tired. Another area of change concerns antisocial working hours. At the moment, core working hours for doctors run from 7am to 7pm on Monday to Friday. Anything else is defined as antisocial which amongst other things carries higher financial compensation. As part of the new contract, the core working hours are supposed to change to 7am to 10pm on Monday to Saturday. The final point of change lies in financial recognition of gained experience. At the moment, pay increases each year to reflect this gain of experience. This is supposed to change to a promotion-like system where pay increases upon completion of training milestones."

Response Analysis:

This is a good response as it aims to address the different changes suggested in the new contract and tries to put them into context with regards to their impact on the individual doctors. It is important to stay as neutral as possible as the question does not ask about opinions, but rather only about the changes suggested in the new contract.

Overall:

This is an important issue as it will eventually affect everyone in the medical profession. Given that this is a rapidly developing topic, it's absolutely paramount that you keep yourself updated by reading the news (BBC Health, BMAT, and Student BMAT). Avoid getting drawn into a political argument about governmental health policies or critiquing the Health Secretary (Jeremy Hunt) – that's not the point of this question or the interview.

57) How would you control the TB problem in the homeless population?

This question has several components to it. On one hand, it tests the student's understanding of an infectious disease and on the other hand, it addresses the understanding of the interaction between health and population as well as ethical issues regarding healthcare. It is important to address each individual component of this question in part in order to gain maximum points. The more holistic the answer, the higher you will score.

A Bad Response:

"In order to control the TB problem in the homeless population, if one exists in the first place, the easiest way is to force every homeless person to receive the TB vaccine. We could use police patrols to detain every homeless person they come across that has not had the TB vaccine and then give them the shot, whether they agree or not. In order to ensure that people are not vaccinated more than once, we can hand out pieces of paper confirming the vaccination status of the individual."

Response Analysis:

Generally, a bad response ignores parts of the question or only providing superficial and judgemental points. This answer is bad in several aspects. It shows very little insight into the complexity of TB and also some serious ethical issues. Detaining an individual and then forcing them to be vaccinated ignores with fundamental principles of freedom and consent to treatment. Consent is a particularly important aspect of this question with regards to a medical interview.

A Good Response:

"TB represents an important problem in the homeless population but also for public health in general. Therefore, control of this problem has a direct positive impact not only on the health of the individual but also population as a whole. In order to control the problem, it is the most reasonable to attack it on several levels. Firstly, there is the TB vaccine. Whilst it has a limited effectivity of 60 – 80%, it still provides an important starting point for the control of the problem. Ultimately, though, the best way to control the problem is by getting the homeless off the street and into secure housing. This requires financial support from the government and establishment of necessary support structures providing general medical care as well as food and addiction support. Due to the general immunocompromise associated with alcoholism, poor nutrition and other drug addictions, providing help for this will also provide a good starting point."

Response Analysis:

This is a good answer that attempts to address all components of the question and also manages to remain non-judgemental. It also provides an idea of some insight into the interaction of infectious diseases with the individual as well as lifestyle and treatment. Also, points out the connection between individual and the population.

Overall:

A complex question always requires a complex answer as there are no easy solutions for complex problems. Making sure to consider the individual as well as the population and the impact of lifestyle choices will always improve the quality of an answer.

58) *What speciality are you interested in?*

Whilst it is certainly not a pre-requisite to applying to medicine, having a few ideas about what speciality you might be interested in and explaining yourself clearly can really impress interviewers. However, it is also important to realise that you have not seen or experienced most of medicine and, therefore, need to explore the field a lot more before deciding.

Some people apply to medicine with already pretty fixed ideas about what they'd ultimately like to do, but still, try to approach this question with an open mind when answering. If you have no idea that's fine too, but maybe have a few specialities and their pros and cons in your head in case you get asked this question. A good place to start could be the specialities you came into contact with during work experience, or specialities you have personally come into contact with (NB if you're going to mention personal contact with health services, then be prepared to talk about it!).

A Bad Response:

"Ever since I was 8, I have known that I want to become a paediatric surgeon. I shadowed a paediatric surgery team for a week of work experience and was totally blown away by the doctors' skills both in theatre and in communicating with patients and their parents. I know that surgery is a very demanding job but I believe I have the passion and drive to see me through the long training. I think it would be a very rewarding role and one that would also suit my personality well."

Response Analysis:

This response doesn't show that you've really thought about it – more that you've seen this speciality and liked it. Knowing what you don't know is half the battle here, try to be more open-minded and maybe preface your answer with, "I have had very limited experience so far but from what I've seen…". It is also a good idea to have done some research on the specialities you might mention and appraise them in your answer. For example, saying what you like about the speciality and why you think you'd be suited to it but also what the downsides to that speciality are or what you might find challenging.

A Good Response:

"My experience of different specialities is very limited as I have only done work experience placements in general practice and anaesthetics. At this stage, I'd say I'm not sure what speciality I'd like to go into and would hope that along the course something would spark my interest. If I had to decide now, based on the very little exposure I've had, I might consider obstetrics, which I saw briefly whilst shadowing an anaesthetist. From my research and brief discussion with the obstetricians I met, I think this speciality has a lot of patient contact, often at a happy and healthy time in their life. It is also a mix of medical and surgical skills which appeals to me. However, I do appreciate that the speciality training for obstetrics is very demanding so it would have to be something I'd see if I like after actually experiencing it."

Response Analysis:

Starting off by framing what you're hanging your answer on may be a good idea and it also demonstrates to the interviewer that this is not an opinion you've simply generated on the spot to answer the question. This response considers both how the speciality is suited to you and the bad points. It is very reasonable to say that you're still not sure and indeed knowing when you will have to decide (apply to training schemes during foundation years), this will also show that you have a good understanding of the profession. If possible, showing that you acted on your interest is great. For example, in this response, finding obstetrics interesting and then discussing the speciality with the doctors on that training programme.

As in this response, if the speciality you did on your work experience did not grip you then try to frame it positively or simply gloss over it in favour of something you're more interested in. Obviously avoid dismissing or shunning any specialities, even if you didn't enjoy your experience of them so far and know you wouldn't want to do them.

Overall:

Try to demonstrate that this is something you have considered but be mindful of your lack of experience and exposure. It's perfectly okay to be interested in one thing or have no idea but try to find out about a few things that you think you might be interested in. If you can get some work experience in your preferred speciality, then that's great but take any opportunity to talk to doctors.

This is a very personal question so don't be tempted to research the speciality of any of the interviewers and say you want to do that simply because they are interviewing you. Speak honestly about your interests and impress them with your consideration. However, don't be afraid to acknowledge that this is too early for you to choose a speciality and you may change your mind as you get exposed to different specialities.

Interviewers know that you won't have a lot of experience of different specialities and that a lot of people change their mind many times during medical school and training anyway! So they won't be looking to admit you purely for your enthusiasm for a specific thing. Instead, you should look at this question as a chance for you to demonstrate your insight into the medical profession and show that you are well-read as to the demands of medicine as a subject and job.

59) What is the EWTD? What is its significance?

The EWTD is the European Working Time Directive. Most of your answer should be based on the latter question; what is the EWTDs significance? In answering this question, it is important to show your understanding of the working environment of doctors, the importance of ensuring that working conditions do not compromise the work of doctors, and the significance of working hours of doctors to the quality of patient care. You should be able to identify the priorities of a doctor in accordance with doing the best job they can with respect to patient welfare and health. You should aim to keep the answer to this question relatively short; you don't need to include much detail in your answer and it is enough to show a basic understanding of the EWTD and the demanding working conditions of doctors.

A Bad Response:

"The EWTD is the European Working Time Directive. It is in place to make sure doctors don't work too hard. Doctors are placed under too much stress as it is. They have endless amounts of work and the work is often very emotionally draining. Doctors should not be forced to work for long hours without a break as this risks causing doctors to burnout and consequently, they will be more likely to quit. The EWTD is an important directive that is a key factor of why many doctors find their jobs bearable."

Response Analysis:

The candidate provides a very excessively pessimist viewpoint of the working life of doctors. The candidate fails to identify any reasons as to why working as a doctor is a valuable or rewarding job. This can cause the interviewer to question the candidate's belief in his/her own decision to study medicine. The candidate mentions the emotional toll of work on the doctor; this is an important and sensitive issue that should be addressed with caution. A doctor needs to be able to cope with the emotional stress that their job carries with it in a healthy manner so that they can process difficult situations without such experiences influencing their judgment or competency.

A Good Response:

"The EWTD is the European Working Time Directive. It limits the number of working hours of doctors in the UK and specifies when rest periods and holiday periods should be given and how frequently they should be taken. The directive is in place to protect both patients and doctors in order to not overwork doctors or cause them to burnout. The importance of the EWTD is great as without safe and fair working hours, we would have tired doctors who are more likely to make mistakes and, hence, endanger patients and compromise their care."

Response Analysis:

The answer identifies that the major issue here is the threat of long working hours reducing the quality of service doctors delivering to patients. Any risk of potential harm caused to patients is a very serious issue and something that must be avoided at all costs, and this is what the European Working Time Directive aims to avoid.

Overall:

The details of the directive do not need to be stated but you should have a good idea of what they are (see the EWTD page earlier in this book for more details).

60) Should a doctor need consent to be able to perform a procedure?

Consent is essential in medical practice as it is the basis of autonomy; one of the core principles of medical practice. In order to achieve appropriate consent, the patient has to be provided with all relevant and significant details of the procedure and be given all the relevant information related to the procedure. This includes the risks & benefits of the procedure and details about what the procedure involves.

A Bad Response:
Consent is just a formality. What matters is that the patient agrees verbally in a conversation with the doctor. Any doctor can get consent from a patient and he does not have to be able to perform the procedure himself. The doctor also only needs to give the patient a rough idea of what is going to happen during the procedure. Details are only necessary on a somewhat limited level, as long as the patient is happy to undergo the procedure. In general, consent needs to be achieved, but it is sufficient to give the patient a general overview of the procedure.

Response Analysis:
This response is inadequate as it has several inaccuracies and shortcomings. This is an issue as it puts the student in a bad light regarding his overall understanding of medical practice. Consent is one of the core values of medical practice and being aware of all the implications associated with this is vital. The student generally displays an overall lack of appreciation of the important information about the consenting of a patient.

A Good Response:
Consent is vital for medical practice. Doctors can only perform procedures that have been given informed consent by the patient. Any violation of this is battery which is a criminal offence. When consenting a patient, a good understanding of the procedure itself as well as of the risks associated is important in order to tailor the information delivery to the individual patient. In addition to this, an understanding of the procedure will allow the doctor to answer any question the patient might have in full and with enough detail to allow the patient to make an informed decision about the procedure. Ultimately, that is the basis that needs to be satisfied in order for consent to be valid. In general, a doctor should only consent a patient for a procedure that he/she is familiar with, as only then will he/she have the necessary appreciation for the exact processes underlying the procedure.

Response Analysis:
This is a good answer as it gives a good degree of background information about the process of achieving consent as well as about the different factors influencing consent and its validity. The student demonstrates a good grasp of what it means to consent a patient for a procedure and the importance of valid consent for medical practice.

Overall:
The aim of this question is to analyse the student's ability to think about medical core ethical principles in a more clinical setting. There is not really a right or wrong answer, but the student needs to demonstrate an understanding of the relevance of consent in the overall practice of medicine and what place consent and the information provided holds within clinical medicine. It also gives an indication of the student's approach to medical practice from a legal perspective and the implications this has on the delivery of care. The necessity of this is two-fold; on one hand, this is to protect the patient and on the other hand, this also protects the doctor from litigation. An understanding of the safety concerns associated with medical care is central for any prospective doctor.

61) Should the NHS be run by doctors?

The NHS is the supplier of the vast majority of medical care in the UK. Due to the nature of the NHS as a government institution, the input into the managing structure is very diverse and includes a high proportion of non-medical professions. In the light of the recent junior doctor contract conflict, the question of NHS leadership and management is very important.

A Bad Response:

The NHS should most definitely be run by doctors. Only doctors are able to understand the complexity of medical care and what it means to deliver this care every day. In addition, it seems that doctors would be more trustworthy than politicians with the latter only being out for power and control. Doctors do the job they do in order to help people and should, therefore, be put in charge of the organisation that was established to help people.

Response Analysis:

This response is a bad one as it is very one-dimensional and does not appreciate the complexity of the issue of leadership. Whilst a doctor may be a great physician or surgeon, that does not necessarily mean that he/she is a good manager with the ability to control and efficiently guide a large body of employees. The student ignores that. The comment on the morality of doctors may or may not be an appropriate representation of the truth, but most importantly, it does not provide a valid judgement of the ability of the individual to perform the specific task at hand.

A Good Response:

The NHS as an institution is very important and very high profile. It is the largest single employer in the world. This necessarily makes its administration very complex. This needs to be reflected in the leadership. Whilst the argument can be made that doctors are able to understand how medical professionals work and how healthcare is provided in the hospitals, this falls somewhat short of an appropriate justification for the superiority of doctors' leadership. Due to their special knowledge of medical realities, doctors should be involved in policy making and long-term decisions in the NHS, but so should nurses and other health care providers as they ultimately work in the same environment. It is also important to underline that only because somebody is a good doctor, they might not be good managers. And efficient management is centrally important in running an organisation as large as the NHS.

Response Analysis:

A good response as it is very diverse and attempts to address the underlying issues surrounding the administration of the NHS. The complexity of the NHS as an enterprise is very important to recognise, so is the appreciation of limited abilities as a manager. This answer also addresses limitations of the question by pointing out that there are more healthcare providers in the NHS than just doctors.

Overall:

This question is relevant at this moment in time as it addresses an important issue with the NHS. Due to its size, an efficient administration is very challenging and appropriate allocation of resources is as well. Having first-hand experiences of healthcare provision will facilitate an understanding of what areas need the most support in terms of money etc. and what aspects demonstrate the biggest shortcomings. It is vital for students to have an opinion on questions like that. Having an understanding and a founded opinion on the questions such as this one is an excellent way for a student to set himself or herself apart from the rest of the applicants and it will make for a very positive and mature impression.

62) What is the "obesity epidemic"?

Obesity is an escalating global epidemic and affects virtually all age and socioeconomic groups. It is no longer limited to developed countries and millions suffer from other serious health disorders as a result. Obesity poses a major risk for diabetes, hypertension, stroke, and certain forms of cancer. Its health consequences range from increased risk of premature death to serious chronic conditions that reduce the overall quality of life.

Obesity levels in the UK have more than trebled in the last 30 years and, on current estimates, more than half the population could be obese by 2050. Income, social deprivation and ethnicity have an important impact on the likelihood of becoming obese. For example, women and children in lower socioeconomic groups are more likely to be obese than those who are wealthier. The car, TV, computers, desk jobs, high-calorie food, and increased food abundance have all contributed to encouraging inactivity and overeating.

A Bad Response:
"More people in the world are gaining in weight which is causing an epidemic. The US is a particular culprit. This weight gain is primarily due to our heavily sedentary lifestyles and high-fat diets."

Response Analysis:
The response itself is correct and contains all true information but it is lacking in detail. "Gaining in weight" is non-specific; a better answer would have included the Body Mass Index as an objective measure of obesity (BMI greater than 30 is classified as obese). The answer also discusses the US. While it is true that America is a key example of the obesity epidemic, it is important to remember that the UK is not innocent. Talking about the UK would be more relevant and could lead nicely into a discussion of the burden on the NHS. The last sentence is also scientifically correct but ignores factors such as genetics and epidemiological factors, e.g. socioeconomic background.

A Good Response:
"The obesity epidemic describes the rise in cases of obesity globally. Obesity is defined as a BMI greater than 30. This rise is not limited to certain areas or ages; we are now seeing children as young as eight years old classified as obese. Obesity comes with a large variety of disorders, including diabetes mellitus, cardiovascular problems and some cancers. This is particularly troubling due to the increasing burden on the NHS which already faces multiple challenges. In the current political climate, the escalating obesity epidemic places great pressure on an already strained NHS."

Response Analysis:
This answer clearly defines obesity which shows us that they know this topic well. Obesity in children is a very hot topic in media and health so by mentioning it, the candidate has shown that they are aware of the key issues on this topic. The increasing burden this places on the NHS due to its various co-morbid conditions is also an essential part of this topic and shows that this is a strong candidate. The last sentence briefly touches on current news – "current political climate" clearly means Jeremy Hunt, the junior doctor debate, and the possible privatisation of the NHS. It also gives the interviewers something to grab onto so you can direct them to a topic you know a lot on (make sure you know about the Jeremy Hunt situation before you do this!).

Overall:
A good answer will look at the impact of obesity on the NHS and draw on current health news. Common follow-on questions to this would be: *"Should obese people be offered weight loss surgery?"* Or *"should doctors be obese?"*

63) How do you think the role of a doctor has changed over time?

Over the years, the role of doctors has changed within the NHS on many fronts:

Change in Responsibilities: Other healthcare workers are now able to do many tasks initially performed by doctors, e.g. Phlebotomists, specialist nurses, etc. This has freed doctors to take on different roles, e.g. management.

Long Hospital Stays: It once was common for a woman to spend 10 days in the hospital after giving birth, rather than today's more standard 24-hour turnaround. Other health care services also came with long hospital stays, now the surgery is performed on an outpatient basis. Some examples include pacemaker implantations, tonsillectomies, and cataract extraction. Technological advances drove many of these changes. Some patients with kidney disease today can bring home a dialysis machine, for example. Laparoscopic surgery, which uses very small incisions allows patients to heal faster. The trend toward moving patients out of the hospital is important to the bottom line. Discharging patients sooner tended to be better for the patient as well. Staying in the hospital for a long time can be detrimental to a patient's health because it increases their exposure to bacteria.

Patient Empowerment: Informed consent and patient autonomy are two ideas that have become key in medical ethics today. Caregivers tend to be transparent with patients about diagnostic information, risks, and treatments in order to establish shared decision-making.

Evidence-Based Medicine: When decisions are made about the care of individual patients, they are made on the basis of the most up-to-date, solid, reliable, scientific evidence. This has formed what is now known as evidence-based practice.

A Bad Response:
"The prestige of being a doctor has declined. Often, patients have researched things on the internet and it is difficult to explain the best options for treatment due to their preformed ideas."

Response Analysis:
The response itself is correct and contains all true information but it is quite negative. By mentioning prestige, this answer brings into question the student's motivation for applying to medicine. Do they only care about prestige? It is important that care of the patient is foremost in your answer. Placing a negative tone on patient self-research implies that the student does not realise the importance of having an informed patient – this will reflect badly.

A Good Response:
"The NHS now offers a patient-centred healthcare approach which is very different from the paternalist medicine from the past. It is important to keep patients involved in the decision-making, so informed consent is essential. Evidence-based medicine has allowed safer research and medical techniques to be put into practice. The NHS has also grown exponentially since it was founded in 1948."

Response Analysis:
"Patient-centred" is a key buzzword and really fitting for this question. "Evidence-based medicine" is also a buzzword and very topical at the moment. Use of these words shows that you are knowledgeable about the NHS and current topics. Use of "informed consent" also shows that the student is aware of the ethical implications

Overall:
A good answer will drop in buzzwords such as "patient-centred care" and "evidence-based medicine". A poor answer will be negative in tone – it is important to show that you know that medicine is moving forward and the patient experience has improved.

64) What do you understand by the "postcode lottery"?

The postcode lottery is shorthand for the countrywide variations in the provision and quality of public services. Where you live defines the standard of services you can expect. So if you live in the "wrong" area, you may get a poorer service than your neighbour or you may not get the service at all and have to pay for it privately. The postcode lottery is a big issue in the NHS.

In practice, there are geographical variations in almost all aspects of care. Recent examples include variations in charges for disabled people's home care; availability of NHS in-vitro fertilisation services; waiting times for NHS treatment; and access to NHS cancer screening programmes. Generally speaking, the lower the socio-economic background, the worse your care and access to it are likely to be. This is known as the "inverse care law". It also shows the variation in spending between GP Practices – both overall and on types of disease.

Although some variation is warranted because different populations have different levels of need, the postcode lottery highlights the need to impose basic minimum standards of acceptable care across the UK. The Government argues that rationing within the NHS is necessary to ensure that resources which could be spent elsewhere are not wasted and that patients receive only treatments which have real clinical benefits.

A Bad Response:
"The postcode lottery means that some people do not get the same healthcare as others. However, it is important for the Government to regulate healthcare provisions to ensure the most healthcare is provided for the most people. This follows the "justice" principle in ethics."

Response Analysis:
The first answer is the worst possible one. Be sure to research key issues in the NHS. The second answer shows a poor understanding of what the postcode lottery is. Although the information is correct, the answer fails to grasp that the widespread inequality caused by the postcode lottery goes against the ethical principle of "justice".

A Good Response:
"The postcode lottery describes the inequality in the provision of healthcare based on where people live. There are differences in access to NHS treatment throughout the country and this can affect the quality and availability of NHS services you can expect. The increase in rationing within the NHS has led to an increase in the effects of the postcode lottery, in determining which patients have access to certain treatments. This has affected waiting times, cancer treatments, and most notably, in vitro fertilisation therapies. I understand that it is important to ration healthcare due to limited resources but there should be a clear agreement on the basic standard of care across England, and even the UK."

Response Analysis:
This answer is very well constructed. It begins by succinctly defining what the postcode lottery is and how it can arise. "Important to ration healthcare due to limited resources" shows that the candidate clearly understands the justice component and thus the other side of the argument. The answer concludes with a strong statement using key information (included in the background) that shows the interviewer that they truly understand the topic.

Overall:
A good answer will show understanding of the topic. Begin your answer with a definition and then go into the causes. Be sure to give a balanced view to show you understand both sides of the discussion.

65) What health problems do doctors face?

As a doctor, looking after your own health is just as important as looking after your patients. Medicine is a challenging and stressful profession. While making care for the patient a priority, it is important to appreciate that doctors can be susceptible to health problems too.

Stigma: There is a large amount of stigma that surrounds illness in doctors. The expectations that doctors place on themselves is likely to contribute to the problem. The myth persists that good doctors do not make mistakes and that illness, particularly mental ill health, is a weakness. Taking time off work is letting colleagues and patients down; showing vulnerability may lose the respect of others.

Stress: Doctors report that stress has an impact on their ability to provide high-quality care, this can be reflected in GMC referrals. Medicine is a stressful profession; sources of stress may include: work pressure, poor support, high demand workload, investigations, complaints and court cases, and trauma of dealing with suffering. There is extra stress for some groups – for example, women with small children have to manage the competing tensions of work and home life.

Mental Health: A third of doctors have some kind of mental disorder. Yet for many, it is a shameful secret because of the deep prejudice towards mental illness that still exists in the medical profession. Doctors often have significant mental health problems before they seek help. Many doctors work long hours and have heavy workloads, which can cause severe depression and lead to suicide attempts. Suicide rates have also increased, particularly in female doctors, anaesthetists, GPs and psychiatrists.

Substance Misuse: Over 5% of doctors will have a substance use problem during their lifetime, using it as a way to cope with stress. Doctors' access to prescription drugs plays a part in their risk of substance use and suicide, as well as making it easier to treat themselves rather than seeking help.

A Bad Response:

"Doctors are people too and they have normal health problems like everyone else. It is important that they seek help but this may be difficult due to their long working hours."

Response Analysis:

The response itself is good in that it mentions that doctors are human so can suffer illness. It also recognises the difficulty doctors face in seeking help. However, it fails to grasp the most complex details of this issue which shows this is a weak candidate. Mental health in doctors is a key issue and a hot topic in the news so would be fitting for this question.

A Good Response:

"Doctors can suffer from poor mental health. Being a doctor is a stressful job which can predispose to mental illness. The personality of people who wish to be medical students can also lead to poor mental health. Media and doctors themselves place a great deal on doctors to act as an infallible guide to health, this can make doctors think they "are not allowed" to be ill. There may be alcohol misuse as a way of coping with stress or a lot of depression. I feel it is important that doctors know how and where to seek help."

Response Analysis:

This answer clearly grasps the most complex issues surrounding doctors' health and shows that this is a strong candidate. Mental health in doctors may be a sensitive topic but it is important to show that you are aware of the darker side to medicine. Any awareness of the pressure on doctors and the myth of the all-knowing infallible doctor shows knowledge of the current news. A better answer would have included the effect on patient safety.

Overall:

A good answer will show understanding of the more complex side of doctors' health. It will also include the potential negative effects on patient safety.

66) What is public health and why is it important?

Public health is defined as "the science and art of promoting and protecting health and well-being, preventing ill-health and prolonging life through the organised efforts of society". This means that it aims to protect the health of populations. These populations can be as small as a local community or as big as an entire country or region of the world.

The National Health Service is a public funded healthcare system that provides healthcare for the UK, so has a vested interest in public health. A large part of public health is promoting healthcare equity, quality and accessibility. Public health professionals try to prevent problems from happening or recurring through implementing educational programs, recommending policies, administering services and conducting research - "prevention is worth more than a cure" – so it works to promote healthy behaviours. Public health also works to limit health disparities.

Public health is heavily influenced by a number of social factors and is, therefore, continually adapting. Although sanitation and vaccination are still key; it has now broadened to include smoking cessation, the harmful use of alcohol, nutrition, obesity and physical inactivity, and multi-drug resistant bacteria.

The work of public health professionals is important because public health initiatives affect people every day in every part of the world. It addresses broad issues that can affect the health and well-being of individuals, families, communities, populations, and societies—both now, and for generations to come. Public health programs help keep people alive. These programs have led to increased life expectancies, worldwide reductions in infant and child mortality, and eradication or reduction of many communicable diseases.

A Bad Response:
"Public health is about the health of the public. It is concerned about the main diseases that can affect England. It is important because it works to reduce the incidence of disease in England."

Response Analysis:
It is important to remember that public health is a worldwide thing e.g. the Ebola epidemic was managed by the World Health Organisation which deals with global public health. The definition does not mention "specific populations" which is key in public health – different populations have different health needs. A specific example of a type of public health initiative would have demonstrated that the candidate had real knowledge on this topic, however, this is lacking.

A Good Response:
"Public Health is concerned with looking at the health of populations and the different diseases that may dominate in a particular population. They look at prevention, which can include screening programmes, for example, the National Chlamydia Screening Programme (NCSP) is an NHS sexual health programme that forms part of public health initiatives, along with the provision of free condoms. The NHS is a public health service so public health plays a key part in its role."

Response Analysis:
This answer has a clear definition of public health. Vaccination is often the example of public health most candidates know so by providing something different this highlights the candidates as someone of interest. This answer also cites the NHS, making it relevant to becoming a doctor.

Overall:
A good answer will add detail and give an example of a current public Health measure, such as the National Chlamydia Screening Programme or smoking cessation clinics. It will also relate the question to the NHS and comment on the importance of public health.

67) Why is antibiotic overprescribing a problem?

Antibiotics are medications used to treat and sometimes prevent bacterial infections. They can be used to treat relatively mild conditions such as acne, as well as life-threatening conditions such as pneumonia. However, antibiotics often have no benefit for many other types of infection.

Bacteria can adapt and mutate to survive the effects of an antibiotic. The chance of this increases if a person does not finish the course of antibiotics they have been prescribed, as some bacteria may be left to develop resistance. This means antibiotics are losing their effectiveness at an increasing rate. The more we use antibiotics, the greater the chance bacteria will become resistant to them and they can no longer be used to treat infections. Antibiotics can also destroy many of the harmless strains of bacteria that live in and on the body. This allows resistant bacteria to multiply quickly and replace them.

Using antibiotics unnecessarily would only increase the risk of antibiotic resistance, so they should not be used routinely. Antibiotic resistance is one of the most significant threats to patients' safety in Europe. It is driven by overusing antibiotics and prescribing them inappropriately.

Antibiotic resistance has led to the emergence of "superbugs". These are strains of bacteria that have developed resistance to many different types of antibiotics. They include Clostridium Difficile and MRSA which are large problems in hospitals. These types of infections can be serious and challenging to treat and are becoming an increasing cause of disability and death across the world.

The biggest worry is new strains of bacteria may emerge that cannot be effectively treated by any existing antibiotics. To slow down the development of antibiotic resistance, it is important to use antibiotics in the right way – to use the right drug, at the right dose, at the right time, for the right duration. Antibiotics should be taken as prescribed, and never saved for later or shared with others. Often doctors feel pressured to give in to a patient's request for antibiotics. Most infections physicians see in their clinics today are viral and do not require antibiotics. Instead, physicians should be willing to engage in dialogue with their patients and to not be afraid to say no.

A Bad Response:
"Antibiotics are given to treat infections. If too many are prescribed it can lead to resistance so they are less effective. This can lead to disease that cannot be treated by antibiotic drugs."

Response Analysis:
The response lacks a key fact: antibiotics are given to treat BACTERIAL infections. The issue arises when patients ask for antibiotics to treat a viral illness, such as a cold, which is not cured by antibiotics but provides a selection pressure.

A Good Response:
"Antibiotics are used to treat bacterial infections. However, overprescribing can create a selection pressure that results in antibiotic resistance. This can create superbugs such as MRSA, which are a big issue in hospitals. It is important for doctors to explain this to patients when they demand antibiotics for viral infections."

Response Analysis:
This answer explains why antibiotics are prescribed and their role in antibiotic resistance. By discussing the pressure patients place on doctors for prescribing, the candidate shows a great understanding of a key issue within the NHS. "MRSA" is always a topical issue in medicine and it highlights the candidate as a competitive applicant because it shows they are aware of this issue.

Overall:
A good answer clearly explains the proper use of antibiotics and how antibiotic resistance occurs. It will also relate the question to the NHS and comment on current health news, e.g. superbugs.

68) What is a DNA-CPR? Why is it so important?

A Do Not Attempt Cardio Pulmonary Resuscitation order (DNA-CPR) refers to a decision, usually made between doctors and a patient approaching the end of life, not to attempt cardiopulmonary resuscitation on that patient in the event of cardiac or respiratory arrest. This question, therefore, includes the end of life issues and you will stand out if you can answer it sensitively and with empathy for those patients reaching the end of life.

The best way to impress an interviewer with your answer is to show your insight into how these decisions are made, who they are made between and why they are made. Lots of applicants will be able to state what DNA-CPR stands for and that these decisions are often made as patients approach the end of life. The most impressive interviewees are those who show awareness of what real life CPR is like (as opposed to CPR on TV) and understand why patients might not want to undergo CPR.

A Bad Response:
"DNA-CPR is a decision made by doctors not to attempt CPR on a patient in the event of cardiac or respiratory arrest. It means that doctors do not spend time and resources trying to resuscitate a patient for whom CPR is unlikely to be successful."

Response Analysis:
This answer shows a lack of understanding that these decisions are usually made by doctors in conjunction with their patients and, therefore, also misses the reasons why it is important for doctors to discuss the DNA CPR with their patient. However, it is important to acknowledge that doctors do have the power to decide upon a DNA-CPR without patient involvement and patients cannot demand doctors to carry out treatment against their clinical judgement.

A good point is made that DNA CPRs are often made for patients for whom CPR is unlikely to be successful but it shows a lack of sensitivity with its reasoning. These decisions are not made to save time and resources for doctors but instead are made with a patient's best interests in mind, i.e. it is not advisable to perform CPR on a patient if it is not likely to be successful. CPR is often traumatic and invasive.

A Good Response:
"DNA-CPR refers to a decision, usually made between doctors and a patient approaching the end of life, not to attempt cardiopulmonary resuscitation on that patient in the event of cardiac or respiratory arrest. The decision is usually made because the chances of successful resuscitation are very low and, even if successful, many patients will suffer broken bones and brain injuries. A large number of patients with DNA-CPRs are those with terminal illnesses. In this case, it is important to discuss a DNA-CPR early so that patients can think about their decision and discuss with their family. This is also important in patients with dementia who will gradually lose the capacity to make their own decisions.

In reality, CPR is not as it appears on TV. It is a traumatic and invasive procedure with only 5-20% success rates and explaining this to patients will assist them in making decisions regarding the end of life. For many people, the most important factor in death is dying with dignity and not performing CPR allows patients to die peacefully and with dignity. This also allows patients to choose a preferred place to spend their final days/hours by avoiding emergency admission to hospital. It is important that patients know that having a DNA-CPR does not mean they will be denied other treatment and pain relief as they approach the end of life."

Response Analysis:
This is an excellent answer which addresses medical reasons why CPR may be refused and also personal issues surrounding the end of life. It clearly demonstrates an understanding of the implications of attempting CPR and also the reality that CPR is most often unsuccessful in patients who have reached the end of their natural life. Mention of a DNA-CPR in patients with dementia shows a wider awareness of issues surrounding capacity and decision-making.

Overall:

The best answers to this question address the needs and concerns of both the patient and the doctor. In medicine, your patients will often have a different agenda to you as the doctor and, therefore, to be an effective doctor, you must show an ability to understand your patients' concerns and find a way to reach an optimal outcome for both of you.

The key point with DNA-CPRs is to remember that although it is a clinical decision, it is good practice to involve the patient and their family (especially if the patient's capacity is an issue).

Now that you understand more about the reasons behind a DNA-CPR, think how you might respond to a follow-up question asking, "How would you react to an angry relative of the patient who disagrees with your DNA-CPR decision?"

69) You witness a doctor fill in a DNA-CPR with the patient, but without consulting with the patient's family. What issues do you see with this?

There are two main issues. Firstly, how do DNARs work, and secondly, to what extent should a patient's family be involved in a decision that is primarily the concern of the doctor and patient.

A Bad Response:

"This doctor is clearly breaching his professional obligations. End of life questions such as resuscitation orders always have to be discussed with the patient's family in order to make sure they adequately represent their wishes. Ignoring the family's wishes would be both unlawful as well as unethical. Every patient is entitled to all necessary treatments to maintain their life. This includes resuscitation at all cost."

Response Analysis:

Whilst this answer is in part right, it also has significant flaws. It is always preferable to consult with the family of a patient, especially when dealing with questions such as resuscitation, but ultimately the decision lies with the doctor as resuscitation is a treatment like every other. The decision to withhold or deliver treatment should be discussed with the patient, but once again, the ultimate decision lies with the doctor. In general, the doctor must always keep in mind the patient's best interest and this might include the decision to withhold resuscitation.

A Good Response:

"If the patient wishes to discuss their end of life plans without involving their family, then the doctor has to accept this. Whilst ideally we would like to involve the patient's family, it is ultimately the patient's decision and ignoring this would represent a breach of confidentiality."

Response Analysis:

This is a good response as it delivers a short & succinct answer whilst acknowledging the finer points surrounding DNA-CPR. Remember that like with many ethical questions, there is no clear-cut correct answer.

Overall:

This is a challenging question with many both ethical and legal components. It's important to acknowledge the ethical challenges as you will almost certainly face them in your future medical career. It's important not to get carried away by your own opinions about end of life care. Not only will this impair the quality of the answer, it might also be misunderstood and reflect badly on you. Remember, medicine is not just about curing the ill – it is also about palliating those we cannot cure.

70) What is clinical governance? Why is it important?

Background:

Clinical governance is one of the most important principles in the NHS but you may not have been aware of its formal existence. It refers to the systematic approach used by NHS Trusts to maintain and improve the quality of patient care within the health service. Prior to the introduction of clinical governance, NHS Trusts were responsible only for the financial management of their organisation and it was the responsibility of individual health care professionals to maintain high standards of care. Nowadays, each trust (alongside the individual clinicians) is responsible for maintaining the highest possible standard of care and doing so in the safest possible manner. The best answers to this question will demonstrate how effective clinical governance is achieved and in doing so will explain its importance.

A Bad Response:

'Clinical governance is the process by which NHS Trusts ensure that their health care provision is delivered in the most efficient way. In a time when cuts to healthcare budgets are commonplace, trusts have to find new ways to cut spending while still providing an appropriate level of care. The cornerstone of clinical governance is finding the most cost-effective methods to serve the local population.'

Response Analysis:

This answer shows a lack of understanding of clinical governance. Clinical governance refers only to the process by which trusts ensure the highest standard of clinical care. Cost-effectiveness of treatments may form part of clinical governance but financial factors are not the focus of clinical governance. It should be noted that trusts are under increasing pressure to control spending but this is not the same as clinical governance.

A Good Response:

"Clinical governance is the systematic approach used by NHS Trusts to maintain and improve the quality of patient care within the health service. It comprises several different components. The trust and clinicians are together responsible for continued professional development so that all professional knowledge is up to date. The trust must commit to clinical audit in which clinical practice is reviewed, altered and reassessed and also to make decisions surrounding clinical practice based on clinical effectiveness. Effectiveness can take into consideration things like value for money and QALYs. Trusts also commit to evidence-based medicine and to find ways to introduce new research into practice in a way that reduces the lag between new discoveries and a reduction in associated morbidities.

In order to ensure proper clinical governance is possible, trusts commit to collect high-quality data on their processes and to allow this data to be openly scrutinised in order that bad practice cannot continue unnoticed.

Ultimately, clinical governance is important in creating systems in which bad practice is stamped out and excellent practice is able to flourish."

Response Analysis:

This is a very thorough answer which explains the mechanisms by which clinical governance is achieved. Crucially, this answer demonstrates an understanding that every mechanism is put in place with the top priority of achieving the highest standard of clinical care.

Overall:

Despite being a concept you may not previously have been familiar with; clinical governance is very easy to get your head around. To summarise, clinical governance is about the NHS trust taking appropriate steps to provide 'right care to the patients, at the right time, by the right people in the right place'. This is done by ensuring that staff remain up-to-date, regular audits, implementing evidence-based medicine and learning from mistakes.

71) How have technological advances changed medical practice?

This is a question related to current affairs, and your awareness of and how much you keep up-to-date with advances in the medical world. There are many ways in which technology has impacted medicine; including more efficient methods of patient record storage, endoscopy, laparoscopic surgery, the use of simulators in training, and advancements in scanning equipment used. Genomic sequencing also allows the identification of particular gene mutations in a patient's DNA, which is important in diagnosing patients and also tailoring treatment to fit their particular needs.

A Bad Response:
Technology has an important role in medicine, which can be seen in how much laparoscopic surgery has taken over when operating. This allows the surgeon to operate without completely cutting a patient open and therefore minimise scarring. A disadvantage of this could be how difficult it is to use, and there may be more errors when performing this type of surgery.

Response Analysis:
The candidate has not fully described what laparoscopic surgery is, how it is performed, or the contexts or types of surgery for which it might be used. Although they have presented both an advantage and a disadvantage, they have provided incomplete arguments for both. The disadvantage argument also comes across as rather weak as it is a guess and the candidate has not taken the time to read up on or briefly research the answer – are there really more errors when performing laparoscopic surgery? The overall impression given is one of incomplete knowledge and understanding of the procedure.

A Good Response:
I think something that is gradually changing the way medicine is practised is the smartphone. There are more and more apps being developed to serve as a quick and easy way to diagnose patients, such as apps to take blood pressure and ECGs (using an attached sensor), and also to interpret the results. Another example is insulin dose-recommending calculators for diabetic patients. These devices could take a load off the number of consultations GPs have to deal with daily. This could also have very positive implications in poorer areas of the world where more sophisticated scanning equipment is not available. Also, video consultations via laptop or smartphone are becoming more and more popular, and serve as a good way for doctors to communicate with patients who are too far to visit or to save a patient time if they are at work or unable to travel to a clinic. The subject has even been reviewed in literature, showing how important it is likely to be in the future of medicine. A possible danger of this is patients relying too much on technology rather than seeing their doctor – perhaps the use of these apps should be regulated more.

Response Analysis:
The candidate has chosen to talk about something very current and relevant, which is having an increasing impact on the day-to-day practice of medicine. The candidate has offered some relevant examples of how the smartphone can be used in diagnosing patients (although perhaps a bit more research/detail is needed) and has mentioned how these can influence the practice of medicine. The advantages are listed, and a disadvantage is also mentioned, as well as a possible way of combating this problem.

Overall:
Technological advances are designed to improve medical practice, so in all likelihood, you will be focusing on the pros rather than cons when giving an answer. Give examples of a situation where and how these technologies can be used rather than just listing. The more recent the advancement(s) you reference, the more up-to-date with the medical world you'll seem.

72) What is the most important medical breakthrough of the 20th and 21st centuries and why?

This question is testing your general interest in the field of medicine. Interviewers won't expect vast amounts of specialist knowledge, but it is a chance to show off any extra reading you've done and also to demonstrate your understanding of how medicine has developed over the last century. There is no right answer to this so feel free to mention several significant breakthroughs and then pick one to explain why it was so important. Examples of significant breakthroughs include ABO blood typing, blood transfusions, the discovery of vitamins, insulin, antibiotics, DNA, radiotherapy/chemotherapy in cancer, MRI, heart transplantation, IVF, humanised monoclonal antibodies, human genome project, etc.

Bad Response A:
"The most important medical breakthrough of the last one hundred years is undoubtedly the discovery of the structure of DNA. Watson and Crick used x-ray crystallography images to unearth the double helical structure of the molecule in 1953 and later won the Nobel Prize for their work. No other breakthrough can compare to this discovery and its legacy."

Bad Response B:
Antibiotics were the most important advances in medicine in the last 100 years because they are used to treat so many different diseases and have saved so many lives'.

Response Analysis:
These answers describe the discovery of the structure but offer little more. The most important part of this question is justifying why you think that particular breakthrough is the most important. With regards to DNA, the understanding of the mechanism of inheritance has arguably been just as important as the structure since it has allowed further work to be carried out; such as the human genome project. This has helped us to discover the gene variants involved in certain disorders.

Good Response A:
"It's impossible to say that one medical breakthrough in the last hundred years has enormously outshone the others. Significant milestones include the discovery of DNA's structure and its mechanism of inheritance, however, we probably can't know the full legacy of this event yet as we are still making huge genetic discoveries each year.

In my opinion, though, the most impactful discovery of the last hundred years is that of penicillin and subsequently the full range of antibiotics we know today. Antibiotics quite literally changed the world we live in. In the pre-antibiotic era, infections like meningitis and pneumonia were often fatal - now they can be easily treated. Antibiotics have also paved the way for surgery which would be a much riskier affair if we did not have a way to treat infections arising from surgery. Antibiotics have saved millions of lives to date but the golden era of antibiotics may soon be coming to an end. Misuse of these drugs has led to drug-resistant bacteria and only time will tell what the legacy of antibiotics may be in another hundred years."

Good Response B:
'The development of a huge array of antibiotics since the discovery of penicillin is perhaps the most important medical advance in the last 100 years. This is because bacterial infections are so common and, before antibiotics, even very small infections could develop to be life threatening. The discovery of antibiotics represented a paradigm shift in medicine whereby a huge number of very harmful infectious diseases (such as tuberculosis, diphtheria, typhoid) became treatable. Furthermore, antibiotics made surgery a lot safer by reducing the risks of post-operative infection. This is why the spread of multi-antibiotic resistant bacteria will present such a severe problem in the future. Of course, there are several other advances that could also be argued to be similarly as important, such as the development of population-scale vaccination.

Response Analysis:
These are well thought out answers that show the candidate has considered an extensive list of triumphs in medicine and their impacts when coming to a conclusion. The answer offers a clear explanation why antibiotics were chosen as the most important breakthrough but adds a very valuable point that this legacy might change as we continue to misuse antibiotics. This broad and well-justified answer demonstrates a strong interest in the field of medicine generally.

Overall:
When given free rein on a question like this, make sure to answer on a topic you know. Do not worry about guessing what the interviewer thinks is the right answer. The most important thing is to be able to justify your answer. An interviewer may be particularly impressed by a candidate who can discuss the detailed impact of a less well-known medical success, e.g. discovery of insulin.

There is no single right answer for this question; you just need to give something reasonable and be able to rationally justify it. Think about whether you mean 'importance' on a global scale or only in the UK. Try to keep it simple, broader, and something that the mass benefit is known. The key to answering this type of question is to be knowledgeable on the subject and be able to explain why you think this is a revolutionary discovery. This does not have to be something in the "Top Ten" list but something that would not look absurd when you justify your answer.

73) What can you tell me about the current NHS reforms?

Background Analysis:

The biggest reforms within the NHS currently are probably the attempted transition to a '7-day NHS' and the general move towards more privatisation – the outsourcing of NHS contracts to private sector companies. This is well worth reading about and there have been dozens of articles written about this over the last few months alone. It is also worth having a general idea of the changes that came through the Health and Social Care Act in 2012, not just for interviews but because it involved changes in the NHS that are important for anyone who is hoping to be a doctor.

A Bad Response:

"There have been reforms recently in the NHS that means the NHS is getting closer to being privatised. This is a bad change because privatisation means the NHS is going to become much more unfair – like in the United States where the private health care system means that some people simply cannot afford healthcare."

Response Analysis:

While it is good that this candidate identified the issue of privatisation, they did not demonstrate any deeper knowledge of the process by which this is happening or the arguments for or against the reforms beyond a somewhat simplistic level. Despite these reforms, massive differences remain between the NHS and the insurance-based system in the United States. The changes since the Health and Social Care Act (2012) extended a market-based approach to the NHS, meaning that healthcare services could be more easily provided by private companies. While this is controversial with arguments for and against the changes, the Act made no overt moves towards any insurance-based system or upturning the principle of an NHS which is free at the point of delivery to patients.

A Good Response:

"The most recent reforms that are trying to be made to the NHS are about introducing a '7-day NHS'. As I understand it, this is the ambition to extend current weekday services – such as access to GPs, specialist clinics and more senior staffing – over the weekend. These changes have partially been based on statistics claiming that there is a higher mortality rate for patients admitted into hospitals on the weekend, though, there have been criticisms that the original research for this is being misrepresented. There is significant resistance to these changes with critics claiming that there is no way they can be brought in without either significantly impairing the quality of care from the NHS or spending an unaffordable amount of money on even more doctors and other NHS staff. Meanwhile, the government says it has a mandate to pursue the changes and that they will ultimately benefit patients."

Response Analysis:

This candidate has shown a good understanding of the controversy surrounding the suggested '7-day NHS' reforms while maintaining quite a balanced standpoint. It can be good to express an opinion as this shows you have really engaged with the arguments and thought about them, but make sure you can support it with good reasoning and bear in mind that the interviewer is likely to have an opinion on the matter and it could well differ from your own so try not to be dogmatic with these controversial problems.

Overall:

NHS reforms are in the news almost daily, so interviewers are likely to expect you to have shown an interest in them and be able to discuss them briefly. These reforms are largely controversial, so when discussing them remember to show that you appreciate that there are two sides to the argument.

74) Name 3 famous doctors and their contributions to medicine.

You should have a basic level of knowledge about medical history before coming to the interview. Consider going out of your way to have a few discussions with teachers or peers or watching a few documentaries if you feel your general medical knowledge is poor.

Person	Discovered	Person	Discovered
Godfrey Hounsfield	CT Scan	Jonas Salk	Polio vaccine
Wilhelm Rontgen	X-rays	Willem Einthoven	ECG
Charles Best	Insulin	Raymond Damadian	MRI
Robert Koch	Tuberculosis	James Thomson	Stem cell treatment
John Gibbon	Heart-lung machine	Rene Laennec	Stethoscope
Rune Elmquist	Pacemaker	Inge Edler	Medical ultrasound

A Bad Response:
"Well, I can think of two doctors who really have had a massive impact on medicine; Edward Jenner and Hippocrates. Edward Jenner developed the vaccine as a medical intervention, which has now prevented millions of people around the world from developing infectious diseases. Hippocrates developed the Hippocratic Oath. This Oath has formed the basis of medical ethics and philosophy for hundreds of years"

Response Analysis:
Bad responses are those that are factually incorrect or do not fully answer the question; i.e. the candidate is unable to think of three doctors, names people who are not doctors, incorrectly states their contributions to medicine etc. The above response is factually accurate but only mentions two doctors. More specific details could be given to impress the interviewer but are not strictly necessary.

A Good Response:
"Edward Jenner invented the vaccine. He did this by discovering the smallpox vaccine, which involved administering pus derived from cowpox to patients. Jenner's discovery is arguably one of biggest in medical history as vaccines are responsible for saving the lives of millions of people and make up an essential component of modern medicine.

Hippocrates is known as the father of Western Medicine. The Hippocratic Oath is taken by doctors to swear that they will do no harm to their patients. It underlies some of the most fundamental facets of medical ethics and has played an important role in laying the foundations by which doctors are perceived as trusted and respected professionals by the public.

Joseph Lister developed antiseptic. He observed that many patients after undergoing surgery would die. He showed that using antiseptics reduced patient mortality. Joseph Lister helped to transform surgical practice by introducing new standards of cleanliness."

Response Analysis:
This response is well organised, specific, and relates back to modern medicine in each example. The answer is fully and completely answered. The answer is concise and covers a lot of detail in a very succinct manner.

Overall:
This question presents a good opportunity for you to share any historical medical figures that have inspired you or who you have learned about in school and taken a particular interest in. The interviewer is likely to appreciate one named, relatively unknown doctor, if you have specialist knowledge, this would be a good method of setting yourself apart from other candidates. You should be able to discuss the achievement and its impact on medicine.

75) In addition to well-known health professionals, can you suggest other industries which play a critical role in the delivery of a multidisciplinary healthcare system?

This question aims to challenge the student to consider the wider players in the delivery of healthcare. Questions concerning the theme of 'multidisciplinary' tend to revolve around work experience and seek reflections on interactions with nurses, physiotherapists and other allied health professionals. However, for this question, students may not be able to immediately draw from work experience. A good approach would be to consider recent news articles which present exciting developments or improvements to current practices. The industries which are at the forefront of these developments are usually external to direct healthcare provision so are not often considered; this would allow the student to quickly reach an answer which can be expanded upon. An alternative approach would be to analyse the journey of a specific patient, including inpatient stay, treatment, and follow-up care to find out what their needs are. Consequently, this will allow students to trace back to the industries which meet these needs and provide the infrastructure to support patients during their journey.

A Bad Response:
Histopathologists are a good example of healthcare providers who are not often considered when discussing multidisciplinary teams. They are vital in the diagnosis of diseases such as cancer by examining tissue samples using microscopy. Although their work is primarily carried out in the laboratory, histopathologists work closely with nurses and other staff. My work experience shadowing various doctors in the pathology department showed me how important the role is.

Response Analysis:
Overall, this is not a poor answer. However, it is important to notice that it is not a good response to the question that was asked. Firstly, regardless of how well-known the speciality might be, histopathologists are doctors. Therefore, this already contradicts the first part of the question ('well-known health professionals'). Secondly, this student would do well to expand upon the 'other staff' that histopathologists encounter as they may list an individual from an industry which answers the question. This ambiguity is not encouraged when answering interview questions. Lastly, for the same reasons, it would be beneficial to expand upon the experiences from work experience, giving insight to the team members and patients encountered and the need for multidisciplinary teams.

In this instance, as the student has already begun discussing something which the interviewer is **not** looking for, a fully well-rounded answer may put the student in a more favourable light than the answer given above.

A Good Response:
A possible industry involved in both the delivery and progression of healthcare is that of bioengineering. These scientists often have an engineering background so are key in the design of new medical devices to improve quality of life. One example might be the prosthesis. This aids restoration of motor function for patients, thereby making daily tasks much easier. I recently read a very interesting article which explained how newer prosthetic devices can allow patients to regain some sensory function as well, such as the new bionic finger which allowed a patient to feel the roughness of the surface. Clearly, the engineers who designed this device would be working closely with other staff, such as surgeons and occupational therapists, to ensure it functions effectively in the real world.

Response Analysis:

A detailed, yet concise answer. It is clear that this student has carefully considered the question and thus has given a well-structured answer. The chosen topic is relatively obscure and likely not one that most students would be able to suggest. The student has done a good job of explaining how the industry relates to the patient. The use of a specific example tells the examiner that the student is confident and the use of literature indicates that the student is genuinely interested in medicine and associated fields. However, if students have not read literature which relates to the answer, it would be useful to try and link in any relevant work experience or news topics. There is some mention of other team members, but again, this could be expanded upon if the student has other ideas. It is important to note that due to the detailed and structured nature of this answer, the interviewer is provided with many options for follow-up questions, which could allow the student to further guide the interview.

Overall:

This is a challenging question and thus can be used as a way to push candidates. The students who perform most successfully will be those who think outside of the box to consider industries which may often play a minor role, or whose role is many steps away from direct healthcare provision. Nevertheless, it is important for students to give a detailed and well-thought out answer which clearly explains how their chosen industry impacts patients and (if relevant) possibly how they believe the role may change over time. The use of current research can further enhance the answer. Some examples to consider are genetic engineers, blood sugar monitoring equipment, suture making industries, prosthetic manufacturers for hip replacements etc.

76) What would you consider the bigger challenge for the NHS, diabetes or smoking?

This question asks you to evaluate two big public health challenges and contrast their impact on the NHS. We need to consider the cost incurred due to smoking & diabetes as well the ethical issues such as stigma, especially because self-inflicted diseases can be seen as a burden on the general public.

A Bad Response:

"Diabetes and smoking represent both very important issues for the NHS. For this reason, cigarettes should be made significantly more expensive through the use of taxes in order to make them less attractive to buy. If cigarettes are more expensive, fewer people will buy them and, therefore, fewer people will smoke overall. The increased income of the taxes can then be used to pay for other things like roads etc. The price increase would be particularly effective as smoking is most prevalent in lower social classes who will be less able to afford buying cigarettes when they are more expensive."

Response Analysis:

This is a poor response as it is judgemental towards specific parts of the population, i.e. lower income households. This is ethically unacceptable. The answer also does not actually address the question but rather goes into detail on how to reduce smoking in a population. Whilst this is an interesting concept, it does not have much to do with the question and will not provide any benefit in the interview.

A Good Response:

"Smoking and diabetes both represent major challenges to the healthcare system. They both affect a significant amount of the population and they both have significant implications for the individual's health prospects. Before addressing them in some further detail, it is important to stress that diabetes is an actual diagnosis, whereas smoking is a lifestyle choice. An additional fact to consider is the fact that diabetes is limited to the individual, whereas smoking has a significant effect on the other individual as well through passive smoking. In general, both factors represent equally great issues for the NHS, though on different levels. Whilst diabetes is a chronic disease requiring continuous treatment, smoking has implications on the future health of the individual. Due to the inherently different nature of the two issues, it is difficult to make a judgement on which one of the two is more severe."

Response Analysis:

This response is good as it takes into account several different aspects of the question and also provides detail about the background of the question. This is important as it shows the individual's train of thought. The latter is particularly important as the student ultimately does not make a choice between either.

Overall:

This question is very complex and addressing the complexity is essential. Any attempt to simplify the question will ultimately cause the answer to be insufficient. In general, being aware of public health issues such as this is very important for any prospective medical student as this demonstrates their awareness of medical developments and the impacts of medical care on the individual. There is always a chance that there might be a question asking about evaluations of impact on the whole of society and common public diseases such as diabetes offer themselves for this type of question.

77) What do you think about the role of GPs in the NHS?

GPs play a vital role in the NHS. In a way, they provide a triage system for patients allocating them to the individual specialities through referrals if necessary. At the same time, GPs are increasingly becoming a bottleneck in the NHS as they have to deal with ever-growing patient loads and continuously reducing numbers of GPs. As waiting times for appointments increase, patients will be more likely to seek help at A&Es, increasing an already enormous strain on these facilities even further. The interaction between GPs and the hospitals is an area medical applicants should be familiar with.

This question is classic and belongs to a family of questions with variations; how important are nurses, or porters, or midwives in the NHS? It's important to have the facts right here explained with the role of GPs both in direct medical interventions but also in Clinical Commissioning Groups. It can't hurt to also throw in some anecdotes as well.

Bad Response A:
GPs are becoming increasingly irrelevant in the NHS. Waiting times have gotten so long that it is easier to simply go to A&E or call an ambulance when unwell. This is further encouraged by the NHS 111 service that gives advice to people. The main responsibility of GPs is to refer patients and to treat easy, chronic cases not requiring any specialist input. With the way medicine is developing, i.e. by becoming increasingly specialised, GPs often are far out of their depth anyway. Having to make an appointment with your GP to have specialist investigations is a nuisance to many patients as it prolongs the process unnecessarily.

Bad Response B:
"From my experience, GPs are the pillars of the NHS. They are the first line of interaction with patients so for many people, they are the public face of the NHS. GPs are effectively the first filter to further treatment. They are the ones who divert patients to specific departments via referrals to the hospital. It is up to them to decide that a patient is sick enough to warrant hospital attention, so they yield a great deal of influence over how patients get treated."

Response Analysis:
The student demonstrates a significant lack of awareness of the role of GPs in the NHS. Underestimating the importance of primary care in healthcare reflects very poorly on the student. GPs play a very important role in the delivery of care in the community and represent a necessary intermediate between specialist care and the patient. The student does, however, raise a relevant aspect of the reality of GP's roles in the NHS: there is too much demand for too few doctors.

The second response is incomplete. For the most part, the response is accurate. The comments about being the public face and first line of interaction are indeed correct, as is the idea of them being the means to accessing further treatment in hospitals. However, this response fails to acknowledge the relatively new role of GPs in clinical commissioning groups since the abolishment of Primary Care Trusts. The response is good but by failing to mention this, it shows a lack of awareness of the current state of the National Health Service.

Good Response A:
GPs play an important role in the NHS. Originally conceived as a gateway and distributor of the patients between community and speciality care, GPs take a sort of triage function as well as providing care for non-specialist cases. GPs also are vital in ensuring the continuation of care beyond the hospital stage and are the main provider of health care in the community. They play a very diverse and complex role in the NHS. The general shortage of staff, however, has an impact on GPs as well. The lack of GPs overall makes it difficult for them to efficiently fulfil their roles. Long waiting times and general overload with patients contribute to the problem of high A&E presentations that could be avoided. All in all, GPs have not lost their importance, but like most other parts of our health service, they are spread increasingly thin making their job very difficult.

Good Response B:

GPs are the public face of the NHS for a great number of patients, especially those who don't go onto secondary care. They effectively operate as the first point of contact for almost all patients in the NHS and fulfil the basic healthcare requirements for many patients. Beyond straightforward ailments, they are also the means by which patients interact with many other NHS services since GPs – by means of referrals – are the ones who direct patients with specific ailments to secondary care. GPs are effectively the ones who conduct initial investigations for patients to accurately target them to the correct treatment. On top of all this, GPs have also become the ones who determine what services are offered by the local NHS trust via Clinical Commissioning Groups since Primary Care Trusts with dedicated managers ceased to exist. The idea behind this is that, theoretically, GPs know best as to what services would suit their patients, but whether this works in practice is open to debate. Personally, it seems like we're asking a lot of GPs given their already heavy workload.

Response Analysis:

This answer attempts to not only outline the role of GPs in the NHS but also tries to provide insight into the challenges experienced by GPs and the consequences this has for the whole of the NHS. This is important as it demonstrates the student's ability to develop an argument and then apply it to a different situation. It also shows that the student has spent some time thinking about the issue and is also up to date with current issues surrounding the healthcare service.

The second response is better with a larger and more detailed overview of the roles and importance of a GP in the current state of the NHS. As in the bad response, this response covers the work of a GP as the first point of contact, but it goes further and touches on the role of CCGs. By mentioning both CCGs and PCTs, it shows that the candidate has engaged in current affairs and is aware of problems in our healthcare system – a trait often neglected by many candidates. Although you should also be wary of coming off as too politically charged. If your interviewer doesn't agree with you, that can be awkward.

Overall:

This question is an important one as the role of GPs in the NHS is a complex and very important one because they represent the first instance of patient contact. Also, since most applicants will have had some form of work experience in a GP practice, it can reasonably be expected that they have some understanding of the GP's role in the healthcare system. If being asked this question, a direct reference to first-hand experiences will result in a more complete answer.

This is no doubt a broad question, but it's important to try and get as much in as you can with sufficient detail. This question presents an opportunity to show off your extended reading and is a perfect chance to show that you've engaged with materials that many candidates often neglect. Doing well on questions like these will help you to stand out from the crowd.

78) How is the nurses' role in healthcare changing?

The NHS is increasingly training nurses to do some jobs that doctors have historically performed. This gives them more responsibilities and more opportunities for training and has given rise to some becoming Nurse Practitioners; an invaluable member of the team in GP practices and hospital clinics. Nurse Practitioners typically see the less complicated patients (e.g. routine check-ups) on their own but have access to a doctor if the patient's situation is more complex than anticipated. This reduces the burden of routine appointments on doctors' workloads. Nurse Practitioners are usually well-liked by patients as their extensive experience gives them excellent interpersonal skills. Nurses also teach and help patients learn about their disease, empowering them to manage it better. Working well with nurses is absolutely essential for a medical student, so this question is designed to seek out any underlying prejudices against the nursing staff or misconceptions about their roles.

A Bad Response:
Nurses are being given more responsibilities to the point where they are starting to take over the doctors' jobs. This means that people will be confused about the role of doctors and will lead to patients respecting the doctors less, and there will be fewer jobs for doctors.

Response Analysis:
Firstly, as outlined below, the roles of nurses and doctors remain different (and equally important!). This answer implies (by saying that people will respect doctors less) that patients think that jobs done by nurses must be easier, i.e. that nurses are less intelligent. The answer also shows a preoccupation with commanding respect as a doctor and completely misses the mark – whilst respect can be an important asset in communication skills, the priority should always be patient care. Does the broader role of nurses improve patient care? If so, that should be the overriding conclusion.

A Good Response:
In order to save money in the NHS, nurses are being encouraged to train to be able to take on more responsibilities and perform more procedures, therefore, freeing up the doctors to focus on tasks that nurses aren't qualified to perform. This has led to some concerns over the nurses "taking over the doctors' jobs", but in reality, whilst there is beginning to be some overlap between roles, the nurses remain responsible for the daily management of the patient whilst the doctors provide more targeted intervention. This is a good allocation of resources – nurses have excellent practical and interpersonal skills from years of experience with patients, whereas doctors have good knowledge and understanding of pathology from studying medicine. For example, specialist epilepsy nurses are able to adjust dosages of anti-epileptic drugs- they act as a go between patient and doctor. This reduces the amount of time doctors need to spend per patient. Whilst there are kinks that need to be worked out, better integration between healthcare disciplines can only be a good result for patient safety and care.

Response Analysis:
This response shows some insight into recent trends in the NHS. The candidate also shows that they understand that nurses and doctors have different and equally important roles, skills, and abilities (and they could potentially expand later upon the important parts of patient care the nurses are involved with). The candidate acknowledges that the transition has not been perfect but more importantly looks at the big picture with the patient as the focus. This shows that the candidate has their eye on the most important person (the patient) rather than getting involved in interdisciplinary squabbling.

Overall:
As working with nurses is so important, medical students who carry prejudices against nurses or who have unrealistic expectations of their roles and responsibilities will find this doesn't help them in clinical practice. With increasing overlap between roles, understanding everyone's jobs and responsibilities is essential.

COMMUNICATION SKILLS

79) Tell me about a time when you showed good communication skills

Communication is a very important part of a doctor's job. Most doctors work within teams and so will need to be able to effectively convey important information to many different members of staff who have different expertise. Communication is therefore essential for an effective integrated approach to patient care. Additionally, in order to ensure that the patient's autonomy is fully utilised, the patients themselves must be fully informed of all the details of treatment plans and procedures. This often requires excellent communication skills.

Bad Response A:
"I was the editor of my student newspaper and was responsible for ensuring the content of the paper was appropriate. I would often have to make guesses as to what the student body would like and then implement this into the paper. Often I felt that my writers didn't accurately convey what I wanted to be published in their articles, which was a real disappointment for me."

Bad Response B:
"Erm, once when I was working with a student I was tutoring, I had to explain how to calculate gradients since she wasn't understanding how the teacher was explaining it, so I sat her down and explained it to her. After going through it a couple of times, eventually she got it."

Response Analysis:
This candidate has identified a role they had where they potentially could have developed very sophisticated communication skills. However, the candidate suggests that they have not effectively communicated with their writers in order to get the most appropriate articles. Additionally, it would have been far more impressive had they said that, instead of guessing, they spoke with the student body to gain a consensus of opinions as to what the paper should be publishing. Instead, the candidate comes across as having approached the paper from an individual angle when good communication with different groups of students would have been more appropriate.

In the second response, the filler word "Erm" is poor form. It can be tough under pressure but avoid filler words. It's better to take your time and speak a bit slower if it means not using so much filler. Filling is not good communication! It gives off a tone of a lack of understanding. Moving on to the bulk of the response, the anecdote is a bit weak. The underlying narrative of helping a fellow student is a powerful one, but this response suffers because it lacks detail and it really sells the candidate short. Also, a note on the anecdote itself; saying things like "I sat her down" comes across as patronising. This is not the tone you want to project.

Good Response A:
"As part of my fundraising ventures, I organised a large ball to be hosted at the local town hall with a number of different aspects to the night including an auction, live musical performances and food. I needed to effectively coordinate my team so that everything ran smoothly. This entailed ensuring that there was sufficient press coverage of the event, arranging the logistics with the catering company and gathering goods to be auctioned. The night was a great success with plenty of money raised."

Good Response B:
"I currently work as a GCSE Maths tutor and often I have to explain difficult concepts to my students in a new way since their teachers' approaches often fall a bit short. An example where I feel I was particularly effective at communicating a concept was recently when I had to explain the idea behind gradients of straight lines. I tried to go at a pace appropriate for the student's ability and I kept an eye on the student's body language so I knew when I'd lost her and I could backtrack and isolate the bits she found most confusing."

Response Analysis:

This candidate has demonstrated an impressive ability to put on a major event, which has apparently entailed communicating with individuals from many different professions. The ability to maturely communicate effectively with so many different individuals to deliver a coherent and successful end product is very impressive. Despite this example being apparently far removed from medical practice, the candidate has effectively demonstrated that they hold fundamental communication skills that are widely applicable for the rest of their life, including their future medical career.

Response B is a considerably better response. Notice the lack of filler words. Here the key is also specificity. This is a good point to ensure that the anecdote you tell is actually true! Giving the specificity of the above response lends itself to belief. It's important to pull from real experience and the confidence of pulling from your actual experience will be evident in your own body language, and will yield a better outcome.

Beyond the details of the anecdote itself, this response is good because it actively highlights what the candidate actually did as far as good communication skills are concerned. The bad responses did not do this. The points about going at an appropriate pace and observing body language are absolutely essential to get across in your response because it shows that you actually know what the interviewer means by good communication skills.

Overall:

Whatever the example you use, make sure that it shows you have developed or are developing good communication skills. At the end of your example, it would then be useful if you could demonstrate an awareness of why communication in medicine is so important, e.g. communicating tests results to the patient or breaking bad news (diagnosis of cancer).

Ultimately, this question is all about the details. Both the good and bad responses used similar anecdotes, but the good response has the level of detail necessary to succeed. There is, of course, a balancing act between giving enough detail to sound reliable and going so far as to become esoteric and alienate the interviewer. Crucially, it's important to highlight what actually counts as good communication skills. Don't fall into the trap of just assuming that both you and the interviewer know what good communication skills are. It's a nebulous term, so going out of your way to specify what qualities it includes is a valuable thing to do.

80) Do you think communication skills can be learned?

Effective communication is a key skill for doctors to possess. Good communication leads to more satisfying interaction with colleagues, enables better time management, and it also makes you a more effective team leader and member. However, the number one reason for complaints in the NHS is due to poor communication. The interviewers here, therefore, want to ensure that you have had a little think about the importance of communication in clinical practice.

Communication can be verbal and non-verbal. Many medical schools have 'communication sessions' which involve role-playing with actors and receiving feedback on the effectiveness of your communication. This means that communication skills can be fine-tuned, if not learned. We may be great at explaining things to patients in simple terms and communicating with our friends and family, but there will be certain circumstances which we may never have faced such as breaking bad news- which has its own format to approach and a skill you will definitely be taught at med school

A Bad Response:
"Communication skills cannot be learned. It is something that an individual is either good at or not. It is not like science or maths where you can learn facts and apply them to practice. And isn't that why the interview process takes place? To see if you have the ability to communicate effectively- this should sieve out the applicants who are weak at communication and only hold on to those who show good communication skills. This then leaves you with people who only need to concentrate on developing other skills such as analytic skills and presentation skills."

Response Analysis:
Whilst it is entirely appropriate to state that communication skills cannot be learned, this candidate was rather harsh in his/her approach to answering the question and the candidate could have followed on by stating that there is scope for improvement. The candidate may, therefore, be followed up with a question asking them about why they think communication sessions take place in medical schools. The counter-answer to that may become difficult.

A Good Response:
"Communication is a very hot topic in medicine and I am glad you asked me this question. I think that whilst many components of communication such as body language and eye contact are difficult to learn and be taught on, I think people can definitely improve the way they deliver information. We have already been taught at school, for example, that we deliver information at an appropriate level to our audience. This way, we are being taught and subsequently, learn how to communicate effectively. Furthermore, whilst eye contact and body language cannot be learned, if people pick up subtle things about how you communicate non-verbally and feed this back to you, you are more aware of it yourself and will make a conscious effort to modify it and better yourself."

Response Analysis:
This response understands the importance of communication. The candidate also provides a comprehensive answer by discussing verbal and non-verbal communication. There is an element of open-mindedness as the candidate has taken on board what has been taught to him/her at school and the feedback he/she has received about his/her non-verbal communication, utilising the information to improve his/her communication skills.

Overall:
Interviewers will want you to understand that communication is central to becoming a doctor. They will want to know how you think/do not think communication skills can be learned. Using personal experiences where you improved/couldn't have improved on your communication skills will strengthen your answer. The BMJ has published a number of articles on communication skills and whether they can be learned and it is advisable to read some of these prior to your interview.

81) How would you tell a patient they've got 3 months to live?

This is a very testing question; it tests your ability to cope well under stress. It is important that you do not panic. When you enter an interview, you should be expecting the unexpected and be broadly prepared for everything and anything! To answer this question well you will need to think logically and work through your answer step-by-step. You are not expected to know any formal protocol on how to deliver bad news to a patient. You should be aware that the interviewer will be looking to see evidence of your empathy skills, your problem-solving skills and your ability to think on the spot. A good answer will be based around the keyword in the question – "tell"; i.e. how will you articulate, communicate or disclose this information?

A Bad Response:
"I would ask the patient to sit down. I would then use a very serious tone of voice. I would try not to show any emotion in my facial expression and be very factual with the information I was passing onto the patient. I would not keep the patient in suspense; I would tell them as soon and as quickly as possible."

Response Analysis:
This answer is too short and not enough thought has been put into it. The candidate has not explained the intended impact of his actions of the patient. If he had, he may have realised that he would have come across as rather cold. The answer also suggests that the candidate would rush this interaction with the patient rather than taking his/her time to deliver the news. The candidate has not identified why the information he is disclosing to the patient is important and seemingly skirts around the fact that he is revealing to a patient that he/she has a terminal illness. The interviewer needs to know the candidate is able to talk about difficult issues in a mature and sensitive manner. The answer above does not demonstrate this.

A Good Response:
"I would be very aware of the patient's current position; the level of awareness and understanding the patient currently has about his condition, available sources of support for this particular patient – for instance, family and friends, religious circles, specific support groups – and the current anxiety and distress the patient is feeling as a result of their poor health. I would adapt the specifics of what I would say as appropriate for an individual patient. But most fundamentally, I would use clear and simple communication and a very professional manner. I would give a thorough background explanation of what has led the doctors to reach this conclusion. I would check throughout the conversation that the patient has understood what I have said before I move onto the next point. I would openly show my empathy and sympathy to the patient by letting the patient know that I am terribly sorry that they are in this situation and by offering my support and patience, and inviting them to ask any questions they have."

Response Analysis:
The candidate shows exceptional empathy skills; they seek to understand more about the patient to understand more about how they will feel and how they can potentially cope with the information they are about to receive. The candidate understands that this consultation is a very personal and sensitive interaction between patient and doctor. This response shows awareness of the importance of good quality communication and understanding of context to help the patient make sense of what is helping them and how they can cope with this life-changing event.

Overall:
The interviewer will want to see that you realise you are doing much more than simply communicating a fact to a patient. They will want to see that you understand the significance of this information to the patient and hence the significance of the style of (well-informed) communication you use.

82) You are a junior doctor on colorectal surgery. Your consultant in charge turns up on Monday morning smelling strongly of alcohol. What do you do?

Situational judgement questions aim to assess your approach to complex scenarios which you may encounter in your workplace. They are designed to test your potential across a number of competencies. In this case, this question tests your ability to deal with a senior colleague whom you suspect is drinking alcohol and has turned up to work smelling of alcohol. There is usually a pattern to follow when answering these questions: try to approach the person in question to gather a bit of information- are they, in fact, drinking alcohol? You may have been mistaken and it would, therefore, be wrong to take any further action. Next, you should try and explore the reason behind their behaviour- is it a transient and short-lasting event that has caused the consultant to drink? If so, hopefully there shouldn't be a long-term issue here. Thirdly, the interviewer would like to hear that you are taking steps to ensure that patients are safe. This may involve asking the consultant politely to get some rest and go home- clinical errors or prescribing errors due to alcohol consumption is dangerous. Lastly, you may want to suggest the consultant seek some help.

A Bad Response:
"Smelling strongly of alcohol at your workplace is, in my opinion, unacceptable. The consultant, although a senior figure, should know better and I think his behaviour should be reported promptly. The consequences of having a drunken consultant in the clinical area are unsafe and it also tarnishes the doctors' reputation as a whole. I would therefore ask my registrar to have a word with the consultant and hopefully, the matter will be escalated to the medical director who can then decide the best course of action."

Response Analysis:
This candidate is rather rash in his/her approach to the situation. Firstly, there is only a suspicion that the consultant is drinking alcohol- it is thus better to sensitively explore this first before discussing the situation with anybody else. Reporting somebody without first getting the facts straight is inappropriate. Lastly, whilst you can seek help from your registrar who will be senior to you, the answer here sounds more like you are passing the buck to the registrar and asking him to sort the situation out rather than seeking advice and acting on the advice yourself; interviewers will appreciate you being proactive and sorting matters out yourself.

A Good Response:
"This is a complex scenario. As there is only a presumption here that the consultant has been drinking (he smells of alcohol only), I would tentatively approach him and politely ask him if he has been drinking any alcohol. I would next offer to explore his behaviour by asking him what has led him to drink alcohol and be so out of control that he still smells of it when he comes into work. I would then suggest he takes the rest of the day off after ensuring his shift is covered by explaining that patient safety may be compromised if he practices medicine under the influence. Lastly, if I believe that this may be a long-term problem, I would suggest to him that he seeks further help, either by going to his GP or going to occupational health."

Response Analysis:
This answer takes a calm and measured approach to the situation by following the 'usual' steps for this type of scenario. The candidate is information gathering rather than reporting the consultant straight away. There is also an awareness that patient safety may be at risk, and the candidate provides a solution to tackle this and understands the need to be sensitive here.

Overall:
Situational judgment questions will be difficult and the key is to take a measured and calm approach to the situation. Reporting individuals straight away before attempting to resolve the situation between teams is often not the right approach, but interviewers would rather you to talk to the person in question yourself and take it from there. But remember that patient safety is the most important aspect here and if the consultant were to refuse to go home and continue seeing patients under the influence, you may then need to escalate the situation to someone more senior to you to ensure that patients are not in danger.

83) You're on a busy A&E call with your registrar who tells you that he feels 'fed up and just wants to end it all'. You know he has gone through a difficult divorce and is on anti-depressants. What would you do?

This is a situational question which aims to assess your ability to take the correct steps to effectively deal with a complex scenario. Approach this situation like the other situational questions in this booklet: discuss the person in question's feelings, ensure patient safety is maintained, and advise the person to seek help.

A Bad Response:
"This is a rather tricky question- I'm not sure exactly what I would do- perhaps I would like to ask my fellow colleagues what they would do if they were in my shoes. I am quite concerned that the registrar wants to 'end it all', but it is a busy A+E shift. I think he should have called in sick if he didn't feel like working today. I could speak to the consultant about him because he is in charge and, therefore, should be able to deal with the situation effectively. Or perhaps his medication has not been titrated enough? Maybe I can advise him to increase the dose of his medication and see if that makes him feel better?"

Response Analysis:
It is important to support your colleagues through difficult times and act compassionate towards them, just like you would with any patient. Therefore, try to listen to them and help them out rather than worry about how busy A+E is. Whilst asking fellow colleagues for advice is good practice, it may be that the registrar has come to you in confidence and would not want you to discuss his situation with others. Also, remember that it is better for you to suggest for the registrar to raise the issue with their consultant rather than you raising it- the registrar will be in a much better position to explain his/her situation than you will. It is dangerous to ask him to increase the dose of his medication- this should be left to the person who prescribes the medication, as they will have information about his other medical conditions and know if it is indeed safe to increase the dose. In this way, it may have been more appropriate to ask the registrar to seek help from his/her own doctor.

A Good Response:
"This is a difficult situation but this is how I would approach it. I would firstly suggest to the registrar to move to a quieter room to explore his feelings further. Before doing this, I would ensure there is adequate staff cover on A&E and inform the nurses of our temporary absence on the ward. From the scenario, it seems as though his low mood has been poorly controlled on the current medication and I would, therefore, advise him to book an appointment to see his GP. Furthermore, I would advise him to discuss his issues and concerns with his educational supervisor, as he will be experienced in dealing with pastoral care issues."

Response Analysis:
This answer demonstrates a good understanding of the necessary steps to deal with a complex scenario. It shows that it is important to discuss the registrar's feelings with him, not only to provide colleague support, but also to understand how severe the low mood is in order to establish whether he is able to continue with work and not compromise patient safety. It also nicely highlights that communicating with the nurse and ensuring the shift is covered is very important. The answer also provides longer term management options and offers the registrar further advice on who to turn to for further help.

Overall:
Situational judgment questions will be difficult and the key is to take a measured and calm approach to the situation. Try not to discuss sensitive issues with your peers but rather try and discuss it with the registrar. If you cannot find a solution, then ask him/her to escalate to the consultant in charge. Remember, patient safety is very important here and if the registrar is too depressed to work, he/she will need to step out of the clinical area. Lastly, remember there are a number of people in the hospital which are present to help doctors with these types of issues.

84) You are faced with a patient's angry relatives. The patient is sleeping poorly and complains staff are ignoring her; she is very tearful. What do you do?

Sometimes hospitals can fail in their care and complaints are made. This is more common than you think and a normal part of working in the NHS. Lack of time and attention paid to patients means that serious mistakes can be made. Medical staff may not have enough time to deal with them so patients' full medical and emotional needs may not be met. Patients are left in a high state of anxiety because staff do not talk to them enough. Patients can be very tearful after surgery and they need emotional support and staff need the time to deliver that.

It is important to take a holistic approach to patient management (this mean developing the whole person including physical, emotional, mental, and, at times, spiritual); there is a whole person sitting there - not just a medical condition. It's also easy to forget that patients frequently suffer from numerous medical problems and that treating one of them might exacerbate the other.

However, hospitals were under huge pressure to deliver a service. Pressures include understaffing, an increasing number of inpatients and emergency admissions, and the financial constraints on the NHS. Hospitals often struggle to cope with the increased number of elderly admissions, especially in winter.

The key skill needed for dealing with angry patients or relatives is communication. It is important to listen to concerns and receive feedback to improve future service.

A Bad Response:
"I would apologise profusely and make time to spend with the patient.

"I can understand why the relatives were angry. However, I would explain that the staff are very busy and would assist the patient as soon as they were available."

Response Analysis:
In the first answer, the candidate does not understand the workings of the NHS. To simply say they would "make time" misses the complex nature of the situation. Doctors are often time-pressured and carving out time is not that easy. The second answer is almost the opposite. It is likely to anger the relatives. The lack of apology and the rush to defend the service gives an impression of lack of empathy. Empathy is an essential quality in a doctor and it is important to acknowledge and address the relatives' concerns.

A Good Response:
"Good communication skills are key to fulfilling a doctor's role. This includes listening. I would first listen to the relatives concerns and try and find out more about the situation – is the patient more concerned about the lack of attention or the reduced sleep? I would then work with the relatives and patient to address the patient's primary concern – partnership between healthcare professionals and patients is important in order to produce a patient centred culture in the NHS."

Response Analysis:
This answer is very well constructed. It begins by very quickly getting to the point of the question – interviewers want to know about your communication skills. By acknowledging this early, the interviewers know you are aware of the key issue in this question. The candidate also shows a caring and reflective nature by realising that there may be more than one reason for the patient's emotional state ("is the patient more concerned about the lack of attention or the reduced sleep?"). Using the phrase "partnership between healthcare professionals and patients", shows the candidate is aware of the need for patient involvement in their healthcare which is essential in the modern-day NHS.

Overall:
A good answer will show empathy and showcase your communication skills. It is important to remember that healthcare professionals work together with patients to deliver optimum care.

85) You are a GP and an elderly patient comes to you saying they are suffering and want to end their life, and they have heard of a place in Holland where they can do this. They want your help to refer them. What are your next steps?

When approaching this question, you need to be aware of several things. Firstly, you should understand what euthanasia is the act of deliberately ending a person's life to relieve suffering. Secondly, you should be aware that euthanasia is illegal under English Law, hence, you cannot advise or help patients in ending their life. Thirdly, regardless of whether you know the previously mentioned facts, your main focus should be on the fact that you have a patient in front of you who is considering ending their life; thus they are in need of serious help. As a doctor, your role should be to protect and promote the health of patients with a focus of ensuring a good quality of life for all patients.

A Bad Response:
"I would express my sympathy for the patient and try to understand how they are feeling. I would listen to them and try to dissuade them from carrying on with their intended plan. If I were unable to change their mind, I would make it clear that they still have a full right to make a decision and I must agree with whatever they decide to go ahead with. Hence, should they still wish to end their life, and though I disagree with euthanasia, I would write the referral letter to the clinic in Holland."

Response Analysis:
This answer involves being empathetic but still referring them or giving advice on how to access the facility in Holland. Many candidates make the mistake of going through some initial steps of trying to dissuade the patient, but then stating that it's the patient's decision at the end of the day and you have to agree with what they wish to do, hence, would refer them to the service in Holland. Whilst this would apply to many other situations, in terms of end of life care, due to the law, you cannot refer them to the service in Holland. This answer is poor because the candidate is not aware of the law for euthanasia.

A Good Response:
"I would attempt to explore the issues around why the patient wishes to end their life whilst respecting their privacy. I would try to understand and empathise with the patient whilst remaining sensitive and sympathetic. I would make it clear to the patient what my role and capacity is, and ensure they are aware that I am not legally allowed to offer any advice or referrals regarding this. However, I would make it clear to the patient that there are other options that may improve their quality of life such as pain-alleviating medications or referring them to specialists such as counsellors. I would state that I'd be willing to work with them and I would treat the patient with respect and try to gain their trust. I would end the consultation reviewing what we've discussed and offer to refer them to a counselling service and arrange a follow-up appointment if they are willing."

Response Analysis:
When answering this question, it involves you being aware of the law on euthanasia. This answer involves being empathetic, considerate and aiming to understand the reasons behind the patient's feelings whilst making it clear that you are not allowed to refer them to the facility in Holland.

Overall:
In summary, in questions regarding difficult or sensitive issues such as end of life, it is always important to realise and think about what you can do in the moment to help the patient, i.e. aim to relieve suffering and increase their quality of life. Realise that you have a patient in front of you who needs help and act sensitively and considerately. It is wise to learn about the laws regarding topics such as euthanasia, abortion, and disclosure of patient information as these are likely to be asked about in interviews, as they are very topical.

86) You were minding your neighbour's dog when it ran away, got hit by a car and died. How do you break the bad news?

This is to see how you are able to handle difficult situations as well as being able to admit to your mistakes and deal with the consequences. You are likely to have patients who are angry/upset at a mistake you have made. Also, you may have to explain to someone that a relative has died while under your care. It is a test of your empathy and ability to communicate. Some universities may even put you in a role-play situation where an actor will play your neighbour.

Your neighbour is likely to be angry/upset; make sure you are as tactful as possible when speaking to them. It is important to remain calm; never say "I understand how you feel" unless you actually do, as this can anger people further. Don't be too blunt as this is fairly heavy news, but break it as gently as you can.

The answers below are just guidelines; in the case of role play, there will obviously be a dialogue with the actor or with the interviewer if they ask you to role play the situation with them. Otherwise, you would just have to relate how you *would* take on the situation.

A Bad Response:
"I would try and say as calmly as possible that her dog had died. I would say that I did the best I could but the dog ran away from me when I wasn't looking. I would offer to help buy my neighbour a new pet to replace the old one I was partly responsible for losing. If she got angry, I wouldn't shout back but would keep quiet and say that I understand. I would stay with her until she had stopped crying."

Response Analysis:
The candidate does not fully accept the blame, saying they are 'partly' responsible and partly blaming the situation on the dog. Although they perhaps think they have come up with a solution to the situation, the candidate shows very little tact in offering to buy their neighbour a new pet when their old one has just died! Saying "I understand" does also not necessarily show empathy – the neighbour may get very angry ("No you don't! How could you understand?"). This phrase is, therefore, best avoided unless you actually have been through the situation yourself.

A Good Response:
"First, I would make sure she was sitting down. Then I would try and break the news to her slowly so she could prepare herself: 'Mrs Jones, I'm afraid I have some bad news. It's about your dog. When I wasn't looking, he got hit by a car.' Mrs Jones is likely to be angry or very upset; I would admit that it was my fault as I was responsible for looking after him and that I feel terrible about it. I would tell her I had stopped the driver and gotten his details if I could have, and I would ask if there was any way I could make up for it, e.g. by helping with the gardening for a month. I would ask her if she needed anything right then, such as a cup of tea, though, if she just wanted me to leave her alone, I would understand."

Response Analysis:
Shows foresight and prepares the situation well by making sure the neighbour is sitting down. The neighbour is prepared for the bad news rather than being told bluntly, showing empathy. The mistake is admitted to rather than passed off, showing the candidate is not afraid to take responsibility. A sense of actually caring and a real desire to deal with the situation is shown in chasing the driver up and in offering to help in some other way to make up for this mistake. Kindness is shown in offering a cup of tea, but the candidate is not pushy in their need to be forgiven, understanding that how the neighbour feels is more important.

Overall:
Be tactful and empathic, showing care for your neighbour. Admit to your mistake and try and come up with a solution to the problem (that isn't buying a new pet!). Work your own experience in if relevant to show empathy ("my pet died last year and I know how devastating it can be").

87) You work in a leisure centre and have double-booked the badminton court for two groups for the same time slot. How do you go about turning one group away?

This is similar to other questions where you were asked to deal with a difficult situation with potentially angry or upset people. You will have to deal with this often in the medical field, e.g. if two patients have accidentally been booked in for the same appointment and you have to tell one of them to wait. The patient will often be less than pleased. Just like with the others, you could be required to role-play this station with an actor.

It is important to keep calm at all times and not become angry. It is also important to admit to your mistake. Show initiative and try and come up with a solution to the problem. This is also partially an exercise in conflict resolution in the case of the two groups possibly confronting each other, or if someone from the group you are turning away asks you why the first groups get to go in and they don't.

A Bad Response:
"I would explain that I had double-booked them and ask them to wait for the next time slot. If they got angry I would just have to explain that there was nothing I could do and that I was sorry. I would suggest that they could always find somewhere else if they didn't want to wait. If they asked me why the other group got the hall and not them, I would say the other group got here first so they were now the ones using it."

Response Analysis:
The candidate may anger the customers further by asking them to wait; this does not really present a solution to the problem. The candidate seems unwilling to find a solution by saying there is "nothing I can do"; the solution offered (i.e. finding somewhere else) is non-specific and not very helpful, and seems a bit like the group is being kicked out of the building, which is unlikely to help their anger. Also, any potential conflict with the other group is not resolved.

A Good Response:
"I would start out by apologising and then explaining the situation in full and say how it was my fault. I would try and fix the problem by offering them another time slot of their choosing or by suggesting a few alternative venues in the local area which might be free at this time. If asked why the other group got access to the hall at that time and why they were the group being turned away, I might explain that the other group had booked the hall first and were thus entitled to it; if this made them angry, I would explain again that it wasn't the other group's fault but mine. If they had paid any money in advance for the booking (after checking with my manager) I would offer them a full refund."

Response Analysis:
The candidate acknowledges their mistake in the situation. A practical solution to the problem is offered in the form of other venues that are nearby and could serve as alternatives. Conflict between the two groups is addressed in the case that it should arise. Foresight is shown in trying to resolve all the reasons why the customer might be unhappy (e.g. money paid in advance) with the candidate not making unfounded promises on their own but addressing their supervisor first.

Overall:
Stay calm, accept responsibility and try and come up with a practical alternative solution. Do what you can to make the group feel they are being attended to and their needs are being met. Make sure any potential conflict between the two groups is resolved.

88) A patient with a needle phobia needs to have blood taken but is very nervous. How would you go about persuading them to have it done?

This patient is afraid to have their blood taken although it is necessary to test their blood, perhaps to check if they have an infection; if their body is responding well to an infection; if they have anaemia etc. As with similar situations, you may be required to role play this with an actor.

This is a test or your ability to remain calm and empathic towards a patient and not lose your patience, and also your ability to communicate and persuade. It is important to be able to ensure patients are fully informed when it comes to what kind of treatment they should receive but also to acknowledge you can't force a patient to undergo treatment as they need to provide consent.

A Bad Response:
"I would tell the patient that the procedure is absolutely necessary for them to get the care they need and that it won't hurt very much. I would tell them that even little children go through it and end up fine so it can't be that bad! I would tell them it would be best just to do it now and get it over with."

Response Analysis:
The candidate is quite pushy in convincing the patient to have the blood test. The candidate tries to reassure the patient, although saying the procedure doesn't hurt 'very much' is subjective and not very helpful. Also, the comment about children going through the procedure may be reassuring to some, although it could also be interpreted as belittling to the patient, implying that they are acting worse than a little child in refusing to have blood taken. The last point about just getting it over and done with is not bad, although it is phrased in a way that is rather pressurising to the patient.

A Good Response:
"I would start by asking the patient why they are afraid – sometimes verbalising fears helps rationalise them. Also, it is important for a patient's fears to be listened to and not dismissed. I would then explain why the blood test is needed and how the hospital staff can't provide the best care possible without the blood test. I would say that it would be over very soon and I take the utmost care over the procedure – if I wasn't the one doing it, I would say I would be there the whole time to offer support if needed."

Response Analysis:
The candidate starts by just talking to the patient about their fears, showing empathy towards them and taking them seriously. The situation is explained to the patient in a way that isn't pushy or coercive, with attempts made to reassure the patient. Further empathy and care are shown in how the candidate promises to do the procedure as best they can, as well as willing to stay and offer support if the patient needs it; making them feel valued as a patient.

Overall:
Show empathy and kindness to the patient and persuade them without being pushy. Don't belittle their fears but talk to them about it and help reassure them. If you bully the patient into it and they have a bad experience, they may not return for future treatment.

89) A woman comes to you seeking an abortion. What do you do?

It is important to have some background knowledge as to the law regarding abortion as it is often the subject of ethical scenarios. Abortion is only legal in the UK under certain circumstances:

➢ If the child will suffer from a serious disability.
➢ If the birth is likely to cause serious physical harm to the mother.
➢ If the pregnancy is likely to in some way affect the mother's existing children.
➢ If the child/birth is likely to cause serious psychological harm to the mother.

The majority of abortions that are carried out are based on the last reason. If an abortion is being performed for the third or fourth reasons, it can only be done up to 24 weeks into pregnancy. There is no time limit if the abortion is being performed for the first two reasons. The partner also has no say in whether or not the abortion goes ahead. It is perfectly acceptable to object to abortion and not consent to carry out the procedure yourself – however, you are obliged to refer the woman to a colleague who can help her in your place.

A Bad Response:
"I personally do not support abortion so I would tell the woman I would not be able to treat her. I would make sure she knows the consequences of what she is about to do and would make sure her partner knows. I would tell her to seriously reconsider undergoing the procedure."

Response Analysis:
The candidate is very pushy in their personal opinion regarding abortion and is allowing this to influence the standard of care they are giving the patient, which is very unprofessional. The patient is likely to feel very judged in this circumstance. Although it is of course fine to recommend that the patient tells the father if they are together, it is also a betrayal of the patient's trust to inform their partner in this instance, where they are not obliged to know as officially they have no say in the matter. The candidate has also shown no knowledge of what the law allows and is instead totally concerned with their opinion. They have also not recommended the patient to another colleague on refusing to treat them.

A Good Response:
"First, I would make the patient feel comfortable, then talk to them about why exactly they want an abortion as it is a very serious procedure which they may regret later. I would also ask her if she is still with the child's father, and if so, whether or not he knows. I would definitely recommend her telling him if they are still together. I would also find out how far along she is to see if she is still eligible for the procedure. As I myself object to abortion, I would refer her to my colleague, but I would make sure I didn't put this to her in a way that would make her feel ashamed or small. I would also assure her that I would keep being her doctor after the procedure and would make sure she had support in recovering from the procedure."

Response Analysis:
This is a very good answer. Many people will look at this question from a detached and objective point of view, forgetting the fact that you are theoretically talking to an *actual patient* who is thinking of undergoing a very serious procedure. Initially, establishing a rapport with the patient and finding out why they wish to have the procedure, as this candidate has done, is very important. Although the partner *officially* has no say, the candidate has rightly advised to inform them if relevant. This candidate objects to the procedure, which is perfectly fine, but has revealed this to the patient tactfully and has referred them to a colleague. The candidate could perhaps demonstrate more knowledge of the legal circumstances when an abortion can be done (otherwise, this may come in a follow-up question).

Overall:
Show some understanding of the law behind the matter, including when an abortion can be carried out and whether the partner needs to know. It is perfectly fine to object if you refer the patient to a colleague who can help her. As well as showing your knowledge of the legal side, make sure you show care and compassion to the mother during this difficult time.

90) If you could interview one person in the world, who would it be?

This question is not to try and trip you up or test your situational judgment but is essentially trying to find out more about you as a person. It's often asked towards the end of the interview and is a chance for you to speak about something you are passionate about, stand out, and make yourself a memorable candidate.

A lot of people will think the interviewer expects them to give an answer that is a famous scientific or medical figure, but this is by no means necessary. If you do not know very much/have just memorised some facts about them, it is likely to come across as clichéd. As long as you do not say someone and only provide very superficial reasons (no reality TV stars), you can potentially talk about anyone you like. Someone who inspires you is best as they are likely to be someone who has done something worthy of note, and worthy of interviewing.

A Bad Response:
"I would interview the Prime Minister to see just what it's like to run the country and how he plans on managing the healthcare system. I would also see what foreign policy is like with other countries and what the Prime Minister's plans are regarding immigration. I would also discuss the world economy and whether or not it looks like the country is going to approach another economic downturn and how we would deal with that in terms of budget cuts."

Response Analysis:
This is likely one of the most overused answers. For one, there are *plenty* of available interviews to watch where these questions have been addressed, and also, there is no passion or feeling in this response whatsoever. The questions are vague and non-specific and thus likely to elicit similar answers. This is a very forgettable answer and the candidate has wasted the opportunity to show a bit of their personality to the interviewer.

A Good Response:
"If I could interview one person in the world, it would be David Attenborough. Nature documentaries are something many people think of as boring, but he is incredibly engaging and never dull to watch and always genuinely passionate about what he does. I haven't had the chance to travel very much – it would be fascinating to be able to talk to someone who has explored such a broad range of places in the world. Aside from narrating nature documentaries, I'm sure he has many a story to tell about his experiences while he was exploring. He actually inspired me to try out wilderness medicine and to travel abroad on my elective, should I get the chance. He also has such an iconic voice – it would be quite something to be able to hear it in person!"

Response Analysis:
The candidate is speaking passionately about someone which they mention inspires them and whom they would genuinely like to meet. They also reveal a bit about themselves here in that they are excited by the prospect of travel and exploring, and enjoys watching documentaries depicting other parts of the world. This turns them from just another application form into a 'three-dimensional' person, making a welcome change from what may well be very fixed or rehearsed answers to previous questions. The answer is enthusiastic and, therefore, much more memorable than the previous answer, making them stand out in the eyes of the interviewer.

Overall:
This is not a trick question! Don't just tell the interviewer what you think they want to hear – give a genuine response and it will seem more natural and memorable. Avoid giving a superficial (e.g. a movie star) or clichéd (e.g. the Prime Minister) response. Talking about someone you genuinely want to meet is likely to be a lot more engaging and memorable.

91) What do you think is more important, spending money on hospital beds or on community care? Why?

One of the biggest challenges in hospitals these days is the discharge of medically fit patients into the community. This is particularly relevant for the elderly that are not able to care for themselves but have no medical conditions requiring hospital care. As they cannot be discharged into an unsafe environment, it is not uncommon for patients to spend a long time in the hospital, even though there is no medical need for them to do so. This binds important hospital resources, is very expensive for the health service, and also puts the patients at risk of acquiring further morbidities, including but not limited to infections by multi-drug resistant pathogens.

A Bad Response:

"Hospitals are more important than community care. Waiting times in A&E are ever increasing and this is in large part due to the overall lack of hospital beds. The provision of more hospital beds is essential in alleviating this. This is particularly true as the patients presenting to the hospital are generally ill and in need of actual medical care whereas the cases in the community are less relevant. Therefore, money should go to hospitals."

Response Analysis:

This answer fails to appreciate the connection between hospital care and community care resulting in vital shortcomings in the answer itself. It furthermore fails to appreciate the complexity of hospital admissions and presentations. Whilst it is true that some people presenting to A&E will be very unwell and needing hospital care, a proportion of people presenting will not. Effectively, it is not possible to judge one more important than the other as there is a very close interaction between both spheres.

A Good Response:

"Availability of hospital beds represent a great challenge in the NHS. In the view of bursting A&E departments that are unable to find space for presenting patients, this message is particularly obvious. It would, however, be wrong to assume that a simple increase of hospital beds at the cost of community care will necessarily alleviate the problem. There is a very fluent exchange of patients between community care, in particular, care homes and hospitals. It is not uncommon for patients that are medically fit for discharge to remain in the hospital occupying beds simply because they have nowhere else to go. This, in turn, produces other issues such as increasing rates of hospital-acquired infections as well as an overall poorer long-term prognosis due to prolonged hospital stay. Not to mention the high cost associated with an occupied hospital bed. In the light of this, it is, therefore, important to spend money on the improvement of both factors: the amount of hospital beds available as well as community care."

Response Analysis:

This response is well-balanced and well-argued, providing a good overview of the complexity of the issue of hospital beds and community care. It gives a precise and justified answer and makes intrinsic sense. It also provides an additional perspective by addressing the consequences of unnecessarily prolonged hospital stays.

Overall:

A very relevant issue to be aware of, especially considering the overall limitations in availability of hospital beds in the UK in relation to the population (237/100 000 in 2011). In the prospect of ever shrinking social care budgets and increasing amounts of council budget cuts, it becomes an even more pressing issue. Furthermore, a good answer to this question demonstrates the student's understanding of the interaction of different levels of healthcare and the interface between these levels and the patients. Different healthcare environments have different requirements in regards to funding, but all are highly relevant for the overall delivery of care that in the end spans all levels of care provision.

92) If you had a patient who only spoke a foreign language, how could you improve communication with them to ensure they had a good understanding of your explanations?

This question is examining your ability to take initiative and be aware that each patient is individually unique and has different needs. When approaching this question, you should acknowledge the fact that patients who speak another language may require more assistance and help to ensure that they reach an equal level of understanding as an English-speaking patient. Think of a variety of ways to help the patient. Many cities in the UK are home to people from a range of ethnic backgrounds, especially in cities such as London, hence it is important to demonstrate the ability to communicate with all patients. Communication skills are very important in medicine and often, medical interviewers will try to examine your ability to demonstrate good communication skills.

A Bad Response:
"I would speak in very slow English to see if they can understand the basics of what I am saying. If this does not work, I would request for the patient to come back with someone who spoke English if possible so that I could explain everything to this other person to ensure the patient received all the necessary information. Similarly, if there was a doctor fluent in the specific language, I would try to transfer the patient to this doctor."

Response Analysis:
This answer involves attempting three different methods in trying to improve communication with the patient. Whilst some are good suggestions, most of the options involve trying to utilise someone else to improve the communication. Whilst beneficial, the use of translators has been shown to reduce rapport built up between doctors and patients. It would be beneficial to suggest other methods that also involve yourself. Furthermore, sending the patient home and telling them to return with someone who is English speaking shows poor commitment and determination, and also it may jeopardise the patient's health and decrease their trust with you as a doctor.

A Good Response:
"Patients who cannot speak English may not receive the same quality of care as those that do speak English. It may affect the doctor-patient relationship if the doctor is unable to communicate with the patient. I would request the help of a translator, but ensure that I take an active role in still trying to build rapport with the patient by using visual cues for example, and with the help of the translator, finding a way to check the patient's understanding such as showing a 'thumbs up'. This would allow me to create somewhat of a relationship with the patient to ease their comfort."

Response Analysis:
Though similar to the poor response, this response suggests several methods involving the doctor such as finding a way to check the patient's understanding or using visual cues. The answer also starts off by stating the effects of language barriers between patients and doctors and their awareness of the difficulties language barriers can pose. This answer is better as the candidate tries to build rapport with the patient and make them feel more comfortable.

Overall:
This question aims to test your creativity and patience with patients. This kind of scenario may be commonly encountered as a practising doctor in various cities in the UK and abroad of course. By suggesting a variety of ways to help in improving communication with patients who cannot speak English, you will demonstrate your ability to take initiative and consider the fact that patients may have different needs.

93) What do you think about the use of statistics when discussing treatment options with patients?

This question has no right or wrong answer. These kinds of questions are asked to test your ability to create a balanced argument by looking at both sides of a question, for and against, and coming to your own conclusion. You will not be marked down for your opinion as long as you can show an ability to rationalise and think from different viewpoints. As a doctor, you will encounter situations where you will be required to rationalise topics and think from various viewpoints, hence why these types of questions may come up in interviews.

A Bad Response:

"I think the use of statistics when discussing treatment with patients are good as they give the patient an approximate idea of the success of various treatment options or the chances of risks occurring. Giving statistics to patients makes options easily understandable and comparable. Without statistics, patients may understand the use of phrases such as 'very good' or 'high risk' differently. Therefore, I think the use of statistics is beneficial and necessary when discussing treatment options with patients."

Response Analysis:

This answer discusses reasons for the beneficial use of statistics when discussing treatment with patients. The reasons are valid and good, however, a balanced argument has not been demonstrated, and no points against the use of statistics have been stated. It would be a better answer if a balanced argument was created and points for and against the use of statistics were discussed.

A Good Response:

"There are several reasons why the use of statistics when discussing treatment with patients may be beneficial. Firstly, they give the patient an approximate idea of the success of various treatment options or the chances of risks occurring. Giving statistics to patients makes options easily understandable and comparable. Without statistics, patients may understand the use of phrases such as very good 'or' high risk differently. However, there are some reasons against the use of statistics. Firstly, patients may take the statistics literally. If a patient is told that their treatment has a 90% success rate, they may be certain that their treatment will work. However, they may be less aware of the fact that there is still a slight chance of treatment failure. Using statistics may give patients a false sense of hope or worry. Overall, I think the use of statistics is beneficial for patients as it gives an approximate idea of success or risk, however, doctors should ensure patients are aware that statistics may not guarantee certainty."

Response Analysis:

This answer is much better as it demonstrates an ability to create a balanced argument. Though the candidate has their own opinion, they mention several points for and against the use of statistics when discussing treatment options with patients, and then conclude with their own opinion. This demonstrates the ability of the candidate to rationalise and think from various viewpoints. The reasons for and against the argument are also valid and well thought of.

Overall/:

In summary, in medical school interviews, it is common to get asked questions that require your own opinion about a topic or ethical scenario. Interviewers tend to look for your ability to generate points for and against a topic, as well as demonstrate your ability to form an opinion. It is common in the practice of medicine to have to think from different viewpoints, and answering a question in the structure mentioned above would show the interviewer that you are capable of this.

94) You are a GP and a 16-year-old patient comes in, accompanied by her mother. You wish to speak to the patient alone as part of the consultation, however, the mother refuses to leave. What do you do about this?

When treating children, the majority of the time you will have to also communicate with their families and interact with them as they may play a key role in their care and decision-making. A question like this may be asked to test your ability to act politely but in the patient's best interest too. In medicine, you may be faced with difficult circumstances where you may be worried about being rude or offending someone, with both patients and relatives of patients. It is important to find a balance between being polite and also doing what you believe is right for the patient with their best interests in mind.

A Bad Response:
"I would ask the patient what their own opinion would be, whether they would like their mother to leave the room or not. If the patient wishes for her mother to leave the room and her mother still does not comply, I would tell the mother that even if the mother refuses, her daughter has the right to be consulted alone and that I am suggesting this because I think it would be beneficial for the patient, in their best interest.

Response Analysis:
This answer is poor, firstly because it involves asking the young patient what they would want. Though this can be beneficial, if the patient is withholding information by saying they would like their parent to leave the room, it may draw attention to this, hence they may refrain from agreeing with their parent leaving. It may put the patient in an uncomfortable position. Also, the way in which the mother is dealt with, by forcing her to leave may create a bitter relationship with the family, especially if there are other children in the family and this may deter the mother from returning to the same GP.

A Good Response:
"In a calm manner, I would suggest that according to standard protocol, I would like to see the patient alone. I would say that I am simply following protocol and this is not unusual with patients of this age and that I believe it is in their best interest. I would allow the mother to discuss her concerns with me about leaving the room and offer her the chance of also having a separate discussion afterwards to allow her to discuss her own concerns about her daughter's health. To prevent this from happening again, I would begin my future consultations by telling patients of a specific age and their parents about the standard structure of consultations with a joint discussion to begin with, followed by a separate discussion with the patient and then with the parent alone should they wish."

Response Analysis:
This answer is much better as it shows the ability of the candidate to be polite whilst taking initiative and simply stating that it is standard protocol with patients of this age to be seen alone as well as with their parents, should they wish. Offering the mother a chance to be seen alone is also a good idea as it shows concern for both the patient and the parent. This answer finds a good balance between being polite and doing what you believe is right for the patient.

Overall:
In summary, when asked these types of questions, it is always important to demonstrate politeness and avoid actions that may damage rapport built between the patient/parent and the doctor. It is important to acknowledge that this is in the best interest of the patient and that no offence is intended to the parent.

95) You are a doctor and your patient requests to instead be seen by another doctor for an unspecified reason. What do you do?

According to the NHS, unless you require urgent or emergency treatment, the patient has the right to be able to see any consultant-led team, or be treated in a specific hospital of their choice for a procedure (provided the team provides this treatment). This choice is offered at the point of referral and is a legal right. If the patient does not wish to be seen by a particular doctor, then they can choose to be seen by another. This question is asked to assess how well you approach the scenario and whether you are able to handle the situation in the most professional manner possible. It's important not to take their refusal personally.

A Bad Response:

"Firstly, if I have been assigned as the doctor to a particular patient then I would have to explain to the patient that I am their doctor and they must be seen by me. However, I would make sure I understand why the patient wants to be seen by a different doctor in the first place."

Response Analysis:

The statement is factually incorrect and is not the best way of handling the situation. The patient has a right to be seen by another doctor and you must respect their wishes. If they have been referred from A&E, then this may not be possible and the answer would somewhat apply. However, in other circumstances, e.g. wards and clinics, this is not the case. The only redeeming quality of this answer is trying to understand the reasons for the patient wanting to see a different doctor.

A Good Response:

"It is my understanding that the patient has the right to choose their consultant-led team and the hospital in which they receive their treatment, given that this treatment is provided by that team. If a patient was referred to me from A&E, I would have to explain to the patient why their request would not be possible. However, I would try and understand the reasoning for why they would like to change doctors and address their concerns. Additionally, I would ask whether there is anything I can do to make them feel more comfortable. If they have been referred to me from their GP, then I would once again try and understand their reasoning but oblige their request and ask a colleague (my consultant) to examine the patient instead."

Response Analysis:

This is a much more in-depth response and has a good insight into the rights of a patient. It also gives an example of a diplomatic method of handling the situation. The bad response involved stating that you would understand their reasoning, but the good response has a much more *active* approach and attempts to address their concerns. The ultimate solution, in this case, is to ask a consultant to see the patient instead as this is what the patient requested. These sorts of questions have a scenario and must be approached in three steps: action, reason, and outcome.

Overall:

The important part of this question is to address the patient's concerns in an active manner. Simply stating your action without a reason and why you chose it is insufficient and requires further depth. What distinguishes between a good and bad answer is not only what you say, but how you say it. The bad response is blunt and lacks empathy. On the other hand, the good response promotes an element of understanding (by asking what the problem is) as well as addressing the problem if it cannot be rectified.

96) As a doctor, when can it be useful to be silent?

Communication can be split up into verbal and non-verbal communication. Verbal communication is often emphasized at the expense of non-verbal communication, but it is vital to remember that it is just as important. Silence, on the other hand, doesn't really fall into either category and can be an incredibly powerful tool that doctors can use when speaking to a patient. For example, when a doctor asks the patient to describe their situation or symptoms, in a moment of silence, the patient will normally try and fill it by giving more information. This could be incredibly useful, especially when a patient is very reserved and may not be giving the full picture. Normal questions ask about either verbal or non-verbal communication but this assesses your ability to think outside the box.

A Bad Response:

"A doctor should rarely be silent as it would make the patient feel uncomfortable. However, it may be appropriate to remain silent when a doctor is writing things down or thinking about what the diagnosis could be. This is because it could be hard to multi-task (talk and think/write at the same time) and may affect their ability to make an accurate judgement."

Response Analysis:

This response, while it may be true, is very short. Secondly, it doesn't really demonstrate a good ability to think about this communication skill in depth. The response could be improved by providing another example and mentioning why it may be important (as explained in the background). The response also provides an example of where it is almost necessary to be silent, as most doctors will be at that stage of the consultation. However, it does not explain why being silent is useful or appropriate in certain circumstances.

A Good Response:

"It is my understanding that there are two types of communication skills: verbal and non-verbal. Silence does not really fall into either of the two categories; at a glance, it may appear that it does not fit into a consultation. Obviously, a doctor should remain silent when a patient is speaking and not interrupt them. However, during times of silence, someone will often attempt to fill the gap and so by a doctor leaving a moment of silence it could help get the patient to speak. This may be advantageous if a patient is particularly reserved and will not reveal much information. Therefore, silence may in fact be appropriate and somewhat more effective than asking further questions. I appreciate that being silent too much is also a disadvantage as it may lead to the patient feeling uncomfortable, so a doctor should only remain silent when appropriate."

Response Analysis:

This is a much more well-rounded response. Firstly, it outlines the two basic forms of communication which demonstrates an understanding of the topic. Secondly, it very clearly gives a realistic example of why silence may be advantageous during a consultation, but only by giving a background of the situation. Finally, the response acknowledges why being silent is not always a good thing as it can be very uncomfortable.

Overall:

This is something that you will be taught more about when learning communication skills in medical school. You will most likely be taught that when listening to a patient's story or situation, you should make sure you are not the first person to speak – remaining silent allows the patient to steer the conversation in the direction they feel most comfortable with. It is only after this initial moment of silence that the questions you have can be addressed. This is something else that can be incorporated into your answer but mentioning the idea of allowing a patient to speak and give more information should be at the forefront of your response.

97) A leukaemia patient is refusing stem cell treatment on religious grounds. Without the treatment, he has a 20% chance of survival. How would you use your communication skills to deal with this situation?

Paternalistic medicine (the attitude that the doctor always knows best) is falling out of favour. It's important to recognise that sometimes, certain lifestyle decisions are even more important to patients than their own health. It would be inappropriate to dismiss these choices even though the doctor's focus is on health. From a communication skills perspective, this question is asking you to demonstrate creativity in how you would use your own interpersonal skills to try to resolve the situation. Reaching a compromise between the patient's values and the physician's goals is a frequent conundrum in medicine, so being able to listen to the patient and figure out what is most important to them is an absolutely essential skill.

A Bad Response:
"I would override his refusal by getting a court order as he clearly lacks the capacity to make a rational decision about his own care. Therefore, I should act in his best interests as I know from my medical training what is best for the patient, and it would be irresponsible of me not to do my best to treat him."

Response Analysis:
Whilst this at first seems like a good answer, the response shows a lack of willingness to engage with the patient on their own terms. The court order is unlikely to lead to treatment being enforced either, especially if the patient has the capacity and is over 18. Whilst it is indeed true that doctors should try to do the right thing for their patients, this paternalistic view would be frowned upon in interviews as it makes the assumption that the treatment is what is best for the patient overall. This opinion suggests that the patient has a 'problem' to be 'fixed', rather than a complex combination of ideas, concerns, needs, and expectations. For example, this patient may suffer severe psychological distress from being forced to act against his beliefs. Therefore, is the stem cell treatment really the best option for his health?

A Good Response:
"I would firstly understand the religious grounds behind his refusal. If there are conflicting opinions within his religion, it might be worth asking a religious representative (e.g. Chaplain or Rabbi) to visit him and discuss his options sensitively. If the patient is a minor and there is reason to believe he is being coerced rather than making his own decision, or the patient lacks capacity, there may be grounds for going to the court to get permission to treat him. However, at the end of the day, respect for patient autonomy must be paramount. If the patient has capacity and refuses the treatment, we must support his decision and instead treat any symptoms and problems he may have as a result of the refusal of treatment."

Response Analysis:
This is a good response. The first part demonstrates a desire to understand the patient's point of view, an open mind to learn about different cultures and backgrounds, and a willingness to use communication (even via a third party) to work through problems and issues. The second part demonstrates knowledge of the process of consent for minors, but interviewees wouldn't be expected to have an in-depth knowledge of the laws and processes involved in this. The third part of the response is the most important point – respect for the patient's decision also involves treating any problems they may have as a result of their (informed, consented) decisions. This is an essential aspect of medical care that many doctors struggle with.

Overall:
Being sensitive to the patient's motivations and concerns is an important part of being a doctor. This sort of question makes sure that the interviewee has the right attitude towards care that is expected of a modern doctor, and that they understand that 'acting in the patient's best interests' and giving the most efficacious treatment are not necessarily the same thing. It's also important to recognise that if a treatment is rejected, the doctor should give their best efforts to support the patient medically through other means, even if the patient experiences problems as a result of having rejected the therapy.

98) You have been asked to go and take a medical history from a patient and discover they only speak a couple of words of English. Talk me through what different techniques you could use to communicate.

This is a common problem faced by doctors and one of the biggest barriers to effective treatment that meets patient satisfaction. This question assesses the candidate's creativity in overcoming barriers to communication. Taking a full history from a patient (i.e. finding out all about their past and current medical problems, social situations, and their family history of disease and medication) is a structured interview that can take at least half an hour and often involves questions and concepts that are difficult to communicate in simple English. It can easily be misunderstood.

A Bad Response:
"I would try and talk as simply as possible to the patient. If they still didn't understand, I would go and find someone who speaks their language."

Response Analysis:
Whilst this response acknowledges that an understanding is essential for the consultation, this response doesn't show much creativity in overcoming difficulties. The candidate also assumes they will be able to assess an understanding without using language – many patients will nod and agree even with no understanding whatsoever, under the assumption that the doctor knows best and they should agree to receive treatment. As discussed below, the candidate should also acknowledge that many people speak more than one language, so they would have more luck finding someone with a common language if they ask what languages the patient speaks.

A Good Response:
"First of all, I speak [language], so I would ask them in [language] if they speak it [quickly demonstrate asking in that language]. However, if we have no common language, there are several other options available. I would first find out what languages the patient does speak so that I could ask one of the nurses or doctors if there is anyone around that speaks any of the patient's languages. If not, there is a translator service available, either in person or over the phone. If none of these are viable options, I may be able to use a combination of techniques to make myself understood. For example, keywords and short phrases may be translated using online translation programs, but this may be not entirely reliable. I could supplement understanding with gestures, touch, and by drawing diagrams and pictures. For example, when assessing a level of pain, sometimes a chart is used with ten facial expressions (from relaxed to intense pain) and the patient is asked to point on the chart to where they sit on the scale."

Response Analysis:
The candidate first of all shows they speak another language, a valuable skill – however, this is obviously not an essential part of the answer, just a bonus to their application! Finding out what languages the patient speaks (not just their main language) is important as it maximises your chances of communication. The translator service is an extremely useful and valued help to many doctors, especially in rural areas.

The candidate then demonstrates creativity by thinking about various approaches they could combine to get keywords across, but also to make sure the patient understands. This multi-sensory approach would serve the candidate well when later talking to patients with other communication difficulties, such as those who have just had a stroke, or those with learning difficulties, or hearing loss.

Overall:
This question assesses overall creativity in communication skills, which can be applied to many areas of medicine, such as paediatrics, stroke, and general neurology. Including the use of pictures and/or diagrams is an important skill that is often under-used by doctors, so be sure to include that in your answer. If you have an additional language, that is a great asset and should also be included!

99) What is more important for a doctor– good communication skills or good clinical skills?

A doctor must, of course, be equipped with both communication skills (e.g. bedside manner) and clinical skills (e.g. phlebotomy). This question is asked to make sure that the candidate understands why both sets of skills are important – the decision made doesn't really matter as long as the response is thoughtful and appropriate. As with any question, a knee-jerk response (particularly one that comes across as lacking insight) shows bad listening skills, so consider both sides of the question carefully. Use this opportunity to show that you can carefully consider a question without immediately disregarding certain points. The temptation is to immediately conclude that clinical skills are the most important (especially as you're applying to a medical school to predominantly study clinical skills!), but it's worth considering why good communication skills may be even more important, and in which situations.

A Bad Response:
"Good clinical skills are more important; communication skills won't fix medical problems."

Response Analysis:
This response shows a lack of understanding of the role of communication and potentially belies poor future bedside manner. Good communication skills can be an essential part of treatment – for example, over half of prescribed medication is not actually taken in the manner prescribed. Ensuring the patient understands why they are taking their medication can often produce a sudden improvement in their blood pressure. The short and blunt answer also shows a closed mind – the candidate hasn't taken the time to step back and reflect on the question before answering. Thinking about the question is an essential skill for a doctor. If an answer such as this is given, the interviewer may prompt the interviewee to reflect on the role of communication skills as a follow-up question.

A Good Response:
"Good clinical skills are obviously required to diagnose the problem and treat the patient. However, communication is also essential as about 75% of a diagnosis is made from the clinical history, which relies on the quality of communication with the patient – for example, a clinical examination can't tell you about the patient's family history of a genetic syndrome. Without good communication, the patient may be non-compliant with medication, meaning that despite good clinical skills, the patient would still not get better. Sometimes symptoms that defy diagnosis can be resolved with good communication skills, such as in the case of Functional Syndrome, where psychological issues manifest as physical symptoms – in the case of this disease, neurological symptoms (which can be severe) can be cured through psychological therapy."

Response Analysis:
This answer successfully shows not only the value of both skills, but also discusses how they relate to each other and how communication sometimes succeeds where clinical skills fail – an important and often overlooked point, even by qualified doctors. Non-compliance is also a huge problem as discussed above. The examples given are very insightful and show off some good knowledge of the diagnostic and treatment processes.

The candidate could then nominate which skill they think is overall more important – but again, reiterate that both skills are essential in a doctor. By addressing both parts of the question, the candidate demonstrates good listening and analysis skills in addition to however they have actually answered the question.

Overall:
In conclusion, an excellent answer to this question can be achieved by playing the skills off against each other to show how they interact and are both essential. The question also tests the knowledge of some underlying aspects of holistic care of the patient, and recognition that 'fixing' the physical symptoms may not be enough in all circumstances. Additional knowledge of situations in which communication skills become more important than clinical skills adds an extra 'edge' to the answer.

100)   You are working at a GP surgery and an elderly lady attends the practice with osteoarthritis. She explains that she feels her current course of prescribed medication is not effective and her friend has recommended herbal remedies that she would like to try instead of her prescribed medication. How would you respond?

This question tests for effective communication skills, and variants of this frequently crop up in MMIs. It's important to remember that how you convey your message is just as important as what you say.

A Bad Response:

"Don't be silly now, this herbal stuff doesn't work at all. You're far better off sticking to the medication you've been prescribed. If you don't like it, we can try something else, but it's pointless spending money on this kind of stuff. You'll probably feel a bit better at first, but it's just a placebo effect. Whoever tried to sell you this is taking you for a fool. They're just preying on your vulnerability."

Response Analysis:

This response is a situation where the candidate is literally speaking their mind. The individual points themselves aren't wrong, but the way they're being conveyed is poor. Saying "Don't be silly now" isn't a good start. It sounds patronizing, which is exactly what medical professionals must try to avoid. We want our patients to see us as their equals, that way they can confide in us without fear of being judged so they can be honest with us. This is what we mean when we talk about moving away from the medical paternalism that dominated the last century of medicine. It also trivializes the patient's concerns. This patient probably wasn't making this decision on a whim, but rather had taken the time to think about this before approaching you. The fact that she's asking you as opposed to just neglecting your treatment shows that she genuinely believes this may be of benefit to her, and by trivializing her concerns you undermine any respect she may have had for you. The rest of the response actually has good underlying points, but poor delivery. It lacks any sense of empathy for the patient's situation and comes across as being short with her. A lot of this is to do with how it's delivered, but generally, a more considerate response is ideal.

A Good Response:

"I would try to explore the reasons for trying the herbal medicine. "Well, what seems to be the issue with your current medication?" "If you're willing to try another treatment, we can help with that." If she seems adamant that she wants to pursue the homeopathic remedies, it's important to address this directly. "Why do you believe this treatment will work?" In response to her concerns, an explanation of evidence-based medicine is useful. Explain that our drugs are tried and tested. We know with a fair degree of certainty that these drugs are relatively safe and do work, however, that safety isn't guaranteed with these alternative treatments. We can keep an eye out on her prescribed medications to ensure there's no conflict, but we can't do that with the alternative therapies because we don't know what's in them. Our concern is finding the right combination of medications to make her feel better. The herb provider is only trying to get her to buy as many herbs as possible. Finally, if I still haven't convinced her and she takes the herbs, she should still come in regularly for appointments to make sure things aren't dangerously wrong."

Response Analysis:

This is a good response for a few reasons. It comes across as far more empathetic with probing questions showing that you've listened. Notice that the core message is the same as in the bad response, but rather than being short with the patient, this response takes the time to actually explain why our drugs work and doesn't trivialise the patient's legitimate concerns. The final remarks about coming in regardless are also important to prevent the patient from becoming disillusioned with modern medicine.

Overall:

This question actually represents a common scenario you may have already encountered in real life. It's important to have a good response here and keep in mind that situations like this are increasing in frequency, at least partly due to the profession moving away from medical paternalism and the internet increasing patient access to information.

101)   If you could propose one policy to reduce obesity in poorer communities, what would it be?

These kinds of questions are difficult to answer, especially if it's the first time you've seen them. Crucially, it's important to remember that there is not one absolute golden response or one concept that is considered correct. Rather, the key here is to present a logical and feasible solution to a serious problem. You are not a government policy maker and your interviewer knows this. The point here is to engage with your further reading to see how much you really understand about current issues.

A Bad Response:
"Fat children are a big issue. The link between diabetes and obesity is well known, and therefore, childhood obesity needs to be tackled. The easiest way to tackle this is to prohibit the sale of junk food and sweets to children. If children do not have access to unhealthy food, they are less likely to become obese. This would solve the root cause of the problem limiting the long-term implications of having too many fat children in our society. You could also have a policy where you make healthy foods cheaper so that more people buy them. That way, more people eat healthily so that they don't become obese. This would probably work because lots of poorer working people are obese because they eat a lot of junk food. So, if you made healthy food cheaper, they wouldn't buy so much junk food."

Response Analysis:
This response isn't actually that bad but it comes across as quite judgemental. The underlying point of making healthy food cheaper is a valid point. But here you'd have missed out on an opportunity to show that you have a greater understanding of how funding works, and why people in poorer communities are obese. It attempts to find a simple solution for a complex issue. Simply making the sale of unhealthy food to children illegal is unlikely to solve the problem and would come with significant challenges regarding the policy itself. It also does not tackle additional factors influencing obesity apart from unhealthy food.

A Good Response:
"I'd propose a government subsidy of healthier food options, funded by greater taxation on less healthy foods. That coupled with the existing legislation that prevents junk food advertising aimed directly at certain communities should help. I think it would work because of the link between poverty and obesity. A lot of the time, parents will feed their children less healthy food, not necessarily kebabs every night, but foods that are high in salts and fat purely because they're cheaper than the healthier alternatives. If you have four mouths to feed on a really limited budget, it makes sense to buy the cheaper option just to make sure your kids get their caloric intake. It's not an active choice to be unhealthy but just a fact of the economics. If the healthier options were cheaper, this problem would be ameliorated."

Response Analysis:
This response is better because it shows a greater understanding of the issues. Now, you might not necessarily agree with the above argument, but at the very least it does sound feasible and is actually proposed by several political think tanks. This response shows a deep understanding of complex issues like the link between poverty and obesity, and a real-world approach to how people in tough situations might behave. It also shows an understanding of basic economics by acknowledging that money for making things cheaper doesn't just come from thin air, but rather from taxation of other products. This kind of holistic approach to problems is important to foster. Whilst the response does not "spell out" a specific policy, it gives solid thought processes that can be implemented.

Overall:
This is a very important question as child obesity is a big problem for the NHS. Don't be fazed if you don't have a unique response to this question. It's important to take a step back and think about this before you answer. Ultimately, if you can show an understanding of the issues (why people make certain food choices) and give details about the implementations of your policy regardless of the efficacy, you'll do well. It may be worth alluding to the sugar tax on fizzy drinks if you really want to shine.

102)   How can a team avoid making mistakes by using good communication skills?

This question is worded difficultly but don't let it put you off. The focus of this question is identifying how mistakes might be made as a result of a breakdown in communications and suggesting ways in which such mistakes could subsequently be avoided. Furthermore, it is key to have a strong structure when answering a question like this, as any answer is liable to becoming simply a list.

A Bad Response:

"One way that stops mistakes being made when communicating is to use simple language. Another way is to ensure you speak slowly and clearly. By doing these things you can save lives in medicine. Another way is to make sure that things are checked over."

Response Analysis:

This candidate does seem to have the basics for some ideas but has presented them in a very poor manner. They do not illustrate their points at all and have not included any explanations or examples. In addition, there is no structure to the answer and it is obvious that the candidate rushed into the question and did not have their answer clear in their mind prior to answering. This is evidenced by the fact that they add in a further point after their summary.

A Good Response:

"Medicine deals with human lives and so mistakes in conveying information, which may be hardly noticed and completely benign in normal everyday interactions, become magnified by the nature of the profession and can lead to dire consequences. Thus, it is paramount that teams of doctors avoid such mistakes.

This can be achieved in two key ways:
One way is to check and confirm that the information is correct and is understood by anyone who receives an important communication. An example of how this can be done is to make sure that the recipient of information repeats back what they think they heard. It is easy to see how doing this can avoid such a crucial mishap as mishearing a decimal place over a poor telephone line.

A second way in which communication errors can be avoided is to make sure they are not made in the first place. One way in which this can be done is to highlight when something important is about to be conveyed. For example, by starting a sentence with 'I have an unusual request and it is important that you take this in'. This will instantly bring a colleague to focus their full attention on listening to what you need to say. This avoids communication errors due to lapses in concentration and due to the making of assumptions about what information is contained within a piece of speech or text. Another way in which mistakes can be avoided in the first place is to avoid the use of complicated jargon and ensure that all speech/writing is at a level that is appropriate for the person you're communicating with. In summary, it is imperative that those in the medical profession do not make errors when communicating. As mentioned above, these errors can be avoided in two key ways; firstly, by repeating and checking information; and secondly, by using techniques that avoid or reduce the number of errors made in the first place."

Response Analysis:

This answer has a very strong opening. They immediately relate their answer to medicine which is clearly what the question was getting at. Furthermore, the introduction powerfully outlines the important implications of their answer.

Overall:

By comparing these two examples, we can see how a strong structure and several illustrative explanations can turn a few basic ideas into a formidable answer. A key learning point is that these 'furnishings' are often formed in the crucial several second pauses between hearing the question and starting your answer.

103)   As a junior doctor you are called to an urgent situation. A patient is angry and is violently threatening the nursing staff. How might you calm this angry patient down?

This question focuses on how you can use your communication skills on the spot and under pressure to bring a difficult situation to a positive conclusion.

A Bad Response:

"There are several things that can be done to calm down an angry patient. Firstly, you could use communication techniques to show that you are not a threat. Secondly, you could use hospital security. Finally, you could explain to the patient that they should calm down as it will not benefit them to be angry. People often fail to realise that their anger only acts as a detriment to the care they might receive in hospital, so it is necessary to explain this to them."

Response Analysis:

This student's answer makes many faults. Firstly, the question asks you to put yourself into the situation, so it makes for a significantly stronger answer if it is delivered in the 1st person. Secondly, the points made are very weak. In questions that involve dealing with some kind of difficult patient, it is paramount that you put yourself in the patient's shoes and try and understand their emotions. Omitting to do this shows a lack of communication skills. In addition, this answer only talks in vague terms and doesn't describe what the student would actually do/say.

A Good Response:

"The most important thing that must be achieved in this situation is to assess what is causing the patient to act in such a way. Is there something they are worried about? Something they are scared about? Or do they think that some kind of wrong has been done to them? Perhaps someone they care about, for example. To do this, it will be necessary to begin an effective dialogue with the patient. It is crucial that I give off a calm and confident persona both through speech and through body language. For similar reasons it is also key that the patient knows who I am, so I would be sure to introduce myself and explain why I had been called. For these reasons, I would begin by saying: "Hi, I'm Nicola, a junior doctor. I understand that there are a few things that you're not happy about. Could you tell me a little bit more about these so that I might be able to help?"

I would make sure that I did not stand in a way that would block the exits and would check that the patient did not have some kind of weapon before I went any closer. If he did have a weapon, I would contact hospital security not only to ensure my own safety, but also for the safety of staff and patients. Upon initiating a dialogue, I would constantly remind the patient that we were there primarily to help the patient and that he/she could leave at any time. After finding out the reason for the angry outburst, I would seek to solve this issue. I would keep in mind that the first concern that the patient raised might be something that was actually mundane which could be masking the real issue."

Response Analysis:

This is a very strong answer. It makes key points and covers all key bases including; identifying the cause of the anger, identifying the need to protect yourself, and ensuring that you identify yourself to the patient. A strong answer should include all of these. Furthermore, the answer uses the first person and illustrates the points with a demonstration of what would actually be said.

Overall:

In questions like this, it's essential to demonstrate that you can put yourself in a patient's shoes and can think on the spot about how to deal with any situation that requires your communication skills.

104)   What issues might arise when using a translator to mediate a patient consultation, and as a doctor, how might you overcome these issues?

This question asks about a part of medicine that is rarely discussed but is of increasing importance to clinical medicine in this country. 'Translators', in this case, could mean official in-hospital translators or could also include multilingual family members who are used for the purposes of translation. Make sure you define this in your answer.

A Bad Response:

"It is bad to use a translator in a consultation. For example, the translator might not be able to translate things fully and so information will be missed. Also, time might be wasted trying to find the translator in the first place and this is especially important for busy doctors. There is a chance that the translator might not know medical terminology and so could struggle to relay all the correct information between the patient and doctor."

Response Analysis:

This is a terrible response for several reasons. Firstly, there is very little structure to the answer. The opening is weak, there is then a list of points that are poorly illustrated, and there is no conclusion that brings the points together at the end. Finally, this student has made the grave error of not answering both parts of the question. This is a mistake that is often made in the pressure of an interview setting. If you are in an interview and hear an 'and' that is joining two questions together, make sure in your head that you set out to answer both parts. You might structure this as two separate answers or combine answers to both into a single argument.

A Good Response:

"In our increasingly multicultural society, the use of translators in medicine is increasingly prevalent and necessary. Many of the usual communication skills and techniques that are used by doctors are rendered useless when the patient does not speak the same language, and a strong patient-doctor relationship can be difficult to establish. Furthermore, in a profession in which strict confidentiality is essential, the use of unofficial translators may be open to abuse and any medical professional should do everything in their power to prevent such abuses.

There is a distinction between in-hospital official translators and when family members are used as translators, as is often the case in clinical medicine. A consultation that requires the use of a translator may not be ideal for either party, however, there are several things that the doctor might do to improve the situation. Firstly, before beginning the consultation, it is crucial that both the patient and translator understand the format of a translated consultation and are happy to proceed. This is especially true when a family member is used as a translator.

Secondly, it is key that all information is correctly conveyed across the language barrier. This can be achieved in several ways. For example, the doctor might use simple language and easily phrased questions. He/she should also only use short questions and wait for the translator to translate each portion. Finally, the doctor could regularly check and confirm throughout the consultation that the patient understands what is being said and indeed that the doctor has understood everything that the patient has said. Furthermore, there are several pitfalls that might occur during a consultation when using translators, and these pitfalls have the potential to be highly detrimental to the patient's welfare.

One potential issue is presented by the identity of the translator. If the translator is a family member or knows the patient personally, something which is quite likely if they come from the same community, then the patient might be embarrassed to present certain pieces of information that may be of critical importance to the consultation. In addition, the same could apply to the translator through their own embarrassment or ulterior motive. For example, if they are wanting to present their community in a positive light, they might not correctly translate information. If any of these possibilities are suspected, then the doctor should seek to repeat the consultation with a different translator.

In summary, there are multiple important issues that arise through the use of translators in medicine. However, translators are an absolute necessity in our multicultural society, and therefore, doctors should be well educated on the possible pitfalls that might arise and should know how these can be avoided."

Response Analysis:
This student's answer starts with a strong opening that describes the importance of the issue. It then goes on to define what exactly the term 'translator' includes in this context. There is a strong structure with each point being well signposted. As opposed to having two separate answers to the two parts of the question, this student has decided to combine the two answers into one narrative. Either is acceptable.

Overall:
Always ensure you answer both parts of a question.

105)   You are asked to gain consent from a patient for a procedure. What do you need to consider to ensure that consent is achieved?

This is a difficult question for a medical school interview. You would not necessarily be expected to know much on this topic but might be expected to think through the possibilities.

A Bad Response:

"Consent is very important in modern medicine; without consent, a procedure cannot go ahead. Consent is achieved when the doctor explains what the risks of a procedure are and has checked that the patient is happy to proceed. The issue of consent has many ethical implications. The Hippocratic Oath states that a doctor should do no harm and should act in the patient's best interests. Modern medicine relies on the fact that patients trust the medical profession to provide the very best service. If this trust is undermined, for example, by not following the Hippocratic Oath fully, then the medical profession cannot as effectively serve the population."

Response Analysis:

The key fault that this student makes in their answer is that they go off on a tangent about the ethical implications of consent. It is easy to fall into this trap as you may have a confident answer to something very much related to the question being asked, so it is tempting to talk about that even if it is not a direct answer. Always make sure that you structure a very relevant answer to the question that is being asked.

A Good Response:

"Consent is a fundamental prerequisite of any procedure in an ethical healthcare system. Before visiting the patient, it is essential that you yourself understand the procedure, why it is being performed on this particular patient, and what the possible risks of the procedure are.

I think that there are four key criteria that must be met to attain consent. Firstly, it is imperative to make sure that the patient fully understands what the procedure involves. For this reason, any explanation of the procedure given by the doctor should not involve medical jargon and should be at a level that the patient can comprehend.

Secondly, the patient must know about the risks involved. Even if a procedure is perfectly explained, this might imply that there aren't possible risks to the procedure and so the patient would not be able to give effective consent. Finally, it is crucial that the patient understands what will happen if they do not have the procedure. They may not wish to undertake a daunting procedure, but this might be by far the better of two options. Therefore, to be able to give true consent, it is necessary that the patient understands this.

However, before one can assess these different criteria, it is necessary to check that they can properly process information and that they can actually retain information. This could be done by asking the patient to repeat what you have said so far at various points during the consultation. Furthermore, we must give consideration to the patient's mental state, for instance, if they are not corpus mentis then consent cannot be obtained. This is because a patient who has a psychiatric condition may be able to appear to give consent but this cannot be accepted from an ethical standpoint."

Response Analysis:

The student gives an excellent answer to the question. There is a strong opening, followed by three clearly structured key points that are a direct answer to the question. The student then goes into further detail by explaining pitfalls that could arise if we just followed the basic formula of consent.

Overall:

A key learning point in this example is to always make sure that you directly answer the question. This is a question about what informed consent is – not an ethical dilemma!

106)   A patient is adamant that they will refuse your treatment and will instead use homeopathic medication. You believe that due to the seriousness of their condition, it is best that you persuade them to follow your treatment plan. How might you go about doing this?

This question is not asking for an ethical argument, instead, it is questioning communication skills and techniques that would be used in the situation to reach the desired outcome for the patient.

A Bad Response:
"I would make sure that I convinced the patient. To do this I would talk to them rationally and would set out in a logical manner why it was necessary for them to have my proposed treatment. I would also show that the benefits of the procedure would outweigh any possible risks."

Response Analysis:
This is a poorly answered question for several reasons. Firstly, most of the narrative is delivered in the first person (notice how there is lots of the use of 'I') and this creates a patronising outlook and shows that the candidate cannot put themselves in the patient's shoes. Furthermore, they have not considered what they would do in this scenario if the patient was still to refuse treatment. This is very important, as again, it shows that the candidate is not putting themselves in the patient's shoes and is not planning for different outcomes.

A Good Response:
"A key pillar of the Hippocratic Oath is patient autonomy. However, if the practitioner strongly believes that a treatment that the patient will not consent to will give the best outcome, then it is his/her duty to try and persuade the patient of their preferred plan.

If I were the doctor in question, before going to the patient, I would read up on the case including the exact treatment option being declined as well as any alternative options. On seeing the patient, after building a rapport, I would try and assess the reasons for why the patient was refusing to accept the suggested treatment. Blunt logical reasoning is unlikely to be constructive in this type of scenario. It is important to show to the patient that I accept and register their beliefs. Simultaneously, I would be trying to assess whether they had an emotional reason as to why they might turn away from modern medicine. This might be an underlying fear or anxiety, or possibly even a previous bad experience.

Next, I would explain to the patient in the simplest language possible why I thought that their homeopathic treatment would not be effective and why the treatment that my team are proposing is going to be effective. I would then proceed to address the possible risks/benefits of the treatment and crucially explain why I thought the benefits outweighed the risks.

Finally, I would address any specific fears or bad memories that I felt the patient might have. It would be key throughout the whole consultation to ensure that I let the patient speak whenever they wanted to raise a point and that I was never overbearing, but instead, always courteous and understanding. I would hope that by doing this I could persuade the patient to accept the treatment. However, if the patient still refused to accept the treatment I would respect their wishes. I would also offer to arrange a second opinion to discuss this further."

Response Analysis:
This is a strong answer for several reasons. There is a strong opening set out for why it is an important situation. There are then several good points that are laid out in a structured manner and are well signposted. In addition, this candidate considers a plan B in case the patient still refuses treatment. Finally, this candidate has gone into extra depth to consider what might be driving this particular patient's beliefs.

Overall:
When answering a question such as this, always try and imagine yourself in the scenario as this helps you to consider what you'd have to say and also what other factors you might have to think about, for example, what to do if the patient continued to refuse treatment as these could be explored in follow-up questions.

107)   *You are just about to finish your work for the day when the ward nurse asks you to talk to the angry sister of a patient who is admitted under a different team. You have a dinner date with your fiancée and drive to the restaurant. What would you do?*

This question is about dealing with an angry relative as well as a nurse who may be left to handle the relative if no one can pacify the relative. It also tests your commitment to medicine and patients, as well as your time/people management skills. Your response to stress will also be assessed. If you don't leave in time, you will be late. Do you get stressed in this situation?

A Bad Response:

"I would say to the nurse that I had finished for the day and as this was not my patient anyway that she should call someone else to speak with the relative."

Response Analysis:

The student comes across as someone who shirks from responsibility and has a lack of empathy. They fail to actually find out what the problem is from the nurse. This is important because simple issues could be quickly resolved, e.g. prescribe analgesia if the brother was in lots of pain. This would mean that the ward nurse wouldn't have to deal with the angry relative. Although it's important that you take your breaks as a doctor and leave on time, it's also important not to neglect your duties.

A Good Response:

"This patient is not on my team but is being managed by Dr Smith's team. What is the problem anyway? If it is something quick maybe I could talk to the relative, and if it requires more discussion I'd advise her to make an appointment to see Dr Smith who is the responsible consultant. I can also bleep someone in Dr Smith's team so that they can explain this to the sister. If this is clinically urgent, I am happy to stay behind but I'll need to make a quick call to my fiancée to explain that I'll be late."

Response Analysis:

Answering this way, you have demonstrated that you are a hard-working doctor that will work well in a team, does not get stressed with unexpected situations, empathise well, and are able to take that extra step for patients' welfare.

Overall:

You will come across this type of situation in your life as a doctor. In such scenarios, it is useful to ensure that your actions don't compromise patient safety (in life and death situations you can't walk away). If someone wants to know about the progress of the family member, you should be able to spend a few minutes if it is a quick discussion to diffuse the situation and offer to get someone else to have an in-depth discussion. It is irrelevant that the patient is from a different team as the on-call doctor may also not be from the same team.

PERSONAL ATTRIBUTES

108)   What are your top three skills?

This question is assessing your understanding of the skills required to be a doctor and your suitability based on those skills. In other words, think of all the different skills you need to be a good doctor and then pick the three skills which you can most easily demonstrate that you possess. Ensure that you provide evidence and state how these skills will help you to become a great doctor.

A Bad Response:

"I am a brilliantly talented pianist and performed my first solo concert at the age of 15. My teacher says she has never taught someone with as much natural musicianship as me before so I would have to say that is my number one skill. In achieving my dream of becoming a concert pianist, I have had to remain extremely motivated in order to fit in rehearsal time amongst my other commitments, I would, therefore, rank my time management as another one of my top skills. I also enjoy musical composition and have received high praise for my work so I would rank my creativity as my third most impressive skill."

Response Analysis:

Whilst this answer demonstrates some remarkable achievements, and even skills which would be very useful for a doctor, e.g. time management and creativity, it seems to miss the point of the question by solely discussing the candidate's passion for music. It does provide good evidence to back up the candidate's claims but it should explain why these skills are useful in medicine.

A Good Response:

"I would say my top three skills are my communication skills, my interpersonal skills, and my ability to work under pressure. I have demonstrated and developed excellent communication skills through the mentoring system in school in which I provide extra teaching sessions for struggling younger students. This work has helped me to develop my patience, my ability to explain things in a simple way, my ability to understand the concerns of others, and my ability to build a rapport quickly with students who are sometimes nervous and intimidated. These skills are directly transferable to the medical consultation in which doctors must be able to put patients at ease and explain scientific concepts in simple language.

I have always considered myself a people person and show a range of important interpersonal skills. I am a naturally caring person, I take interest in other people and find it easy to be empathetic. I interact confidently with people from lots of different backgrounds. I have further developed these skills during my time volunteering in a care home where I enjoyed talking to the residents and getting to know their stories and their struggles. I have become a better listener in particular from this experience. Again, these skills are vital for a doctor and will help me to treat patients holistically rather than just treating their disease. Finally, through my years on the debating team, I have improved my ability to work under pressure and am confident in making decisions quickly and effectively. This skill is of vital importance for doctors treating patients in an emergency and will help me to keep a cool head in stressful situations."

Response Analysis:

This is an excellent answer that shows a clear understanding of the skills required to be an effective doctor. It promotes the candidate's suitability for a place by providing convincing evidence that the candidate possesses these skills and that they can demonstrate the practical benefits of honing these skills.

Overall:

If you are lucky enough to be asked an open-ended question like this, make sure you take full advantage of it. These types of questions give you huge freedom to display your understanding of the qualities required by a doctor and give you an invaluable opportunity to sell yourself to the interviewer. Make sure you back up everything you say with evidence and continually demonstrate why your skill-set would make you an excellent doctor.

109) *Can you describe a time you showed leadership?*

Leadership is a key quality in a doctor. The important thing is to show that with this experience you had to demonstrate qualities such as initiative, decisiveness, organisational abilities and the ability to manage, guide and motivate others. These are skills that are often used in a medical setting.

It may be that you have not had any leadership roles, however, these experiences can be small. If you have ever taken the lead in organising a social event or group activity – a party, group trip, book club – then this can be used as an example. Describe the situation, how you came to be in a leading role, the steps you took to keep things running smoothly, and the result – for example, a successful event or crisis averted.

When answering this question, it is helpful to think of good qualities in a leader and weave them into your answer. Remember that managing a team doesn't necessarily make you a great leader. It's important to choose a story that demonstrates true leadership — stepping up to guide or motivate or take initiative, ideally in challenging circumstances. Do not be afraid to sell yourself!

Bad Response A:
➢ *"I do not often take on the leadership role. I prefer to work as a team member and work together to achieve a collective goal."*
➢ *"I'm never in charge so I never really get an opportunity to show leadership."*

Response Analysis:
Although it is essential that doctors act as team members, they also pay a dual role as team leaders due to the multidisciplinary nature of healthcare. Both answers don't give any example of leadership and are thus poor. It is clear that the candidates don't realise the importance of leadership in the role of a doctor.

Good Response A:
"I am a Charity Officer currently and had to organise the Charity Fair. I scheduled a meeting for the full team to discuss ideas but discovered that four people had dropped out. We had to divide the responsibilities between the remaining team members as a result, people were overworked and morale suffered. I baked for each weekly meeting to demonstrate my appreciation for all of their hard work during a challenging time. I also ensured that I asked them for ideas on how to be more efficient. I made it clear that no idea was stupid and that it was a safe environment for making suggestions. Performance improved and we all worked together to make the Charity Fair a huge success."

Good Response B:
"After having a string of lost games in my school rugby team, I noticed that morale in the team was getting low. To try and counteract this, I tried to lead by example and be as positive as possible and encourage my team-mates to come to training and make sure they knew exactly when and where it would be. I think this was important in stopping some of my team-mates from choosing to drop out of the team and was one of the reasons why we got a win soon after. I know it is only rugby, but I think being able to help organise and motivate a team could be relevant to medicine."

Response Analysis:
The answer shows many key qualities needed in a leader. By baking, the candidate shows that they understand the importance of motivating team members and showing appreciation for their work. The candidate also shows great listening and communication skills.

Overall:
A good answer will demonstrate knowledge of the qualities seen in a good leader such as communication skills, motivating others and inspiring trust. A better answer may relate the skills shown to what they have seen in clinical practice.

110)   *Do you think it's better to lead from the front or from the back?*

This question may be asked to test your ability to argue and defend a point and stimulate further discussion so that the interviewers can get a better understating of your personality. It is reasonable to pick either of the options, however, it would be wise to consider both in your answer. Where possible, try to include examples of leadership you've seen or experienced (not necessarily in a healthcare setting) and analyse the good and bad points about them and how that influences your decision.

You may wish to take a more neutral stance and suggest that leadership is dependent on the goal and team so needs to be tailored to them rather than a particular style. This idea also lends itself to the notion that leadership is a more fluid concept than simply 'from the front' or 'from the back'.

A Bad Response:
"I think leadership is almost always better from the front – setting a good example and explaining what is expected but being able to look back to support members of the team that need it. When doing work experience, this is that style of leadership I saw from one of the consultants who all the juniors liked and respected. They said he was nice to work for as they all know what he expected of them but he was approachable to ask for help if needed."

Response Analysis:
This response isn't terrible; it's just narrow-minded and would almost certainly be challenged by the interviewers with a counter example. Discussing personal experiences would be helpful here too, particularly as during your training and early career you will witness many different leadership styles but it is developing your own that is important.

A Good Response:
"I would argue that leadership is specific to the situation and team it is applied to and, therefore, a good leader will adapt their style accordingly. I saw a good example of this when doing work experience on a respiratory medicine firm at my local hospital. The consultant very much led 'from the front' during the ward round and all the juniors I spoke to said that this was helpful as they knew exactly what they needed to do for all the patients that day. However, at a different time, I saw the consultant lead rather more 'from the back' when he was encouraging his juniors to take the lead in consultations during a clinic session.

In situations where I have led, I have also experienced that the style of leadership needs to be adapted to the team I'm leading. For example, through a programme my school runs where students teach sport to local primary school students, I try to lead from the back when it is a session I have planned. This suits the group of peers I'm working with and also shows us as a united team to the children we teach. However, at my part-time job as a waitress, I very much lead from the front when I am the floor manager as this sets a good example to any junior staff but I am always happy for them to ask me questions!"

Response Analysis:
This response includes both clinical and personal experiences of leadership and demonstrates a good depth of thought into the subject. The neutral stance allows you to put more arguments forward for both styles and shows you're not blinkered by one experience but open to new ideas. When discussing the leadership style of others, it's good to ask the members of the team what the style is like and whether it works for them, as in this response where you say you spoke to the junior doctors. Of course, your own observations are valid and good to talk about too.

Overall:
Leadership is a big part of medicine and this question is a great opportunity for you to demonstrate that you are aware of leadership styles and are already developing your own. Personal examples of either experiences being led or leading are great to include – perhaps a great opportunity to work your personal statement into the conversation that hasn't come up yet.

111) *Would you describe yourself as a leader or a follower? / Is it better for doctors to be a leader or a follower?*

This question really gets at the idea that a healthy balance between these two personality traits is highly desirable in a good doctor. Leadership skills are absolutely essential in being able to coordinate a potentially large team of highly educated and skilled individuals in the most efficient and effective way possible. However, being a "follower" in the sense of being part of a team led by another member of staff is an intrinsic part of being a doctor. Throughout your training right up to consultancy (and commonly even during this period), being part of a team and following instructions is pivotal to ensuring the best possible healthcare for your patients.

This is the kind of question that promotes an immediate knee-jerk response ('leader!') from many candidates, but is actually asking for a deeper analysis of the roles within the interdisciplinary team that doctors work in. A balanced answer is the best approach to this loaded question!

A Bad Response:
"I am a leader because doctors lead their team. I have a very strong personality that has been cultivated from my experiences in leading my group during the Gold Duke of Edinburgh award as well as captaining my school rugby team. I enjoy executing my vision of how a task should be completed and am proud of my ruthless attitude in ensuring that my team complete the job in hand the way I want. I rarely get questioned or challenged, and therefore, I believe that I make an excellent leader, and would be a very decisive doctor."

Response Analysis:
Though it is good that the candidate cites occasions where he has led a team, his explanation of his role is very worrying. He puts far too much emphasis on his personal vision and strongly implies that he doesn't consider the views of his team, but just forces them into executing his plan. Doctors should confer with their team to come to a consensus for a treatment plan given that often "more heads are better than one" and also will build better team morale by considering their views.

This view leaves little scope for the doctor to be humble and learn from others. No one can know everything, so the team members rely on each other to make sure the patient receives the best care possible. For example, nurses tend to know more about how the patient is doing on a day-to-day basis, and are often confided in by the patient when they don't want to interrupt the doctor or 'waste their time'.

A Good Response:
"I would say that I have a healthy mixture of these two traits. When leading my team on Duke of Edinburgh, I effectively sought a consensus of opinion on our group's next move when stuck in a particularly difficult situation. Having every member of the team contributing to the plan led to a collaborative attitude within the team and helped me to fine tune our approach leading to a team-based decision. This was invariably very appropriate. Likewise, I am a good member of my local care home's staff and ensure that I best apply the plan implemented by the management for the care of patients whilst also offering feedback from my experiences as to where things could be improved.

The doctor should be both a leader and a follower depending on the situation. The job involves taking on responsibility and learning to organise and lead a team. However, the doctor is also a follower – always looking to learn from others and better themselves. Having the integrity to recognise and actively work on your failings is very important, so whilst the doctor should try their best and be confident in their abilities, they should also have the humility to learn from their juniors as well as their seniors.

Overall, I would argue that the doctors should be able to make a seamless transition between a leader and a follower to provide the best care for their patients."

Response Analysis:
This response uses Duke of Edinburgh as a parallel for the everyday ward decisions that need to be made by teams of doctors. It shows that the candidate has cultivated crucial team-working skills as both a leader and a follower and accurately assesses the doctor's role in the multidisciplinary team, recognising the importance of learning from everyone around you regardless of hierarchy. It also acknowledges that the doctor should gain confidence in their abilities and take on responsibilities. This dual nature is essential for doctors, so being able to recognise it before beginning medical school shows a valuable insight into the true nature of the profession.

The final part of the response throws a bit of a curve-ball to the interviewer – medicine should always be patient-focused, but whilst discussing hierarchy and roles in the multidisciplinary team, the patient is often forgotten. By invoking the patient, the candidate shows they can think outside of the medical team and focus on what is really important.

Overall:
This question attempts to elucidate a reflex response based on the old paternalistic view of doctors as leaders. A thoughtful and balanced answer to the question can show a very realistic understanding of how a medical team works and the role of a doctor, which are essential qualities in a medical student. Thinking of the patient in this context demonstrates a high level of empathy and patient-focused care.

It is essential that you identify an experience that you've had which demonstrates you as having a balanced approach to leadership. Leadership is an essential quality in doctors, however, the interview answer must not accidentally sway too far the other way and suggest the candidate is arrogant and doesn't consider the opinions of the rest of his team. Likewise, you should appreciate that for large chunks of your career, you will be junior to a doctor or manager, and therefore, should have a healthy attitude to 'following' too.

112)   Tell me something you have done that you are proud of.

This is a simple question with many potential pitfalls. Many will use this opportunity to list all their achievements, often without adding any further depth to their responses and failing to use this opportunity to highlight the qualities they have that would make good future doctors. This question aims to test a candidate's ability to self-analyse. Do not be afraid of picking an achievement that you're worried may seem boastful. Remember, the main point of the question is not to focus on things that you have done but rather the skills you learnt from them.

A Bad Response:

"I am most proud of the academic results I have achieved so far. I was able to get the highest grades in my school for both GSCE and AS levels, which is something I am very happy about. I was also recognised in the local newspaper which was a very rewarding experience. I was delighted to make my family proud, but even more so, I was pleased that my hard work and determination paid off."

Response Analysis:

This answer, unfortunately, lacks any real depth. The candidate failed to explore the skills that they gained from the experience but rather focused on the superficial details. The candidate also needed to highlight more qualities applicable to life as a doctor, and perhaps should have chosen a broader response to develop a more comprehensive answer.

A Good Response:

"One of the most memorable moments that I am proud of was winning the Governor's Award for Excellence at my school. It was an honour, but I like to think of it as a culmination of all the different areas of school life that I contributed to and all the different skills I gained. I was involved in the school's peer mentoring initiative in which we helped pupils in lower year groups struggling in science and maths. It was a great experience and really showed me how effective communication is essential to reaching common goals.

I was also a part of the school's successful athletics and football teams which was great fun and helped to develop my sense of teamwork and accountability in a competitive environment- attributes that I firmly believe apply to the world of medicine. The award was given in recognition of my academic results, which were a product of consistent hard work, a quality that is core to being a successful doctor. All in all, I believe winning the award was a fantastic experience and gave me a lot of confidence moving forward."

Response Analysis:

This answer is a good example of being able to take an achievement and break it down into its component skills and qualities. Not only does the candidate highlight their ability to self-analyse, but they are also able to relate their skills back to being a good doctor.

Overall:

Think of something you have done which incorporates a lot of different qualities, then break them down to discuss individually. It is important that you expand on each individual thing and relate them back to being a doctor.

113) *What is your biggest weakness?*

This question often catches candidates out. A careful balance needs to be struck between not coming across as arrogant and demonstrating a dangerous lack of insight (nobody is perfect!). It is also important not to identify a weakness that may make the examiners worry about who they are admitting to read medicine. The answer needs to identify a weakness and then demonstrate how you are attempting to rectify this.

Avoid the urge to give an answer that is not really a weakness, e.g. "I'm a perfectionist", as a more profound degree of self-criticism will be appreciated more. Instead, by simply changing the phrasing and customising it to yourself, you can say something very similar, e.g. *"my time management can be a weakness, often because I spend too much time concentrating on minor details in my work"*. You would need to develop this by showing what you've learnt from reflecting on your weakness, e.g. *"...so when I am working on a project, I set myself strict targets to meet and try to get the bulk of the task done before worrying about the finer details in the early stages."*.

Showing humility when answering a question such as this is a good way to make you appeal to the interviewer as a person. Some candidates may be tempted to answer this with a joke, however, this is not advisable as it is a very important question for medics.

A Bad Response:
"My biggest weakness is that I'm sometimes quite arrogant. I've always been very successful at most of the things I try and do and so have an awful lot of self-belief. I rarely feel the need to ask for help as I know that I will likely be OK without it. When I fail at something, I get very angry with myself and will often feel down for several days afterwards."

Response Analysis:
This is a dangerous response. Many medical applicants will indeed be very good at lots of things; however, saying that this has made them arrogant is not good. The candidate states that they rarely seek help for things and have an innate belief that they will be good at anything they turn their hand to. It is not possible to be good at everything from the offset, and knowing when to ask for more senior help is an absolutely critical part of being a doctor. In medicine, it's not just that your ego will be bruised if you fail, but a patient's health may be severely affected.

A Good Response:
"I consider myself a natural leader and so my instinct in many situations is quite often to lead the team and exert my authority in coordinating others. However, I appreciate that quite often during my medical career I will not be the most appropriate individual to lead a team. Therefore, I'm working really hard on my skills in working effectively within a team and not necessarily as the leader. In order to improve on this, I've recently started working at my local carpentry shop with little experience, and am therefore very reliant on senior advice."

Response Analysis:
This candidate identifies a valid weakness that, if too extreme, would be a problem in medical practice. However, crucially the candidate has demonstrated insight into this problem and how this could be an issue as a future doctor. Impressively, they've even shown that they are being pro-active in trying to address this weakness (working as part of a carpentry team).

Overall:
Medical practice is quite rightly very keen on quality control and ensuring best practice. Therefore, it is essential that those that practise medicine have sufficient insight to identify where they are struggling and when to ask for help. Be this a surgeon whose struggling with a new procedure or a doctor who fails to take into account the opinions of his team sufficiently. A good doctor will identify their flaws and adjust these so as to prevent the quality of patient care being affected.

114)   How do you deal with stress?

This question is a particularly important one as studying and practising medicine can be very stressful and that might not be the right thing for everybody. Having good mechanisms to cope with stress is essential to function well as a doctor in the long run. This includes two types of stress, the underlying stress when there is a lot to do in little time, and the acute stress of being in an unexpected or particularly challenging situation.

A Bad Response:
"I do not get stressed, so I do not see the need to cope with stress."

Response Analysis:
Any answer that goes in this direction is inadequate. The study of medicine as well as the practice of medicine are both very stressful and will be challenging. For this reason, it is essential to have appropriate mechanisms to deal with stress. Even if you have not felt stressed up to this point, it is very likely that medicine will put you in a situation that you have never experienced before which will be very stressful. You need to be able to demonstrate that you have thought about ways on how to cope with situations like that.

A Good Response:
"Medicine can be very stressful. My work experiencing with the St John's Ambulance service has repeatedly put me in situations where I had to make fast decisions. This has allowed me to develop techniques to keep a clear head in heated situations. I have found that focusing on the task at hand and breaking my duties down in small, logical steps helps a great deal to make a situation more controllable and manageable. I also have a good network of friends that I can rely on and I like to play the Piano which I find very relaxing."

Response Analysis:
This response is a good one as it provides clear examples of situations experienced as well as techniques used. This answer addresses the acute type of stress, but a similar principle can be applied to the general underlying type of stress of being very busy. Providing exact examples of coping mechanisms is important as anything else will remain superficial.

Overall:
Whatever your individual coping mechanisms for stress may be, provide examples of where you have applied them. It will make them look a lot more valid as they are tried and tested and not just made up. Sources for coping mechanism can vary. Competitive sports can be one, playing an instrument can be another. They can also include outlets such as sports. Remember, though, this mainly applies to the underlying stress of being very busy.

115)   What is your biggest strength?

To answer this question well requires a good sense of self-awareness. First and foremost, your answer should be honest. Your biggest strength does not necessarily have to relate to medicine, although it would be advisable to relate your strength back to how it would enable you to be a better doctor. For example, your biggest strength could be creativity, which is very useful in terms of problem-solving and developing and adapting methods of communication to specific patients with special needs, to give but a few examples.

A Bad Response:

"My biggest strength is my ability to think quickly on my feet. I think this is a very important skill for a doctor to have. Doctors think on their feet every day using both their clinical and scientific knowledge and can also be required to rapidly assess the ethics of a situation as well as using past experiences to inform judgement. If an emergency situation arises, there is no time to panic, you simply need to be able to act in the most appropriate manner and think clearly and logically."

Response Analysis:

This response sounds fake. The candidate gives no evidence to support what he is saying. The candidate needs to demonstrate to the interviewer either how he has developed these skills or an example of how he has used these skills. The question is asking for details about the candidate's strength and not about the way in which this strength is useful in a medical career, and hence this answer is lacking much detail. However, this response does show good insight into the role of the doctor which adds value to the answer.

A Good Response:

"I think my biggest strength is probably my leadership ability. I have a lot of experience in leading a range of ages and groups in different situations. I really enjoy getting to know the strengths of the members of a team, define and set aims and objectives for a team, and lead a team efficiently to secure the best possible outcome. With my theatre group, I directed a cast of 20 young people in a performance of an adapted, classic fairy-tale. In year 11, as well as being my form representative, I also led my school's Learning to Lead Energy Team, where I worked with staff, energy companies, contractors, and the school community to reduce the carbon footprint of our school. I know how to communicate effectively with a team, organise a team, and take on a role of responsibility to deliver to a high standard. I also appreciate the value of reviewing and constructively criticising my performance as a leader in a given situation to enable me to develop and improve my leadership skills."

Response Analysis:

This response is focused on a single strength and goes into specific detail to provide evidence that the candidate possesses this skill. Two examples are given to demonstrate the leadership experience of the candidate. The candidate shows knowledge and understanding of what good leadership is and promotes a good reflective attitude towards the way in which he/she works. The candidate also demonstrates a good understanding of his or her own personal development.

Overall:

It shows insight and maturity to have thought about ways in which you can bring your strengths to good use in your potential future career as a doctor, do take some time to do this.

116)   In what way will you contribute to University life if you become a student here?

The interviewer wants to see that you have considered your future life at university and that you are a balanced individual with a variety of interests that predisposes you to be a well-rounded individual. Your answer should be enthusiastic and passionate. You could talk about any societies you want to join that could introduce you to something you have never tried before, or any skills you already have that you want to bring to university life. If you have any ambitions of taking up specific roles of responsibility at university, it would be worth mentioning them in your answer, as well as if you have any ideas of things you would like to discover and explore or start up at the university.

A Bad Response:
"When I get to university, I will work exceptionally hard at my studies. I will aim to achieve top scores in my examinations and represent the medical school as one of its highest achieving medical students. I think I will consider joining some sort of arty society at University if that fits in with my timetable. Or maybe I would consider doing a sport."

Response Analysis:
This answer does not give the impression that the candidate will gain much on a personal or developmental level from University life; it does not show a willingness to get involved with University life. The candidate is very focused on his/her medical studies to an unhealthy extent and also demonstrates arrogance in their answer. The candidate shows very little interest in extracurricular pursuits and appears to have a limited awareness of the unique opportunities university life brings with it. The candidate appears unprepared to start university life and it does not seem as though he/she will make the most of a place at University.

A Good Response:
"I would love to volunteer within the community with the University. Living in a city will be a very interesting experience for me as I have lived in rural areas all my life. I would be interested in getting involved in supporting homeless people or those with disabilities in the city. I am very keen to stand up as an ambassador for the University by supporting the neighbouring communities. I would love to take part in a team sport such as hockey as I feel this would put me at the centre of student life and would be a very healthy break from my studies. I have not had the opportunity to play a team sport before and I feel I would gain some really useful skills from the experience. I am eager to make the most of the clubs and societies and unique student events held at the University, and aim to become as involved as I can with University life."

Response Analysis:
The response is very personal, which makes it stand out to the interviewer as well as marking it as an honest and respectable answer. The answer is not overly ambitious and realises that limitations may be placed on the candidate over the academic year. Nevertheless, the candidate demonstrates motivation to try new things and a willingness to help others and get involved in University life. It shows that he/she can see past the academic requirements of medical school.

Overall:
Aim to show the interviewer that you are passionate, have a lot to offer the University, and that you are excited about the University as a whole, rather than simply just the medical school. Being pro-active is a good trait which shows that you are an independent and capable individual.

117) Name some of the difficulties involved in leading a team, how did you make a difference?

In whatever job you do in the future, it is very likely that you will be working as part of a team. This question is looking for examples in the past when you have worked as a team, but more importantly, the challenges that the team experienced and what you did about those challenges. It is perfectly fine that you had problems working with a team in the past, but the interviewer really wants to see your response to these challenges. This does not have to be related to a medical team (although this can only help the answer) but should show skills desirable in a doctor.

Being a good doctor means more than simply being a good clinician. In their day-to-day role, not only are doctors expected to provide clinical care, but they are also expected to provide leadership. The interviewer knows that you are capable of leading, but wants you to prove it to them. The way to answer this question is to provide them with a strong example of when you led a team successfully.

A Bad Response:
"I do not often lead teams so this question is a little difficult for me. I think I tend to follow the team leader more often, but if no progress is made then I do step up. For example, we were involved in a group presentation and the 'leader' wasn't really leading, so I had a discussion with the other members and it was decided that I should become the leader for this presentation. I was quite uncomfortable with the whole situation but I didn't really have a choice. We managed to get the presentation together after I became the team leader. In this way, I think I did do a good job of leading the team."

Response Analysis:
This answer lacks confidence and assertiveness. These are skills that good leaders should demonstrate when leading their teams. The candidate perhaps did not use the best example of leading from the front as they had not volunteered to be the leader but were coerced into the position. The answer could have been improved by expanding further on how the candidate thinks they did as a leader; did they motivate their peers after morale was low, did they assigns tasks to people?

A Good Response:
"I have developed my teamwork skills over my years at school but this has not been without challenges. I really love tic-tac-toe so I quickly joined my school club in Year 9; however, I was disappointed that the club was not running enough events so I met with the president to discuss my concerns and she offered me a position on the executive committee. When working on the committee to organise an interschool tic-tac-toe competition, I had trouble dealing with the treasurer who was not responding to my emails. I arranged a meeting with him and found out that he was having family problems. I offered to help him with his current situation and further suggested that he talk to our college counsellor. I had to delay some of the payments for the event but it all got sorted after one week. I found that by talking to unresponsive members of the team, the real issue could be understood and this helped to build team unity."

Response Analysis:
This response is significantly better than the first, although, note the similarities in much of the content. The first main difference is the person concentrates on what they did within a team rather than talking about how they led a team. The person also brings in a specific challenge that they faced in this team as well as a suitable way of dealing with the challenge (they also showed empathy in this response).

Overall:
This question may throw a few people because it involves talking about a weakness or challenge, but do not be fooled. You should show your strengths by showing how you dealt with a particular challenge. This will be a common theme in questions that ask about challenges that you faced in the past. The main part of this question lies with how you worked within a team to create a positive impact; any challenges that you faced and how you dealt with them also increase the maturity of the response.

118)   Who do you think is the most important part of your team when you become a doctor?

Teamwork is an important part of medicine, but this question also requires you to understand your own role in the team and the specialist services that members of the team can offer. You can approach this question in several different ways – for example, from the point of view of different situations or from the point of view of your grade through your career. When structuring your response, you may wish to start by exploring exactly what the 'team' at the time or situation you're discussing would consist of, and then, having demonstrated you really understand how much of a multidisciplinary approach medicine is, you can comment on who you think would be the best important part.

A Bad Response:
"I think the nurses would form the most important part of the team for me. They are the people who know their patients best and spend more time with them during the day than the doctors have the time for. During my work experience, I found the nursing staff were very helpful to me and to the junior doctors."

Response Analysis:
This response falls into the trap of speaking before the candidate fully structured their response. This question is so broad that you need to start by narrowing down the situation you are referring to, for example, a situation you witnessed during work experience is a good place to start. When preparing your answer to questions, also try to think about what holes the interviewers could pick in your argument. Here, they could ask you what would happen if there were no doctors, or why have so many doctors if nurses are the most important team members.

A Good Response:
"This is a really tough question because medicine so often relies on the skills of a multidisciplinary team in order to work well. Therefore, everyone is, in a way, as important as each other. For example, during my work experience, I spent some time in theatre where the operation could not happen without the correct patient, a skilled surgeon and assistant, a team of scrub nurses, an anaesthetist, and so on. Missing any one of those people or skills would have meant the procedure would have to have been cancelled.

In some situations, one could argue that the patient is the most important member of the team as the majority of factors affecting their health will be experienced outside the hospital, so they are the one with the most power to make decisions and changes. However, in the case of neonates, not all patients can be educated by doctors in order to make decisions about their health. Overall, I would say there is no 'most important' member of the team provided all the necessary members are there and each situation is highly dependent on the specific patient and their health."

Response Analysis:
This response justifies your opinion well using an example to illustrate a situation common in medicine. Suggesting the patient is the most important person is unlikely to be a novel or exciting response for the interviewers, however, if you reason why you think so and highlight cases where this may not be the case, you have demonstrated a well-thought-through approach to the question. In this kind of question where there are multiple points and situations to consider, summarising your thoughts at the end of your response will demonstrate conviction and will be impressive.

Overall:
This question is definitely worth thinking about and structuring your ideas in advance of attending interviews. You can really impress with a well-thought-through reply that stands out from the 'nurses' and 'patients' the interviewers will have heard a lot of. Any experience you have of teamwork can work well as an example to include in this question or your experience when shadowing doctors. It is also worth considering that this question asks about the future when you will be a doctor so you could consider what you might expect to change about medicine in this time and how that will impact on the important members of the team.

119)   *What have you read recently?*

This is a very broad question and it gives you the scope to tell the interviewers something about yourself. Make very good use of a question like this as you can bring in something that will impress the interviewers-there will not be many questions that allow you to say whatever you want, but this is one of them.

Bad Response A:
"The last book I read was War and Peace by Leon Trotsky; it was a fantastic tale of the Napoleonic wars and really highlighted to me the importance of medicine. To further my medical knowledge, I read the Journal of Thoracic Surgery and the Journal of Underwater Physiology. I really liked the latest article where they talked about... oh I've forgotten what they talked about but it was very good. Finally, I read about the Junior Doctor Strikes in the Daily Mail this morning."

Bad Response B:
"I recently read about a new 15-minute test for cognitive decline, which requires only a list of instructions and a piece of paper and a pen. It said it might increase the rate of diagnosis for Alzheimer's disease and other forms of dementia which would be good."

Response Analysis:
Firstly, War and Peace is written by Leo Tolstoy and not Leon Trotsky. Secondly, the student forgets the name of the article that they read in one of their research journals. Both of these errors suggest that the student has not actually read these and is simply lying their way through the interview. If you are going to pretend that you have read a book/journal, make sure you know some of the key ideas and can talk about them confidently. Secondly, the student is quite vague in both answers. In the first response, the student vaguely mentions that War and Peace somehow relate to medicine and then completely skips over the issue of Junior Doctor Strikes – a great opportunity to show your understanding of the new junior doctor contract. This suggests a lack of interest or unfamiliarity. Answers should always try to provide specific examples and justification. Finally, avoid mentioning tabloid newspapers!

Good Response A:
"The last fiction book I read was War and Peace by Leo Tolstoy, it was very interesting to see the difference in how the doctors treated their patients in that era compared to modern times. In terms of medical reading, I am an avid reader of the Student BMJ; I remember a recent article on carpal tunnel syndrome which was particularly fascinating to me because I met a patient with this disease during my work experience. Finally, I keep up to date with current issues by reading the Telegraph. Today's front page was on the recent strike by Junior Doctors so it was especially relevant to my interests."

Good Response B:
"After my volunteer work with patients with dementia, I was very interested in reading about a new 15-minute test for cognitive decline, which requires only a list of instructions and a piece of paper and a pen. This test is intended to direct people at risk of Alzheimer's disease and other forms of dementia towards primary care. While widespread use of this may be very effective at increasing the rate of diagnosis of these conditions, it did occur to me that its application could be potentially harmful. There is a stigma and fear associated with these conditions that would make false positives particularly harmful. Also, an early diagnosis for a very slow cognitive decline may simply prolong the time for people to worry about their condition without having any treatment options."

Response Analysis:

In response A, the subject is very similar to the previous one but there are some key differences. Firstly, notice that the student provides a useful detail about War and Peace. It is perfectly acceptable to mention non-medical books in this answer. In both responses, the student mentions an article and some form of medical reading; note that although a major journal isn't cited, it is the fact that the student has taken an interest which is important. Finally, the student mentions a reputed newspaper and provides some detail on a relevant article.

Overall:

This question is very useful from the student's perspective. It allows them to shape the flow of the interview and lead the interviewer in a certain direction, e.g. by mentioning the Junior Doctor strikes, the interviewer may pick up on this and ask for your opinion- if you anticipated this and had already prepared a response (but of course make it seem spontaneous), the interviewers will be very impressed. This question will also give the interviewer a good idea of your cultural knowledge- are you one of those people who just read A-Level Biology textbooks, or do you read widely for interest?

It is important to research some contemporary news stories about medicine. The Health section of the BBC News website is a good place to start. The New Scientist's online articles and TED talks are good ways to be quickly briefed on cutting-edge research. Reading beyond the original article to further investigate the topic and offering some small level of criticism/appraisal are good ways to demonstrate your scientific interest. Relating your reading back to your work experience can show how you are interested in the application of what you have read.

You may get asked about an article or controversial health bill in the news and your views on it. It would look good if you can give both sides of the argument on the article and come up with your own views. Remember, you may not know the views of your interviewer so there is a risk that your opinion might be opposite to theirs. Be perceptive, and if challenged on your view, explain it with a good argument (your background reading should have prepared you for that). Some universities like Cambridge will inform you in advance about who your interviewers will be. A search on interviewers can help you in knowing their views.

120)   What extracurricular activities do you do?

This is a very nice question that comes up a lot. Some interviewers may just use this as an icebreaker. However, your response allows you to shape the course of the interview so you should use it to your full advantage.

A Bad Response:

"I absolutely love medicine and everything medicine related. I currently volunteer as the tea maker at my local hospital and this always gives me undulated ecstasy. I have perfected the tea-making technique so this task has become even more enjoyable. I have also recently become interested in astrophysics so I bought a telescope last week and have been looking for stars in the sky ever since. Finally, I play video games in my spare time; my favourite game is World of Warcraft."

Response Analysis:

Please note that volunteering in a hospital is not really an extracurricular activity and they are really asking what you do for fun. Do not worry if your extracurricular activities are not medicine related- they don't have to be. The second interest of astrophysics may be genuine but it has only lasted one week- try to have extracurricular activities that you have been doing for an extended period of time so that you can show commitment. Finally, there is nothing wrong with playing video games but this does not add anything to your answer. Each extracurricular activity you bring up must add a desirable quality to you as a candidate.

A Good Response:

"Outside of medicine, I am very interested in astrology. I have been visiting my local fortune teller since the age of 14. Over the last four years, I have really got to learn about the history behind this field. Although I myself do not really believe in this field, it is fascinating to look at other people's perspectives. I also really enjoy playing video games, specifically World of Warcraft. This game has been a real passion of mine so I have formed a World of Warcraft society at school. We are particularly interested in the graphics behind the video game, so each week, we analyse a portion of the computer code from the game and try to learn as much as possible from it. I think this has really led me to develop my programming skills which helped me create my own heart monitor application. This application allows users to track their heart rate over 30 minutes."

Response Analysis:

 This response is significantly better as each extracurricular activity adds something to the candidate's skill set. Although astrology might seem like a ludicrous extracurricular activity, many patients you see in hospital will rely partially on alternative forms of medicine. The candidate states that it is interesting to see other people's perspectives so this will be particularly useful for these patients. Just like the bad response, the candidate has an interest in video games, however, this time, they have formed a society. This shows both initiative and teamwork skills. Secondly, they learn programming in this society which can only be an advantage in an ever more digital world. Finally, they link these skills to a medical application which ties off the answer very nicely.

Overall:

The question might seem very innocent at first, however, it is very easy to mess it up. You must ensure that each of your extracurricular activities adds a positive characteristic to your profile. They do not have to be medically related but the skills that you gain from them should be applicable to medicine.

121)   What do you enjoy most about your hobby?

This question is an opportunity to demonstrate that you are interested in more than just academic studies. Doctors tend to be well-rounded people and often have other pursuits outside of medicine. When answering this question, focus less on what you have achieved through your hobby and more on how you have developed and how that can relate to a career in medicine.

A Bad Response:

"I play the piano and the saxophone to a high standard and have achieved grade 8 on both instruments. The thing I enjoy most is playing in the school band where we get to try out lots of different music genres and also perform on a regular basis. I have played in the band for many years and am now the 1st saxophone."

Response Analysis:

This response does answer the question, but it also wastes the opportunity to show off achievements, skills, and knowledge. The answer is too superficial and should instead delve into what has been gained from playing in the school band, and whether or not this could be useful for the future. Also, only one element of playing musical instruments is discussed, which is a shame as the others could have demonstrated other qualities.

A Good Response:

"My main hobby is music; I have played the piano and the saxophone for many years and have achieved grade 8 on both instruments. This has taken years of dedication, practice, and commitment. This hard work has taught me to persevere and see something through to the end, because eventually, I would master the piece I was struggling with and would then really enjoy playing it. The sense of achievement and accomplishment is great. Music is something that can be appreciated by many, so I'm incredibly lucky to have been given the opportunity to perform many times which has brought my friends and family together and really heightened my confidence. I also joined the school band, which truly developed my sense of teamwork. However, I play 1st saxophone, so I also have to lead the other saxophonists whilst listening attentively to ensure we all stayed in time and tune together. I think all of these skills I've been lucky enough to gain from something I enjoy so much will really help me to become a good doctor."

Response Analysis:

This response picks one hobby – music, and breaks it down into its different elements which allows for a much more complex answer. This can be done whatever your hobby – e.g. if you are interested in sports you can talk about training, matches, coaching other people etc. For each element, think of something you have learnt from it that you think might be an important quality in a doctor. Although this may sound like a simple question on the surface, it can be explored much deeper to demonstrate that you understand what it takes to make a good doctor. It clearly highlights some of the transferable skills that can be developed in music. The answer doesn't seem to be forced.

Overall:

Pick a broad hobby such as music, sports, or performing arts, and break it down into its individual components. You can draw on what you have gained and learnt while taking part in your hobby and how this can apply to medicine. It is important that you actually answer the question and demonstrate how much you enjoy your hobby!

122) Do you think you will have time to continue your hobby when you start medical school?

Medical school is an extremely demanding and challenging environment with a large workload and plentiful contact hours. This means that time management is imperative for success in the course. However, it does not mean that your life should involve solely your studies and nothing else- this is not a healthy balance to have. Although many students may think that medical schools are focused on the academic side, in reality, this is not true. Universities recognise the need for students to have balanced lifestyles because hobbies are a good stress relief and enable them to develop skills such as teamwork and perseverance which will be beneficial to their future careers. Continuing a hobby also demonstrates good time management skills, which is an important skill in many parts of life.

A Bad Response:

"Although I currently have a few hobbies, I understand that the workload at medical school will be highly demanding, therefore, I might not be able to continue them. I would like to bring my guitar in case I get some free time when I am not working, and maybe play some sports. However, I know that the contact hours will be long so I may not have much free time outside of studying. At the end of the day, I know that the purpose of medical school is to study and if I get time outside of that to continue a hobby that will be great, but if not, it won't be the end of the world!"

Response Analysis:

This response suggests that the student would be happy to just focus on their studies and have no life outside of that. This shows that the student may not have good time management skills. It is also worrying that the student is happy to give up all hobbies, potentially leaving them with no methods of managing stress which can be high at some points during the challenging degree. Therefore, the student may find it hard to cope with the stresses of the degree if they do not do anything outside of their studies.

A Good Response:

"I fully understand and am expecting medical school to be academically highly demanding and challenging, with more contact hours than almost any other course, as well as lots of work needing to be done outside of this. Therefore, I am likely to have less free time available to me than there is during my A-level studies at the moment, during which I take part in many extra-curricular activities including sport, playing the guitar, and being part of the charities committee, all of which have helped me to develop valuable skills such as teamwork which will be beneficial to my future studies and career. Doing lots of extracurricular activities has also helped me to improve my time management skills, which is directly transferable to medical school. Therefore, although perhaps I will not be able to continue all of the hobbies I currently have, I certainly will not stop them all to spend my time solely focused on my studies. Using my good time management skills, I would definitely like to keep up playing sport, probably football but I am also keen to try something new. I strongly believe that to succeed in my future studies and career, hobbies play an important part in maintaining a healthy and balanced lifestyle that will lead to success."

Response Analysis:

The candidate comes across as passionate about their hobbies and will likely use them in a positive way to benefit rather than hinder their studies. The interviewers will be keen to meet well-rounded individuals who are able to manage their time well and develop important life skills which will be necessary during their future career in medicine. It is good that the student has recognised that medical school is not only about the studies, but learning life skills and becoming well-rounded as an individual.

Overall:

Although academia is obviously an extremely important part of the medical degree, it is important to have hobbies outside of your studies. Not only does this demonstrate good time management skills, but also hobbies are often a crucial method for managing the stress of such a challenging course. The universities will want to ensure that you will be able to deal with this stress, and will also be keen for students to get involved with other aspects of university life, thus make a positive impact on the university community.

123) *How will your experience of D of E benefit your future studies?*

The Duke of Edinburgh award is a highly rewarding scheme to get involved with and will look very good on your medical applications. However, it will not necessarily make you stand out from the crowd as a lot of other applicants will have also achieved the award. Therefore, it is important to make sure that you are able to show the interviewers what you have gained from the award, and how this will benefit your future career in medicine.

A Bad Response:

"D of E gave me the opportunity to work as part of a team in some of the expeditions. Teamwork is an important skill which will be useful during my future studies. I also improved my leadership and time management skills. As well as this, through the volunteering, skills, and sports sections of the award, I managed to learn many other useful skills which will help my future studies."

Response Analysis:

This response is too short. D of E is such a diverse award and this response makes it appear as if the student hasn't gained very much from it. If you did the award properly, you should have lots to talk about. Thus, if your answer is short it will suggest that you only did the bare minimum to 'tick the boxes'. This response does not show that the student has really gained some valuable skills from completing the award, and instead, makes it seem as if they haven't reflected on their experiences either.

A Good Response:

"My experience of the Duke of Edinburgh award has been highly rewarding, and one of my proudest achievements to date is completing the gold award this summer. There are many aspects of the award which will benefit both my future studies and career. To start, for my volunteering section I joined the Air Training Corps, which was one of the best decisions of my life. Through this organisation, I learnt many skills from drill to sport, to rifle shooting and orienteering. Learning new skills is something that I will have to do on an almost daily basis whilst studying medicine and during my career, so I think it is important to be able to pick things up quickly. The ATC was also helpful in improving my teamwork and leadership skills, which are important in every aspect of the medical degree. Other activities that I was also involved in as part of the award was playing for a local ladies' football team and starting guitar lessons. Being part of a football team was fantastic for improving my teamwork skills, and is something that I would like to continue at university.

Of course, the most well-known part of the D of E award is the expeditions. I enjoyed these immensely and learnt a lot about teamwork, patience, and hard work. Providing support to other members of my team who struggled from time to time was one of the most positive things to take away from the experience, as this is something that will be important during my studies. I am fully aware that the degree will be demanding and challenging, so it is essential that students work together to help each other through."

Response Analysis:

This response is much better because the student has properly thought about what they have gained from each aspect of the D of E award, and how these skills can be transferred to both their future studies and career. They have shown from this in-depth answer that their experiences of D of E were very rewarding and much more than just ticking off a box. The interviewers would be confident that these skills learned would be beneficial to the future medical studies of this student, and it shows that the student has the type of dedication and commitment that would be needed to succeed in the future.

Overall:

This question looks deeper into an extracurricular achievement which many students these days have, thus it is important for the interviewers to be able to differentiate between them as not all students will have gained as much as others. Therefore, to answer this question well, the student should think carefully about what skills they learnt from each aspect of the process, and how they can transfer these to their future studies.

124)   What is the biggest challenge you faced and how did you deal with it?

This question is aimed at trying to identify those candidates who have the personal attributes to thrive in this often challenging and stressful career. It is important that the example cited by the candidate has some kind of "moral to the story" that demonstrates these attributes. This is the sort of question where it pays to have thought about examples beforehand.

A Bad Response:

"I was working in a nursing home when an elderly lady fell on the floor. She was clearly very distressed and I remembered from my biology lesson that she was likely to have suffered a fracture of the neck of the femur due to her obvious osteoporosis. Everyone in the room was very scared and didn't really know what to do as moving her may cause added pain. Finally, one of the care workers came and called an ambulance and put a blanket on her to keep her warm."

Response Analysis:

Though the candidate has indeed identified a challenging situation, they fail to demonstrate that they performed any sort of active role in overcoming the problem. The candidate has suggested a decent insight into what has medically happened to the elderly lady, but this is not what the question was asking. The candidate should ideally have themselves called for help, fetched the blankets and perhaps calmed the lady and everyone else in the room down. This demonstrates knowledge and an application of problem-solving skills, as opposed to merely watching others perform them.

A Good Response:

"I was captain of my school's 1st XI football team and we went through a very bad run of results right at the start of the season. Team morale was very low and people were starting to have a go at each other on the pitch. This was having a huge knock-on effect on our relationships with each other and our schoolwork. As captain, I had to analyse the situation closely and identify where things were going wrong. Unfortunately, this entailed dropping my best friend from the team and exerting my authority over my peers. Though this was an awkward situation, I feel I dealt with it maturely and my team respected me for that. Sure enough, the team's on-pitch success and morale improved."

Response Analysis:

Though the candidate chooses an apparently trivial matter (a school football team), it is the principles that he garners from this experience that will interest the interviewers. He demonstrates that he has the leadership qualities to successfully improve team performance and is not afraid to make hard decisions for the good of the team overall. These problems are not dissimilar from those encountered by teams of doctors in ensuring the best possible patient care. The candidate would be well advised to then draw the parallel between their footballing situation and real life medical team situations to solidify their point.

Overall:

The interviewers won't expect you to have been challenged with the life or death situations that doctors occasionally face. Rather, they will be impressed if you can identify the necessary problem-solving and leadership skills that are beneficial in doctors and show from a personal experience of any sort that you have these qualities.

125)   A patient has explained to you, a medical student, their concerns about having a CT scan as they have a pacemaker fitted and have claustrophobia. How do you respond?

A large part of being a doctor (or a medical student) is much more than treatment: it involves listening to a patient's concerns and then finding the treatment that is right for them. However, sometimes tests cannot be avoided and are required for an accurate diagnosis. This kind of question assesses your ability to empathise with the patient and involves you realising whether you have limited knowledge on a subject or not. Remember, an interview is generally not a test of your knowledge itself but is about the way you can apply what you do know to a different situation. It could well be that you do not know the answer to a question, but make sure you demonstrate initiative to find it out (in the situation: by asking a doctor or reading up on the topic).

A Bad Response:
"I don't understand why you're feeling this way, there's no reason to feel claustrophobic. We need to get an accurate diagnosis. There are a few things that you can do to keep calm like taking deep breaths and making sure you don't panic. However, I think the pacemaker may actually interfere with the CT scan and a different test may be appropriate"

Response Analysis:
This answer is rather short and doesn't fully explore their concerns. It is good that the answer involves providing one solution to their problems, but it is somewhat limited. Crucially, the answer is factually incorrect. If you are unsure as to whether something is correct or not, it is far more preferable to admit you do not know but will ask someone senior and relay that information to them. Secondly, you must never provide a medical opinion as that is the role of a doctor.

A Good Response:
"I understand your concerns with being claustrophobic. However, I just want to say that the test might be really helpful for us to identify the problem and give you an accurate diagnosis. I assure you that the test won't be uncomfortable as there will be someone there speaking to you the whole time to help you keep calm. We can even provide you with headphones to help pass time more quickly. You could also keep calm by trying to take deep breaths. With regards to your pacemaker, I am afraid I am not sure as to whether it interferes with the test or not. I will give this information to the consultant and get back to you with more information"

Response Analysis:
The reason this response is good is because it gives a multitude of options to help them cope with their claustrophobia during the CT scan, as opposed to only one option in the bad response. The main distinguishing factor between this response and the last is the fact that it involves stating that you do not know a piece of information. It does not provide false information and instead offers a solution by asking a senior member of the team.

Overall:
This question is a chance to demonstrate your knowledge (show that a pacemaker does not interfere with a CT scan) or admit to your own shortcomings, both of which are equally acceptable responses. It is important not to give medical information as this is not the role of a medical student.

VOLUNTARY & WORK EXPERIENCE

126)   How did your work experience change your views of medicine?

This question is essentially giving you an excellent opportunity to present concisely what you learnt from your work experience. There is a need for you to compare your views on medicine before and after the work experience, which is potentially tricky. However, if answered correctly, this question is inherently structured in a way that allows the candidate to easily make the critical observations interviewers look for when talking about work experience. Namely, that the candidate has <u>learnt</u> something from the W/E rather than just observed passively. Therefore, the candidate should aim to identify a particular situation they observed during W/E and how this challenged their preconceptions about medicine, and subsequently usefully informed them about the career. This is how W/E questions should generally be approached, as opposed to merely reeling off a list of things that you saw.

A Bad Response:
"Whilst observing a heart operation, I was shocked by the amazing skill of the surgeons in suturing together two different areas of the heart so that the blood flow around the heart would improve.

Response Analysis:
Identifying the "amazing skill" as something that you've learnt is probably inadvisable. It's not very specific, and it shouldn't really be that "shocking" if you're seriously considering a career in medicine. Additionally, it wastes a good opportunity to talk about something far more insightful and useful to a career in medicine. The second issue with this answer is the very simplistic explanation of what the surgeons were doing during the procedure. It suggests that perhaps you didn't really know what they were doing and didn't <u>actively</u> participate in your learning, and rather were merely passively by-standing.

A Good Response:
"I observed a heart operation and decided to talk to the anaesthetist throughout the procedure so as to have some insight on what was going on. I was fascinated to learn about the difficulties the anaesthetists encounter when trying to maintain the physiological function of the systems of the patients' body whilst the surgeons perform the operation. What is found to be particularly challenging is maintaining sufficient perfusion pressures to tissues in a patient who already has advanced ischaemic heart disease. This also allowed me to appreciate the multidisciplinary nature of medicine, which is so reliant upon good communication between each speciality. Previously I'd seen medicine as consisting of several distinct specialities that each deal with their own problems. But with this complex patient with lots of co-morbidities, the importance of a multidisciplinary approach to medicine is clear."

Response Analysis:
This response identifies two key learning points for the candidate: the more general observation of the importance of multidisciplinary approaches to complex medical problems and also a more technical aspect of physiology that the candidate found interesting. This is ideal as it shows both an interest in the dynamics of medical practice as well as the underlying science. Importantly, the candidate sticks to the question asked and emphasised that prior to his work experience, he didn't appreciate the importance of multidisciplinary approaches to certain complex patients. He also leaves plenty of "carrots" for future questions from the interviewers e.g. why is maintaining perfusion pressure important?

Overall:
When answering questions about "what you learnt from your work experience", you should always aim to show how your views/understanding of medicine has been changed by the experience. This is instead of simply reeling off lists of what you've seen- it's all about quality and not quantity. Organise your thoughts before the interview and categorise different experiences into different learning categories. This will help you to present your thoughts as efficiently as possible.

127) What did you see as part of your hospital shadowing?

The key to nailing this question is to describe what you learnt from your hospital shadowing and not just what you saw. Use anecdotes of your experience to describe what it taught you about the role of a doctor, how doctors interact with their patients, or perhaps what you learnt about the patients' experience of being in hospital. It is important that you can show you have reflected on your work experience. The best candidates will describe what they saw, what it taught them, and why it confirmed that medicine is the best career path for them.

A Bad Response:

"During my work experience, I shadowed a paediatric anaesthetist and, most memorably, I spent some time talking to the mother of a baby with pyloric stenosis. Pyloric stenosis is a condition in which the opening at the bottom of the stomach (the pylorus) becomes blocked due to the thickening of the sphincter. This means food cannot pass from the stomach into the duodenum. Babies with this condition usually present with projectile vomiting soon after eating and often do not produce tears or urine because they are so dehydrated from the stomach blockage. Dehydration and electrolyte imbalances are the biggest danger of this condition and these issues are normally resolved before surgery is undertaken to unblock the sphincter."

Response Analysis:

This answer gives an impressive account of a condition seen during hospital shadowing and demonstrates a level of detail that would not be expected of a sixth former. However, the purpose of this question is not to show off knowledge of pathology but to demonstrate an understanding of the medical career that you are hoping to embark on. This answer shows little insight into the role of a doctor and none of the personal details you would expect from an encounter with a worried mother. A student could gain this information from the internet or a textbook and would receive little credit for offering this in an interview.

A Good Response:

"During my work experience, I shadowed a paediatric anaesthetist and, most memorably, I spent some time talking to the mother of a baby boy with pyloric stenosis. Pyloric stenosis is a condition in which the opening at the bottom of the stomach (the pylorus) becomes blocked due to thickening of the sphincter. This mother had brought her baby to hospital because she was worried that he was projectile vomiting after every feed. The baby looked slightly older than most babies who are seen with pyloric stenosis and so the doctors at first dismissed the possibility of this condition. This dismissal made the mother very distressed and she insisted that there was something seriously wrong with her baby. After further investigations, the doctors established that this baby did have pyloric stenosis and were able to give the baby the treatment he needed. The mother was very relieved.

This encounter taught me that doctors can have a profound emotional impact on the people they work with and the relief and gratitude of the mother showed me that medicine is an enormously gratifying profession. I learned the importance of listening to the patient's concerns, especially when you are dealing with a worried parent who has brought their child to hospital. It showed me that being a doctor is also about treating people and not just the diseases."

Response Analysis:

This is an excellent answer that combines an awareness of the mother's concerns and the impact of a doctor in this situation. Additionally, it raises a very important concept in medicine, 'being a doctor is also about treating people and not just the diseases'. It shows a real insight into the medical career.

Overall:

No matter how much or little work experience you are able to do, ensure that you reflect on every encounter and are able to describe what you have learned from the experience. Showing an insight into the ideas, concerns, and expectations of patients will also help you to stand out as a genuinely compassionate individual and as someone well-suited to a medical career.

128)   What did you learn from your work experience?

This is a question you can almost expect to be asked (and even if you're not, reflecting on your experience is never a bad thing!) so have a few thoughts about what you'd like to say prepared. It doesn't matter whether you shadowed a top neurosurgeon or volunteered in a nursing home – it's what you learn from the experience that really counts, so make sure your answer focuses on that.

This common interview question can actually be a great opportunity to steer the interview towards something you want to talk about – you could answer with an ethical point, practical skills that you learnt, the teamwork you witnessed, or simply how healthcare works in day to day practice. You can also use this question as an opportunity to demonstrate your qualities and personal development, such as how you were inspired to improve your own teamwork work skills after seeing what a vital part of medicine they are.

You may want to structure your answer by starting with what you expected your placement to be like and what you had hoped to learn, then lead into a bit about the work experience itself, and most importantly, what you gained from it.

Bad Response A:
"Most of my work experience was in a nursing home so I didn't actually get to see what doctors do there, but I guess I learnt about communicating with the elderly and how to stay on the right side of the nurses. I also did a week shadowing the doctors on a vascular surgery ward. I attended clinics and saw some operations that they performed. I learnt a lot about the day to day jobs of various grades of doctors and how patients are referred to a clinic, scheduled for an operation, and then cared for by the doctors on the ward during their stay."

Bad Response B:
"I learnt that it is very important to catch and treat a stroke as soon as possible and also how clinics work."

Response Analysis:
Response A focuses too much on the negatives and fails to highlight the key skills developed during the experience – communicating with patients and staff, along with teamwork. It feels too much like a list of the things seen rather than what the experience actually taught the candidate. Instead of listing, try to frame your answer with the context in which you learnt it. For example, "Following a patient from the clinic to their inpatient stay for an operation gave me the opportunity to appreciate the many different professionals involved in patient care and importance of team working..."

Definitely avoid snubbing other professionals. Generally, it's better to assume you haven't seen the great work that they do and not that they don't do great work!

Response B fails to show even a small amount of appreciation for how their experiences give insights into what it is like to be a doctor. They do not expand upon their experiences and how they are going to impact on their own practice in the future.

Good Response A:
"Something that has really stuck with me from my work experience on a geriatric ward was the sense of the patient being at the centre of a team of professionals and that the best care relies on the specialist skills of all the members of that team. I was lucky enough to spend time with several teams during my week - doctors, nurses, pharmacists, and physiotherapists – and I learnt a lot from them about the importance of good communication skills, both with staff and patients. Since my work experience, I have been trying to develop my own communication and teamwork skills by volunteering in the "Buddy" scheme at my local nursing home. Through this scheme, I spend an afternoon a week chatting to and arranging activities for the residents which has allowed me to fine-tune my organisational skills and ability to work in a team."

Good Response B:

'One thing I learnt in my work experience was from an encounter with a very upset patient with inoperable pancreatic cancer. This had a great impact on me. By her own admission, the doctor I was shadowing grew close to tears at the bedside, yet maintained her professional objectivity. This really helped me understand the importance that a doctor remains compassionate while maintaining a level of emotional detachment and how much of a challenge this can be.'

Response Analysis:

These responses really demonstrate that you've reflected on the experience and used what you learnt there to develop your own personal skills. Highlighting a couple of key points and then expanding on them is much better than simply listing off things you saw or facts you learnt. It also demonstrates that you appreciated the role of healthcare from the perspective of other professions.

You could use your response to talk about ethics, for example, discussing a particular ethical dilemma that you witnessed and what you learnt both about the ethics of the situation and your own personal response to such situations during the process.

Overall:

You need to have reflected on your work experience and have a fluent answer to this question. This question can often be a springboard to further discussion depending on what you say, so it's also a good idea to think about what questions they could ask you regarding your response.

Before embarking on work experience, write down what you think you will learn and then keep a diary of things you saw or did so that you can better remember and reflect on them later. Your opinions may change over time with more experience, your personal experience of healthcare, or from things you hear and read in the media – these are also all worth noting and reflecting on for this question.

Finally, don't forget that this will be a spoken interview so practise with someone asking you spontaneous questions. The more practise you get, the better, more fluent, and more impressive you will be.

129)   Tell me about your volunteering work. Did you find it more or less useful than your work experience?

Volunteering is important. It shows the compassionate and caring side to your personality, which is a very important requirement for a doctor. Work experience, on the other hand, demonstrates you have a realistic insight into the profession. This is very important considering the fact that you are committing to a lifetime career. It is important that you have an understanding of the complex nature of a doctor's role as well as being aware of the highs and lows of the profession. The best way to approach this question is to state what duties you undertook as a volunteer. Once you have spoken about what your role was, it is very important to follow this with explaining what you learnt from volunteering. With regards to explaining whether it was more or less helpful than your work experience, it may be a good idea to highlight some of the differences you experienced between both placements and why you found one or the other more useful.

A Bad Response:
"I volunteered at my local hospital for 6 weeks and I was responsible for providing drinks to the patients, talking to them about their stay in the hospital, and cleaning up in the kitchen. It was a good experience overall. During my work experience, I shadowed the junior doctor on the ward and sat in a number of clinics with consultants. I was surprised at how busy it can get. I found both of them equally useful to be honest as they were both placed in a hospital environment"

Response Analysis:
Whilst the candidate outlined his/her roles and responsibilities during volunteering and the activities undertook during work experience, there isn't a follow-on with regards to what was learnt from both experiences. It is just stated that it was a good experience. What interviewers would like to know is how it was good- was it useful because you understood how the ward operates? Or because you learned about how patients feel when they are in hospital?

A Good Response:
"I volunteered for 6 weeks at my local hospital. I served patients drinks and snacks, tidied the ward up, and cleaned the kitchen. During this time, I gained an understanding of how a ward functions and that ward rounds occur in the morning when the doctors reviewed the patients. The doctors then carry out their jobs such as taking blood or ordering tests. Sometimes, there used to be lunchtime meetings when doctors would present a case. I also learned about the role of nurses and healthcare assistants and physiotherapists. It enabled me to appreciate the role of the team as a whole. I understood better what it must feel like to be a patient in hospital as I regularly spoke to patients and their relatives. It struck me as to how terrified some of them are. During my work experience, I shadowed a doctor in A&E where I developed an understanding of how the NHS works and skills that a doctor must possess such as the ability to work well under pressure, communication skills, and perseverance. It was also an excellent way to apply any anatomy and physiology you have learnt during your GCSE/AS levels to patients and their medical problems. In this way, I think work experience better prepared me for life as a doctor as I hadn't appreciated just how long the hours are and how stressful it can get at times."

Response Analysis:
This answer excels in discussing the learning points gained from volunteering and work experience. There is a clear understanding of the role of different healthcare professionals in the multidisciplinary team and the role of doctors in their day-to-day life at a hospital. They also took away learning points from talking to patients on the ward and discovered some of the highs and lows of being a doctor in a busy hospital.

Overall:
We all know that everyone takes a lot away from their volunteering and work experience posts. The key to answering this question is to spell out what you did, but more importantly, what you learnt from it. Reflecting on an event and what you learnt from it is key to being a good doctor and this skill is what the interviewers are looking for here.

130)   You didn't actually do much work experience, why was this?

The most important principle to think about here is '**Quality over Quantity**. If you haven't done substantial work experience, do not worry. You don't need to have done weeks and weeks of work experience to impress at an interview. The best preparation for an interview (and medicine itself!) is to do some work experience and to use it as an opportunity to learn something about the role of a doctor and how doctors interact with their patients. With this question, you therefore want to put forward a strong case that you were still able to learn a great deal about the profession from your experience. Most interviewers will understand that it is often difficult to arrange work experience if you don't personally know a doctor, especially given that many hospitals have strict rules about who can undertake work experience and the paperwork that needs to be completed before you can start.

A Bad Response:

"I was quite disappointed not to be able to do more work experience than I did. My careers teacher was in charge of organising work experience at the local hospital but she missed the deadline for sorting it out and no one at school got to do any hospital shadowing. I was really hoping to do some work experience with an orthopaedic surgeon because that's the speciality I would like to go into, but instead, I got stuck with just a couple of days with a GP and it was pretty boring."

Response Analysis:

The first problem with this answer is that it is immediately negative about the little amount of work experience done. Don't give the interviewer an easy opportunity to give you low marks for this question! Secondly, it makes excuses for the lack of work experience. Instead, this answer should be about the experience you did get and what you learnt from it. And thirdly, don't state that you know what speciality you would like to do before you have even started medical school. It's good to have interests but you will come across as close-minded if you sound too focused. Certainly don't say time with a GP was boring!

A Good Response:

"Whilst I was only able to complete two days of work experience, I feel I still learnt a lot about the working lives of doctors and how they speak to and comfort their patients. My time spent with a GP taught me that doctors do not just treat biomedical disease but rather they treat their patients as people and must learn to understand how a disease affects their patients' lives. I have also spent some time volunteering as a meal assistant on a ward and have been able to talk to hospital patients about their experiences and struggles. This has taught me a great deal about coping with illness on top of what I have learnt from my work experience."

Response Analysis:

This is a good answer because it puts a strong emphasis on the fact that the work experience has been a worthwhile and reflective process. A follow-up question might ask for specific examples of what you saw and what you learned (see later question: 'What did you see as part of your hospital shadowing?') This answer also includes voluntary work and shows that the candidate is motivated to gain more exposure to a medical environment. Important point: if you struggle to organise work experience, it is often easier to arrange voluntary work as a meal time helper on a ward or in a nursing home and you can learn a lot from talking to patients in these situations.

Overall:

As with any question about work experience, it is important that you can demonstrate what you learnt from your experience and how you reflected on what you saw. Interviewers are not impressed by candidates with months of work experience if they cannot explain why it was valuable. Don't panic if you are struggling to organise lots of work experience!

131)   Tell me one thing that you learnt about MDTs during your work experience.

Multidisciplinary teams (MDTs) are an essential day-to-day component of any healthcare system. This question aims to ensure you understand the importance of the MDT in action and to highlight the skills needed to ensure the MDT operates at a high standard in every clinical scenario and setting. The other component of the question is to come up with an example from your work experience – this does not necessarily have to be a poignant, acute situation (where an organised MDT can mean the difference between life and death), so don't panic if your work experience did not involve any emergency medicine. Inter-professional communication is a core theme through all aspects of healthcare provision, from inpatient care through to community services.

A Bad Response:
"I noticed how important MDTs are within the hospital setting as both doctors and nurses come together to provide a high level of patient care in a critical situation."

Response Analysis:
Although the student may only have had hospital work experience, it is important to demonstrate an understanding that MDTs are applicable to all healthcare settings: primary through to quaternary care. This response also fails to mention the other key members of the MDT, which suggests a naiveté as to their importance. This answer needs to expand on the actual function of the MDT and what skills are involved in providing comprehensive care.

A Good Response:
"One thing I identified is the importance of having a profound understanding of your individual role within the team and how this interconnects with other members' skills to provide a cohesive, quality intervention.

For part of my work experience, I was placed on the geriatric ward, which I believe is a speciality that epitomises the importance of a well-polished MDT. On my first day, I sat in on an MDT meeting where I could immediately see the how the different roles contributed to the patient's pathway of care. It was impressive to see just how many different disciplines came together to help a single patient: doctors, nurses, occupational therapists, and physiotherapists. I was lucky enough to follow a patient throughout their entire hospital stay and so witnessed their whole pathway. A frail, elderly lady was brought in by an ambulance having suffered a fall and sustaining a fractured hip. She had input from the geriatricians, the old age mental health team, and the orthopaedic department. She was well cared for by the nursing staff. Her rehabilitation and progression to discharge were smoothly coordinated between the geriatricians, the physiotherapists, the occupational therapists, and the community nursing team.

I believe the cohesive running of this team enabled the patient to go home as quickly as possible whilst minimising stress throughout her stay, which is imperative to a patient-centred approach."

Response Analysis:
This answer demonstrates a comprehensive understanding of the importance of inter-professional communication and its implications in the clinical setting. The answer is backed up by a detailed example from personal experience with the benefits of the MDT acknowledged and understood. Unlike the example of a bad response, this answer shows an understanding that the inter-professional team is not merely limited to doctors and nurses but involves multiple healthcare professionals. The learning points from this answer should be applicable to any situation the student may have witnessed during work experience.

Overall:
MDTs are a foundation to all healthcare provisions, so are important. The answer to this question needs to be a detailed example, rich enough to demonstrate an understanding of the breadth of input into an MDT and the importance of each individual role. It also needs to show that you understand that ensuring high-level patient care requires a cohesive and well-oiled team.

132)   Tell me about a time when you felt sad when doing your charity work

This question wants to ensure you understand that in reality, as a doctor, you will encounter sadness and other emotional challenges on a regular basis. Think about your experiences during charity work, what you have learnt from them, and how you can apply these to being a good doctor.

A Bad Response:

"I volunteered at a day centre for people with advanced Alzheimer's. We would try and get everyone involved in activities, such as singing songs and doing jigsaw puzzles. At the end of the afternoon, the families and carers would arrive to take the patient's home. Often the patients wouldn't even recognise their loved ones or people they see every day, which I found really difficult to witness."

Response Analysis:

Whilst this response describes a clearly emotion-evoking scenario, the answer does not go into enough detail. This answer would be a wasted opportunity to demonstrate an understanding of life as a doctor and the qualities required to overcome its challenges.

A Good Response:

"I volunteered at a school for children with varying degrees of learning difficulties and developmental delays for an academic year. I used to visit for an afternoon each week and join in with maths and music lessons. Over the months, I got to know several of the children well and developed a close bond with them. One girl in particular, who I spent a lot of time with unfortunately got really sick, and later died. It really affected me and I struggled to go back to the school after hearing about what had happened to her. I know that doctors must often face death, but I also know that sometimes it must be accepted that not everybody can be cured, and the most important thing is to think about the patient's best interests and what they want. I don't think it is a bad thing to be emotionally affected by what happens to your patients. Keeping this humane side is essential to maintaining empathy as a doctor, something that I believe to be perhaps the most important quality to building a doctor-patient relationship and providing patient-centred care."

Response Analysis:

It is essential to recognise that you will often face sadness during your medical career. Whilst it may be tempting to act seemingly unaffected by something like this, it is more important to recognise and address these emotions. Relating the experience to becoming a better doctor gives a well-rounded and complete answer. Perhaps during your charity work you did not encounter something quite as emotional as the example given above, but it is important to think carefully about how you can relate your experiences to life as a doctor. Think of the sad event as a challenge to be overcome and learned from.

Overall:

Don't be embarrassed to say that you were emotionally affected by whatever it was you saw during your charity work. It will show that you understand that being a doctor will entail emotional scenarios. What is important is that you discuss how overcoming these emotions would actually make you a better doctor.

133) Compare and contrast your experiences at the GP and the hospital.

Background Analysis:

The answer to this question is clearly very personal as you are asked to draw on your own experiences. Questions like this can often take you by surprise and there is nothing wrong with taking a few seconds to really think about your answer to ensure that you have a clear idea of what you want to say before you start talking. This may seem obvious, but silence in the interview room can seem deafening, so there can be a strong impulse to just start speaking. Try to demonstrate that you have thought about your different experiences and what it is like to be a doctor.

A Bad Response:

"My experiences made me feel like I definitely want to be a hospital doctor. Work experience at the GP mainly just involved sitting through clinics all day whereas, at the hospital, I got to go and see some amazing surgery. I think being a hospital doctor would be much more exciting and interesting and that I am much more suited to that."

Response Analysis:

This response does not really answer the question and suggests quite a superficial appreciation by the candidate of their experiences. The candidate does not seem to realise that a huge amount of hospital medicine – including for surgeons – is worked in clinics and so if clinics are unbearable to them, then maybe they should rethink much of hospital medicine too. Also, lumping all of the hospital-based medicine in with his experience in surgery suggests that the candidate has either not done much work experience, or has failed to recognise how vastly varied hospital medicine is. Secondly, the candidate has potentially given some bad impressions regarding their motivations for why they want to study medicine. Their answer suggests that the candidate prioritises their own personal experiences of excitement or interest over the rewards of helping people and noticing how these interactions differ between a GP and a hospital setting. It potentially also suggests an unrealistic thrill-a-minute perception of hospital medicine.

A Good Response:

"On my work experience and from my volunteer work, I got an appreciation for how different it can be to work as a GP and as a hospital doctor. I also realised how varied it can be for different types of hospital doctors. At the GP, I was struck by the continuity of care element to the doctor's practice – he already knew a lot of the patients and had treated them for many years. This must be a particularly rewarding part of being a GP as you can build long-lasting relationships with your patients which is likely to be appreciated by the patients too. This is not necessarily the case for some hospital doctors who may sometimes only get to see patients once or twice before they are discharged. There was also a huge amount of variation at the GP – in a single morning clinic, the GP was required to deal with problems in cardiology, dermatology, psychiatry, paediatrics, and so much more. There was just as much variation when I had work experience in a hospital A&E, but in other areas of hospital medicine, there was a lot less so. For example, I spent a morning following an orthopaedic surgeon who specialised in hand surgery and mainly just did the same type of operation every day. These specialists had the benefit of seeing some of the most complex and interesting cases, though, and were able to help people who could not be treated in primary care."

Response Analysis:

This candidate has shown that they engaged well with their work experience, were observant, and have thought about their experiences. Showing an awareness of the differences between a GP and hospital from the patient's perspective also nicely showed that they have not lost sight that the ultimate goal of medicine is the wellbeing of the patient and a positive patient experience.

Overall:

Before the interview, think about all your medical experiences and what you have learned about what it is like to be a doctor and also, just as importantly, what it is like to be a patient. Think about how the different areas of medicine that you have seen have varied, and which particular areas appeal to you and why.

134)   You are a medical student observing in the hospital. The doctor forgets to introduce you to the patient and ask permission for you to observe the consultation. What do you do? What would you do if the patient does not want you in the room?

When in the hospital, during your time at medical school, it is highly likely that you will be met with this scenario. This question may be asked to assess how you react to the situation you may well be presented within a few years' time. Often, the doctor can forget to introduce you to the patient, however, it is incredibly important that you introduce yourself so that the patient knows you are part of the team and feels comfortable during the consultation. The second part of the question also addresses another very common scenario whilst at medical school; not all patients feel comfortable when there is someone else in the room especially if discussing an intimate or personal topic.

A Bad Response:
"Although I agree that it is important for the patient to be aware of who is going to be present, if the consultation continues then introducing myself by interrupting may not be appropriate depending on the circumstance, especially if a sensitive matter is being discussed. Moreover, it is the doctor's responsibility to introduce the medical student and if the doctor does not introduce me it is probably for a good reason. Only if the patient asks who I am would I tell them."

Response Analysis:
Although it's easy to see the merit in this response, it is still not the best route to take. It is definitely important not to interrupt *during* the consultation, especially if the doctor is building a rapport with the patient so as to allow them to open up. However, the patient has a right to know who you are and why it is you need to be there. Normally, the doctor will introduce you but if they do not, it is absolutely your responsibility to do so. The response states, 'I will state my name and the fact that I am a medical student' but fails to obtain consent from the patient (whether they permit you being present). It also lacks an insight into why and does not answer the last part of the question.

A Good response:
"It is crucial that the patient knows exactly who is part of the team. Before the consultation was to begin, if the doctor forgot to introduce me I would state my name, the fact that I am a medical student and ask whether the patient is ok with me being present in the room during the consultation. The patient could feel awkward with my presence and would affect how open they are during the consultation. I understand that the patient may feel more comfortable speaking to a doctor rather than a medical student – something that is important when discussing an intimate matter. If the patient wishes for me to not be present, I would fully respect their decision and leave the room."

Response Analysis:
This is a much more empathetic response. It demonstrates an understanding of the relationship between a patient and a doctor and insight as to why the patient may feel uncomfortable with your presence. The response addresses the question in three parts: what the problem is, why it might be a problem and an acceptable solution to the problem. This is the approach which should be taken in all situation-based questions.

Overall:
This question can be used to show your empathetic skills and demonstrate that you understand your sometimes limited role as a medical student.

135) *What was something that you will take away from your voluntary work? / Tell me about an experience from your voluntary work.*

This is a very open-ended question that can be used to get an idea of your values and what is important to you. Did you gain skills or valuable interpersonal experiences from your voluntary work? Remember that whilst paid work is usually about skills, volunteering is often more geared towards gaining valuable experiences.

A Bad Response:

"During my voluntary work, I was in charge of organising a fundraising event for [charity]. This was really difficult to organise because we had some last minute cancellations, but I found a backup and the event continued as planned. Therefore, I gained a lot of organisational skills during my voluntary work which will be useful during my medical training. It was also very stressful but I kept my cool, which shows that I cope well under stress."

Response Analysis:

This is not an awful response – the candidate shows that they have gained skills and experience from their volunteering work and acknowledges organisation is important for doctors. The candidate also successfully brings the question back to why they should be considered for the medical school. However, if the interviewer wanted to hear about organisation or skills they probably would ask specifically (or correct the candidate once they started talking about something not related to this.) – This question is more about reflecting on an important experience than gaining skills to tick boxes.

A Good Response:

"I think I will always remember my time volunteering in the local hospice. Whilst I was too junior to be heavily involved in patient care, I remember meeting one patient who was very near the end of his time and had refused any further treatments. He was completely at peace with his situation and calmly ready. This really challenged my views on end-of-life care and made me reconsider the roles of a doctor, and I think this experience will help me better understand decisions made in palliative care."

Response Analysis:

This is a thoughtful response reflecting on a real and important experience gained during voluntary work. The candidate acknowledges that the experience challenged their opinions and beliefs, showing they have an open mind. By having their beliefs shaped by experiences such as this one, they will likely be a mature and empathetic student when interacting with terminally ill patients; an important skill that can be very difficult to teach. Once again, the candidate brings the experience back to link it into why they would be a good choice for the medical school, using a poignant experience to strengthen their own application. Bringing your response back to answer the question and support your application is a really important and useful interview trick.

Overall:

Medical schools ask for volunteering experience in the hopes that candidates will gain valuable insights and important experiences. Open-ended, vague questions like this give space to assess whether checking boxes or real experiences are more important to the candidate. Obviously gaining skills is useful, but this can be assessed by more closed questions (and if the interviewer meant to ask about that, they can correct themselves once you start talking about the patient that you met). Instead, talking about personal experiences and reflecting on how they impacted you shows that you were emotionally engaged with the volunteering work and that you gained something valuable from it.

NB: It should go without saying - **NEVER** use any identifying features (name, address, strange tattoos!) when talking about a patient. Breaching confidentiality is severely punished in medicine and good habits start early.

136)   How did your perspective of medical hierarchy change after your work experience?

The phrasing of this question might compel you to give an answer that suggests you had some sort of revelation about medicine and an assumed hierarchy following your work experience. That isn't what you need. Rather, this question requires you to take an example from your experience and show that you've learned from it and that your perspective has broadened.

A Bad Response:

"During work experience, once I sat in on a multidisciplinary team that was discussing several cases to do with kidney diseases. It was interesting to hear the doctors discuss the complex issues of patients, even though I didn't understand much. But I saw how doctors from different specialities were working together and it taught me the importance of teamwork in medicine."

Response Analysis:

This response isn't all that bad. It does show that the candidate has learned from their experience, but this response is lacking. Here, detail about the experience isn't all that necessary – you wouldn't be expected to give details about the issues you'd heard about. Rather, it details about how your view has changed. Not necessarily changed to the degree of a massive paradigm shift, but perhaps a slight change or reaffirmation of what you thought medicine and how things worked. This anecdote lends itself to that sort of reaffirmation quite nicely.

A Good Response:

"During my work experience, I was based in the pathology department at Royal London Hospital. The consultant I was shadowing often sat in on multidisciplinary meetings so I was allowed to join. It was a great opportunity to see so many doctors from different specialities working together to consider individual patients at a time. On one particular session, they were discussing a series of patients with various kidney pathologies that I didn't really understand, but crucially I saw how the doctors worked well together and how they opened a dialogue when they disagreed. I think it was a bit of an eye opener for me because up until that point, perhaps foolishly, I had the impression that, yes, doctors worked in teams, but there was always this rigid hierarchy of who could say what and consultants were effectively the leaders who couldn't be questioned, with one consultant never talking to another. But here I was observing consultants working together. The experience really brought home the idea that teamwork is at the core of modern medical practice."

Response Analysis:

Same anecdote, better response. This response is better purely because it directly addresses the question at hand. The candidate has made it clear how exactly the experience has changed their view of medicine and how doctors work in a team. Crucially, the change here isn't a huge shift, i.e. beforehand they didn't think doctors worked in teams but now they do, rather it's a subtle readjustment of the candidate's views about the hierarchy in medicine. By directly addressing the question, by giving both the perspective before the experience and after, the contrast is highlighted and shows that you actually understood the question being asked, and aren't just giving a rehearsed answer. Generally, the difference between the good and bad response is that the good response acknowledged the need to show a change in views whilst the bad response only really showed what had been learned from the experience without much detail.

Overall:

This question highlights the importance of showing that you've actually understood what the interviewer was asking. The anecdote is only half the story. When presented with this question it's important to realise that they're looking for a change in perspective and in your response, you should make it obvious that you've recognised this. The best way to do that is to give the before and after, thus creating a contrast and showing that you've engaged with the materials.

137) *What differences did you see between GPs and hospitals when it comes to patient care during your work experience?*

This question may seem to lend itself to a sort of diffuse response that highlights the difference in care offered by the two institutions, but this is not the case. This question is a relatively straightforward one that should be taken as an opportunity to show off slightly and show that you have a deeper awareness of what goes on. This is best portrayed using anecdotes.

A Bad Response:
"Well when I was working in the GP, I realised that compared to the targeted approach that doctors take in the hospital, GPs were more concerned with the holistic concerns of a patient. Also, the obvious difference in my experiences was the kind of patient I saw come into the clinic. With the GP, I saw the doctors deal with colds and cases of flu as well as diabetes and heart disease, whereas when I was at the hospital, I saw a lot more severe conditions like people with really bad respiratory conditions and people on ventilators, but that was all confined to specific departments."

Response Analysis:
This response isn't actually half bad and would probably provide a decent scoring. However, there are several points where this candidate could improve to give a better answer; for example, when they say "targeted approach", what exactly does that mean? It would be worthwhile clarifying that point. Also, the latter half of the response sort of alludes to the idea of compartmentalization in hospitals and the variance in diversity between hospitals and GPs. That's all fair and well, but it's better to just explicitly talk about that as a contrast – it is a perfectly valid point.

A Good Response:
"When I was shadowing a GP, I saw a rather wide variety of conditions and people, ranging from people simply coming in to be signed off work with the flu to people with multi-factorial issues like a combination of Type II diabetes, dementia and heart disease. Both of those patients were seen by the same GP on the same day. In contrast, when I was shadowing a registrar in the neurology department at my hospital, I saw only people with neurological disorders. Of course, the patients had other problems as well, but the focus was clearly on neurology. So I guess the immediate contrast I've seen between GPs and hospitals is how GPs see a rather large variance in the kind of patients they see, whilst hospitals are compartmentalized, although there is still significant overlap. It does make sense since GPs are the first line of interaction for patients, being primary care. On top of that, I realised that for the most part, GPs tend to be more emotionally involved than their hospital colleagues. I worked at a GP for about a month and saw several patients repeatedly, and GPs got Christmas presents and the likes whereas my registrar didn't really have that kind of relationship with his patients. He knew them whilst they stayed in hospital but not really more than that. Although he did say that sometimes he had, as he called, 'frequent flyers'."

Response Analysis:
A solid albeit long response. It effectively covers two points; the idea that GPs see a greater variety of patients and that GPs have a more emotionally involved position. That's a perfectly valid comparison between the two institutions and the level of detail conveys that the candidate had really learned from their work experience and was able to show that by making valid reasoned comparisons between different healthcare delivery environments.

Overall:
Here, the aim of the game is to convey your differences but avoid giving poorly backed up responses. By providing anecdotal evidence from your experiences, it reinforces your conclusions and makes you more believable. Crucially, it shows that you've learned from your work experience and are able to make valid comparisons.

138) Describe a moment in your volunteering where you made a positive impact on someone's life.

It's worthwhile before going into an interview to prepare in your mind a few key moments from both your work experience and volunteering that could be used as an example for several different criteria if asked. This does not have to be an incredible story; it might be something that was relatively mundane but try and think of how the situation involved criteria such as teamwork, communication, empathy and others.

A Bad Response:
"I once helped an old lady in a home who had become very upset. I organised for her family to come over and visit her. I felt really good for having done that and I think she appreciated it too."

Response Analysis:
This is a particularly poor answer. There is no background given to the story and the description is lacking in detail. This makes it hard for the interviewer to engage with the story and thus holds less weight in an interview setting. There is no explanation as to how this benefitted the old lady's life.

A Good Response:
"There was one moment during my volunteering placement at an old age home that particularly sticks out in my memory.

Janet was a resident who I had come to be good friends with over the course of my placement. I was in the dining room of the home and was helping Janet with her dinner alongside one of the nurses who worked in the home. Janet is very elderly and was suffering from several conditions that reduced her mobility and meant that she needed others to help her eat. While the nurse and I were helping to feed her, Janet burst into tears - she claimed that she did not want to live anymore.

At first, we tried to comfort her but to no avail. It was at that point that I remembered her telling me, the week before, about her three children and how much she loved them. At that point, I decided to talk to her about her children and showed her the picture of them I knew she had in her wallet. This quickly calmed her down. I then pointed out that they hadn't visited in a while and that I was sure that if she asked them, they would be more than happy to come. I messaged all three of them myself on her behalf. In the end, they all began regular visits and this led to a great improvement in her quality of life in the home. I figured that she had become quite lonely in the home and had felt cut off from her family. I will never forget what a wonderful woman Janet is."

Response Analysis:
This is a much better answer even though the underlying story is the same. The answer opens with a brief introduction that is more or less repeating the question. This gives the student time to think and structure their answer so as to improve its quality. The scene is then set by giving background details to the story. The story itself is well illustrated with imagery. The story is brought to a firm conclusion that explains exactly how this benefitted her life and also relates this to the feelings of the student who is giving the answer.

Overall:
It's extremely important to have a powerful narrative here. This includes setting the scene of the story, using imagery to illustrate the story and having a strong conclusion. Including these aspects makes for a powerful and engaging answer to an interview question.

139) Name one powerful moment you experienced during your shadowing.

This kind of broad question might seem intimidating but it really shouldn't. It gives you a wide remit to talk about anything you thought was really powerful. There is no correct experience to draw upon. Rather, the key here is to convey your passion and genuine interest. You may not feel that you saw much, but even so, if you can show that you've learned from the exposure, you'll be fine.

A Bad Response:

"I saw a post mortem examination being done on a homeless man who'd died in a stairwell on a council estate. It was the first time I'd seen a dead body like that and it was really scary. I almost fainted. It was also the first time I got to wear scrubs which was pretty fun. It was quite cool to see how all of the organs were removed and how they figured out what was wrong with him. He'd died of pneumonia and had really bad alcoholism."

Response Analysis:

This response is bad not because of the anecdote, which is a potentially powerful one, but because it fails to attach any real meaning to the experience. The candidate has been candid about his experience, but beyond it being "pretty fun" he hasn't said what he's taken away and learned. If anything, this shows a total lack of understanding of the point of shadowing. This risks projecting the idea that the experience was a waste on you. The response is effectively missing an entire half that details what he's learned.

A Good Response:

"I was shadowing a coroner and one day I had the opportunity to observe a post-mortem examination on a homeless man who'd been found dead in the stairwell of a nearby council estate. The coroner explained that he was looking for the cause of death. It was an entirely new experience for me because up until this point, I'd only ever seen dead bodies on TV. I was terrified as I watched the body being dissected – I almost fainted. I did think it was very surreal as the coroner pulled out organs individually to examine them. It felt like we were detectives. When the coroner examined the lungs, he said that the patient had died of pneumonia and showed me how he knew. It turns out the patient's entire right lung had been badly infected. He would have been in excruciating pain, but he'd used alcohol to self-medicate. We knew about the pneumonia because when we poked his healthy lung, it was bouncy but his diseased lung just crumbled. We figured out his alcoholism based on his cirrhotic liver. I really enjoyed the experience in the end. I'd never really thought about what a coroner did beforehand and I liked the sense of playing detective. I could see myself doing that kind of work in the future."

Response Analysis:

This is a long response, but that isn't a bad thing! This response makes far better use of the anecdote and the level of detail conveys a certain passion that shows the candidate has learned from the experience. That's ultimately the point of the response. The anecdote itself need not be so extravagant. This response is good because it shows interest in what the candidate observed and shows that the candidate is capable of taking a novel experience and learning from it.

Overall:

There will no doubt be a great deal of variety in what the interviewer will end up hearing in candidates' answers, but don't fall into the trap of trying to come up with the most eye-catching story - especially if it isn't true! You should aim to pull from a real experience, even if it's a common one, and just try your best to convey genuine passion and learning.

140) Why is work experience mandatory for medical students? What do you gain?

This is a relatively straightforward question and it's important to be candid. What can make you stand out here is by both explaining why you believe work experience is necessary but also how you have fulfilled the requirements, and how you understand it to be an important experience. Directly addressing the question will likely lead to a lacklustre response.

Bad Response A:
"I think work experience is mandatory because you need students to show a certain level of dedication to working in healthcare and the time commitment of work experience shows that they care enough to deserve a place. It also shows them the kinds of traits they need to develop to succeed."

Bad Response B:
"Medicine is potentially a tough career and the decision to begin medical training should not be taken lightly. Speaking to consultants about their work and the details of the management of their patients has personally confirmed to me that this fascinating career is the one for me."

Response Analysis:
This response isn't great, primarily because the focus is more on the superficial issues of time consumption, rather than any sense of deeper engagement. The risk of a response like this is that it suggests that the candidate only partakes in work experience as a means to an end and had no real intention to engage with what they were doing. Yes, there is mentioning of the fostering of beneficial traits, but that should have been more explicit rather than being tackled near the end.

Response B is unsatisfactory for a few reasons. Firstly, they fail to pinpoint an exact learning point from their work experience that shows that they have reflected on their experiences and are a more informed applicant for it. Secondly, they are focused on identifying the roles of the consultant. It takes many years to become a consultant and much of the day-to-day management of the patients is left to the more junior doctors, who may, therefore, be able to provide prospective applicants with a very good view of what it's like to be a doctor in training in the 21st century. Thirdly, they have suggested that they wanted to gain some knowledge of the precise details of potentially complex patient management. Better would be to identify general principles that broadly inform you of a career in medicine.

Good Response A:
"I think work experience is mandatory for a couple of reasons. The profession we're trying to pursue requires a certain degree of dedication and a passion for healthcare that not necessarily everyone has. I think by insisting candidates have work experience, it helps the candidates themselves to recognise whether or not they fit that bill before they end up regretting their choices later on in life. For example, when I worked in an assisted living facility, if I found the experience to be revolting and didn't want to work with the sick and elderly, I'd probably be forced to rethink my application. On top of that, by directly interacting with the people we want to become, like GPs and hospital consultants, it shows us the kinds of personality traits we either should have already or should develop if we want to succeed. An example is when I sat in on a multidisciplinary meeting and saw just how much modern medicine relies on effective communication skills and teamwork in order to provide the best possible care for patients. Ultimately, I imagine the aim of insisting we have work experience is to show us as candidates what we're in for and see if we actually want what we think we want."

Good Response B:
"Work experience is valuable in helping prospective medical students make an informed choice about the career they wish to embark upon. It is very easy to be swept away in the stream of the popular media representations of the day-to-day life-saving procedures that doctors perform, but in reality, the practice of medicine is far less glamorous and is a tough career. For instance, when speaking to a junior doctor on my work experience, I learnt of the large amount of paperwork that they have to deal with that often precludes their participation in surgical procedures that are important for their prospective career as a surgeon."

Response Analysis:
This is a superior response because it shifts the focus away from the idea of doing work experience purely to meet the entrance criteria – as the bad response suggested – and interpreted the requirement as one necessary to confirm an individual's convictions. This response makes it clear that the insistence on work experience is for the sake of the candidate and is not just done on a whim by the institution. This projects the idea that this candidate is one who recognises the importance of work experience and actively attempts to learn from each opportunity. Crucially, it moves away from the idea that this candidate only does work experience to fulfil criteria; an image you absolutely do not want to associate with yourself.

In Response B, the candidate identifies a particular example of where they have been informed of the realities of being a junior doctor (paperwork and training time issue). This shows a degree of reflection upon their experiences, which is exactly what interviewers want to see.

Overall:
This is the kind of question that really helps to sort out the stronger, more passionate candidates from the weaker ones. It's not a difficult question to answer, but in answering, it's important to suggest the right kinds of ideas. Getting across the idea that you got more out of your work experience than just the ability to confirm you've done some is the key.

The danger here is that the candidate tries to cover too much ground in their answer and doesn't go into sufficient detail. Therefore, this is a typical question that candidates should try and pre-empt (i.e. the importance of work experience) so that they can give a good, concise answer to the question in hand.

141)   Which do you feel was more useful, your volunteering work or your work experience?

This isn't a trick question. It's perfectly alright to say you found volunteering more or less useful. This will depend on what you actually did. Crucially, you should give details about what you did, what you took away from the experience, define what you actually mean by 'useful' and sound passionate and engaged when doing so.

A Bad Response:

"I volunteered at an old people's home after college twice a week for about six months. I served meals and worked behind the admin desk. I think it was probably more useful than my work experience where I just shadowed a GP for a week, although that was fun too."

Response Analysis:

This is a poor delivery of a really good experience. Working at an old people's home is fantastic volunteering experience so it's important to convey a genuine interest, which isn't what comes across in this response. Also, whilst it's good that this candidate has explicitly addressed the question by making the actual distinction between whether the volunteering or work experience was more useful, they haven't defined what useful means! Saying "that was fun" gives the impression that by useful you mean enjoyable which you most certainly do not. And the response misses a trick by not talking about what the candidate has taken away from volunteering.

A Good Response:

"I volunteered at an assisted living facility near my college, twice a week for around six months. My main duties involved serving meals, working behind the admin desk and generally helping the residents get around. I like to think I actually made a small difference in the lives of the residents and tried to maintain a positive attitude at all times, although that could be difficult at times. I think I found the experience as a whole to be more beneficial to my understanding of working in healthcare and the kind of personality traits required when compared to my work experience of shadowing a GP for a week. That was good too, but I think I appreciated my volunteering work more, probably because I was able to be a lot more physically engaged with my volunteering. I was actually able to help my residents in volunteering whereas, since I'm not actually qualified for anything, I wasn't able to offer any support to the patients I saw at the GP surgery."

Response Analysis:

Details about how your volunteering work made you feel, and what you took away from the experience, as described above are what make this response better than the bad one. This response is also considerably better when considering why the choice of which you've preferred was actually made. No clear answer was given in the bad response, but in this response, it is clear that the distinction was made because of the more direct interactions the candidate had when volunteering, compared to the relative lack of input the candidate had when shadowing. This is a common complaint amongst people who've shadowed and is a perfectly valid comment to make. It's important to remember that the question is open to interpretation and that shadowing schemes and volunteering programmes offer considerably different experiences, each with their own drawbacks. It is perfectly valid to offer up these distinctions.

Overall:

Whilst both responses here focus on volunteering as being the more useful opportunity than work experience, don't feel that this has to always be the case. Indeed, if you can make the converse case, by all means, do so. How you approach this question largely depends on both your individual experiences and what you'd hoped to gain from your work.

MISCELLANEOUS

142)   What is the difference between a good and a great doctor?

This question is a very individual one as everybody has their own definition of what makes a doctor good or great. There are two ways to answer this: on one hand, you can use your own experiences with doctors if there is one that you perceived as particularly great, or you can stay on a more theoretical level. Both pathways will require you to provide an explanation for your differentiation parameters.

A Bad Response:

"A great doctor is simply better trained and qualified than a good doctor. In order to be a great doctor, you need to be close to the top in your field, if not the best in your field altogether. Only hard work and training will make it possible to reach the status of a great doctor as it is necessary to perfect all technical abilities to the extreme. Unless a doctor's medical skills are perfect, a doctor cannot call himself great."

Response Analysis:

This answer solely focuses on the technical skills of the doctor. It ignores that doctors need to be more than just very good at knowing the theory of their field. Medical care is a lot more complex than theoretical approaches. Not everybody that knows everything about their chosen field will make great doctors. This answer also ignores the distinction between good and great.

A Good Response:

"First of all, it is important to stress that this differentiation is a very individual one. A doctor that seems great to some might not seem great to others. This is due to the fact that everybody has a different set of values when it comes to the definition of greatness in medical care. However, for me, being a good doctor requires the individual to know their subject and to be able to interact with their patients satisfactorily. In order to be a great doctor, my doctor needs to not only know his subject and be able to communicate it to me appropriately, he also needs to make me feel like he understands me and my fears, like he knows what is making me tick and why I react the way I do. If I know that I can trust my doctor to make the right decision for my care that not only will treat and cure me, but also respect all my wishes and concerns wherever possible, then I can call him a great doctor."

Response Analysis:

This response is a good one as it appropriately reflects the complexity of the question. It also provides examples for the distinction between good and great and focuses on personal preferences. This makes the answer a lot more balanced and gives the interviewer a better impression of the student.

Overall:

This question is a challenging one as it reflects the most basic considerations of medical practice. We all strive to be great doctors to every patient we will ever have. Achieving this, however, is very challenging and requires a good balance of excellent theoretical knowledge and excellent people skills.

143) What is your favourite disease?

This is a great opportunity for you to showcase some of the reading relating to medicine that you have been doing. Give a good answer here and it shows that you are interested in medicine and have made an effort to read beyond your A-Level/IB syllabus in your own time. Showing this sort of commitment is key in showing the interviewers that you have the appetite for this tough and long degree. It also allows you to show off some scientific flare if you like. Generally, I'd advise approaching this answer as saying what you find particularly fascinating about a particular disease.

A Bad Response:

"My favourite disease is necrotising fasciitis as I find it amazing that bacteria can cause so much tissue destruction so rapidly. I think it's cool that such a trivial infection can cause such destruction."

Response Analysis:

On the face of it, this is an okay response. The candidate has identified quite a niche disease (shows wider interest in medicine) and has made a slightly profound point of the bacterial burden not necessarily correlating with the extent of subsequent tissue destruction. However, they fail to really justify why this is their favourite disease beyond that it has cool effects. They should have explained in greater detail that the toxins generated by the bacteria that cause the destruction and possibly link this to some recent relevant research they have read about in relation to diagnosis/treatment of the disease. It just requires better justification that reflects some insight into the underlying pathogenesis.

A Good Response:

"My favourite disease is Parkinson's disease. This is because of the fascinatingly mysterious underlying pathophysiological processes that lead to the wide array of symptoms and, additionally, the different dimensions of treatment intervention that are currently being researched. For example, we can either try and directly modulate the pathological beta oscillations in the basal ganglia with deep brain stimulation or we could consider trying to directly replace the dying nerve fibres with stem cells."

Response Analysis:

This is a good response as it shows that the candidate has genuinely thought and read fairly widely about a particular disease that they have identified as interesting. The extra detail regarding the different methods of treatment suggests that this is a candidate who isn't just sticking to their A-Level syllabus but is interested and engaged enough in medicine to look way beyond this for their own interest. This is important as it blatantly demonstrates your interest in medicine to the interviewers beyond what you've written in your personal statement (potentially under your teacher's instructions).

Overall:

These are the sorts of questions can catch out candidates who haven't done extra reading around their subject. Interviewers won't expect extensive knowledge at all, but merely want a taste of your keenness for medicine. Hence, going into detail about a particular disease is a good way of doing this. Also, if you're going for Oxbridge, then the extra scientific details will show your flare for this aspect of their course.

144)   Is there any question that you wished we had asked you?

This question underlies the attitude interviewers will expect you to have when you come to interview. When you are preparing for medical school interviews, you should have three underlying themes you continue to refer back to:

➢ Knowing what your strengths are as an applicant– other than your academic grades. For instance, do you have work experience from which you gained a lot of understanding into the medical profession, or an experience of having a high level of responsibility, or an independent project you have completed?

➢ Knowing what makes you stand out compared to others – this is slightly different to the previous question. Here you are focusing on your individual skill set and attitudes rather than your experiences. For instance, proactivity, empathy, leadership and the ability to listen well. You should have examples ready to prove that you have these skills.

➢ Knowing what the interviewer wants to hear – you need to be in the interviewer's head, knowing what he/she is really asking you and the underlying tone of the question. Ultimately, the same common questions are asked in interviews but are asked in many different ways to throw you off.

If you are asked this question, this is a golden opportunity to refer back to these themes. Open-ended questions are the best type of questions to be asked. For example:

➢ What are your strengths as an applicant to medical school?
➢ What skills do you have that will make you a good doctor?
➢ Describe a situation from which you have learned a lot.

A Bad Response:
"No, I think I have given you a good idea of who I am and why I want to study at this medical school."

Response Analysis:
To answer "no" to this question is a missed opportunity to show yourself off to the interviewer. If you have a good answer to a standard medical school question that you have not yet been asked, then you could state this question or a more general question that shows you to be a very competitive candidate where you summarise your strengths.

A Good Response:
"Yes. I would have liked to answer the question: 'Why do you think you have the potential to be a good doctor?' I would answer this question by reflecting on the volunteering of caring for special needs children last summer. I worked as part of a team to look after a large number of children with a range of diverse disabilities. This was my first experience caring for children with special needs and I was required to adapt and problem-solve in response to a role of responsibility I had never held before. I learned a great deal through this experience.

I learned that it is important to understand the limits of your competence and the importance of communicating this to the team around you and seeking help from more senior members of the team. I believe I am an individual who is able to adapt very well to new and challenging situations and I am passionate about ensuring the best quality of care while understanding the importance of good communication, teamwork and empathy skills in doing this."

Response Analysis:
This answer shows a constructive reflection of how the student has developed and have compassionate values. Avoid the urge to start answering the question until the interviewers acknowledge your question.

Overall:
Always try and relate your answers to questions back to your understanding of the medical profession; what makes a good doctor and how you feel you would be an asset to the profession.

145)   What does lifelong learning mean to you?

Background Analysis:

A career in medicine inevitably requires a commitment to lifelong learning. Medicine is such a fast-moving field that even the most experienced doctors are required to work to keep up-to-date on recent developments in research, technology and clinical guidelines. This process, termed 'continuing professional development', is not just good practice but a formal requirement throughout a medical career. At medical school and as junior doctors, this is obviously in the form of passing exams. Furthermore, junior doctors are required to complete a portfolio to showcase new skills and experiences such as courses, audits and presentations as they acquire them. More senior doctors are required to go through a process called revalidation with the GMC every 5 years, in which they must demonstrate that they are up to date with modern practices.

A Bad Response:

"Lifelong learning is something you are supposed to do in medicine to make sure that, as medicine advances, you know exactly what the perfect treatment for every patient is. For example, if you learn all the guidelines from NICE, the National Institute for Health and Care Excellence, then you will know what is best for all your patients. I really don't think this will be a problem for me as I had no problem memorising the syllabus for my A-levels."

Response Analysis:

While this candidate shows that they do appreciate that there is a need for lifelong learning in a medical career, there are significant problems with this answer. Firstly, they show very little understanding of what form this learning takes. There is substantially more to it than simply memorising guidelines. In addition, be careful when using terms such as 'the perfect treatment' as this may be taken to suggest that the candidate has an unrealistic understanding of what medicine is really like and can achieve – medicine remains an imperfect science, where sometimes doctors have to accept that there is no perfect treatment.

A Good Response:

"To me, lifelong learning is a critical part of what it means to be a doctor. As well as the learning requirements that doctors are required to go through throughout their careers, such as building portfolios of their skills and undergoing revalidation, I think there is also a much more personal element to lifelong learning. I think it is about honing your clinical practice to try and be the best doctor you can possibly be. This is not just by making sure you are as up-to-date as possible with medical advances and guidelines, but also by reflecting on your own practice to think how you can improve it. I saw this in my work experience at a GP surgery where I helped the GP with an audit on his skin excisions. He wanted to analyse how successful he was at identifying potentially cancerous skin lesions and demonstrated to me the importance of being constantly self-critical in an attempt to improve your practice as a doctor."

Response Analysis:

This candidate has demonstrated a good understanding of some of the elements of continuing professional development while also introducing a thoughtful and more personal response about what lifelong learning means to them. The candidate also shows a realistic understanding that it is not possible to be completely up-to-date with everything in the medical field, but that it is important to do our best to keep on top of the important things. As always, if you have relevant work experience, then this is good to talk about.

Overall:

If you are someone who really enjoys learning new things, then this is the perfect kind of question to talk about that and how you have shown/experienced that in the past. It will reinforce the impression that you really are committed to a career of learning. Furthermore, continuing professional development is a very popular concept in the medical community and so if you are not quite sure what it means or what form it takes, it is well worth looking up to make sure you have a clear idea of what is expected of you in a medical career.

146) Is medicine more of an art or a science?

This is an often quoted stereotypical strange medical interview question. Many candidates assume life as a doctor will be all reading charts and prescribing medications, and underestimate how much communication is involved (between doctors and patients, but also between doctors, for example, chasing blood tests or persuading a consultant to come and see a patient). Doctors who avoid or underestimate communication tasks will not be very good at their jobs!

A Bad Response:
"Medicine is a science subject requiring biology and chemistry, as well as incorporating aspects of mathematics and science. Treatment is chosen according to research and clinical trials rather than unscientific gut intuition, making it safer for the patients. Doctors also often take part in research such as clinical trials, which requires an understanding of how science works."

Response Analysis:
Whilst nothing in this response is incorrect and it acknowledges the key role science plays in medicine, this response shows the candidate is stuck in one mindset and unable to think about why art might be involved in medicine. An important skill in medicine is the ability to take a moment to step back and think about an unexpected question with an open mind and decide what is really being asked. Whilst this candidate certainly understands the role of science, they come across as someone who won't easily be able to consider things from a non-scientific point of view, which is often essential in communicating with certain patients – not everyone is driven by science and logic.

A Good Response:
"Medicine should always have science at its core - treatments should be chosen based on empirical evidence and facts from properly conducted scientific research with appropriate controls and significance. Similarly, using research findings enables NICE to write guidelines to standardise practice across the whole of the UK, which is important for continuity of care between different hospitals and GP practices. Daily life as a doctor involves lots of reading numbers and charts and data analysis. However, there is an artistic aspect to being a doctor, too. For example, whilst the surgeon can read many articles about the best method for an operation, there are nuances and art in the detailed knowledge of anatomy and each decision to cut away a structure, or which direction to suture, for example. Communication skills are also an art – no research paper can teach you how to read a patient's response to bad news and how best to support them emotionally. Overall, I would say that medicine is a science but there are human parts of the job that can't be learnt through bookwork."

Response Analysis:
The first part of the response shows an understanding of why science and evidence are important in medicine, and not just in terms of choosing a treatment – guidelines form a large part of modern practice, so this is very insightful. The second part of the response shows an understanding that books can't teach everything and that experience and skill are also an important part of being a good doctor. Finally, picking a side shows that you haven't forgotten what the initial question was and that you have thought about both arguments and come to a conclusion. Overall, this response has some special insights into the roles of art and science in medicine, and also acknowledges the different types of learning medical students need.

Overall:
Evidence-based medicine is an important pillar of modern practice and doctors are increasingly encouraged to choose treatments based on empirical evidence rather than going by what their superior always did. This means that new treatments are implemented faster and patients benefit from new research sooner. In this aspect, medicine is becoming increasingly scientific. However, medicine is above all else about the patient, a complex entity that requires a holistic view, unlike statistical analysis of data in traditional scientific jobs. Acknowledgement that the job also requires 'art'-like skills in various areas shows that you understand there are many types of learning required.

147)   Could computer technology eventually replace the need for doctors? / Will advances in technology and artificial intelligence render doctors obsolete?

With the advent of WebMD and other such online healthcare websites, patients are increasingly well-informed and often have an idea of a diagnosis before the doctor has even examined them. Having a good answer to this question is also helpful in dealing with patients who have self-diagnosed using the internet and are convinced that the doctor has nothing to offer them other than access to the relevant treatment drugs.

A Bad Response:

"No – doctors have to think about hundreds of different diagnoses for each patient and narrow it down. A computer could never manage that skill successfully; the human brain is much better suited to that kind of task.

Response Analysis:

This answer shows a knee-jerk response to not wanting to lose their dream profession without a thoughtful analysis of the question. A doctor must have an open mind and be open to progress and technological advancement, especially since evidence-based medicine is increasingly focused on. For example, electronic prescribing records are now being trialled in hospitals in the UK and hopefully the addition of certain rules in the programs will prevent common prescribing errors. Whilst the statement is most likely correct, the candidate doesn't explain why the computer wouldn't be able to diagnose, missing the essential point that the computer is unable to examine the patient and take a full history to use past experience and subtle clues to decide which diagnosis is most likely.

A Good Response:

"It is true that there is a lot of information about healthcare available freely online nowadays and doctors are increasingly using apps in their practice. However, such information has long been available prior to the internet in book form, but physicians have endured. There is an argument that programs could emulate the diagnostic process of a real doctor, but so far WebMD has yet to achieve this level! One major reason for this is that the doctor is skilled in clinical examination of physical signs of disease, whereas the patient (or computer!) may misinterpret a rash several different ways. This expertise would be difficult to emulate – a lot of diagnostic skill is in balancing probabilities by looking at many individual factors and the whole clinical picture holistically. Another important role of the doctor is in holistic care – organising teams to look after the various needs of a complex patient, whilst making sure that the patient is involved in clinical decisions and fully understands procedures and treatments. The doctor can also be important for emotional support when they form a relationship with the patient, particularly in General Practice."

Response Analysis:

This is a thoughtful response to the question, where the candidate uses the prompt to show that they understand the holistic roles and responsibilities of a doctor. Organising colleagues (such as chasing up blood results or persuading a consultant to come and look at a complex patient) is a large part of a junior doctor's workday and is often underestimated by medical school candidates. The candidate also shows that they understand recent advances in technology and demonstrates that they would likely be very effective in talking to a patient who has the wrong self-diagnosis.

Overall:

This question tests three aspects of the candidate's suitability for medicine: understanding of the role of a doctor; openness to innovation and technology; and the ability to thoughtfully consider a provoking question and answer thoughtfully, without rushing to a conclusion or knee-jerk reaction. Successfully navigating this tricky question shows proficiency in all three areas. This is an area where a small amount of preliminary reading (for example, on a news website, looking at recent advances in the area) would be of real benefit prior to an interview and also show an interest in keeping up-to-date with medical advances, which is an important aspect of being a practising doctor.

OXBRIDGE

148)   *Why have you chosen to apply to study at 'Oxbridge', rather than another Russell Group university?*

This is a very broad question and one which is simply designed to draw out the motives and thinking behind your application, as well as giving you an opportunity to speak freely about yourself.

A **good applicant** would seek to address this question in two parts; the first, addressing the key features of Oxbridge for their course and the second, emphasising their own personality traits and interests which make them most suited to the Oxbridge system.

It is useful to start off by talking about the supervision/tutorial system and why this method of very small group teaching is beneficial for studying your subject, both for the discussion of essay work and, more crucially, for developing a comprehensive understanding of your subject. You might also like to draw on the key features of the course at Oxford and Cambridge that distinguish it from courses at other universities.

When talking about yourself, a good answer could take almost any route, though, it is always productive to talk about which parts of your subject interest you, why this is the case, and how this ties in with the course at Oxford/Cambridge. You might also mention how the Oxbridge ethos suits your personality, e.g. how hard work and high achievement are important to you and you want to study your chosen subject in real depth, rather than a more superficial course elsewhere.

A **poor applicant** would likely demonstrate little or no knowledge of their course at Oxford/Cambridge and volunteer little information about why studying at Oxbridge would be good for them or why they would be suited to it. It's important to focus on your interests and abilities rather than implying that you applied because Oxbridge is the biggest name or because your family or school had an expectation for you to do so.

149) How did you choose which college to apply for?

This question is a good opportunity to tell the interviewer about yourself, your hobbies, motivations and any interesting projects you have undertaken. You can demonstrate that you have read about the college thoroughly and you know what differentiates your college from the others. The decisive factors can include a great variety of different things from history, alumni, location in the city, community, sports clubs, societies, any positive personal experiences from Open Day and notable scholars.

This is a warmup question – an ice-breaker so just be natural and give an honest answer. You may not want to say things like *"I like the statutes in the garden"*. The more comprehensive your answer is, the better.

A Good Response:
"I chose which college to apply for based on a number of factors that were important to me. First of all, I needed to consider how many other students at my college would be studying the same subject as me; this was important to me as I want to be able to engage in conversation about my subject with my peers. Secondly, I considered the location of the college as I wanted to ensure I had easy access to the faculty library and lecture theatres. Thirdly, I am a keen tennis player and so looked for a college with a very active tennis society. Finally, I wanted to ensure that the college I chose would feel right for me and so I looked around several Cambridge colleges before coming to my conclusion."

Response Analysis:
This response is broken down into a set of logical and yet personal reasons. **There is no right answer to this question** and the factors which influence this decision are likely to be unique for each individual. However, each college is unique and the interviewer wants to know what influenced your decision. Therefore, **it's essential that you know what makes your college special** and separates it from the others. Even more importantly, you should know what the significance of that will be for you. For example, if a college has a large number of mathematicians, you may want to say that attending that college would allow you to discuss your subject with a greater number of people than otherwise.

A **poor applicant** may respond with a noncommittal shrug or an answer such as *"my brother went there"*. The interviewers want to see that you have researched the university and although the reason for choosing a college won't determine whether or not you get into the university, a lack of passion and interest in the college will greatly influence how you are perceived by the interviewers.

150)   Why are fewer human females colour-blind than would be expected from the incidence in males?

[Extremely clear-headed] **Applicant**: *"Well, I know that women are much less likely to be colour-blind than men. Why don't I start by defining colour-blindness and working out why there is a gender difference using Mendelian inheritance, and then think about mechanisms of colour-blindness which may not be accounted for in this method. I noticed you specified females in relation to males, so I'm going to suggest that whatever this mechanism is, it is sex dependent."*

Now being this clear-headed is unlikely to happen when put on the spot, but shows that the question can be broken down into sub-parts, which can be dealt with in turn. At this point, the interviewer can give feedback if this seems like a good start and help make any modifications necessary. The applicant would realise that colour-blindness is inherited on the X-chromosome and the second female X-chromosome may help compensate. Although a single defective X-chromosome would lead to colour-blindness, in having two defective X-chromosomes does not necessarily mean that a woman would be colour-blind as the defects might be opposites and, therefore, cancel each other to lead to normal colour vision. The details are unimportant, but the general idea of **breaking down the question into manageable parts is important**.

The interviewer is not looking for a colour-blindness expert, but someone who can problem-solve in the face of new ideas. Note that this is a question about Proximate Causes in disguise; although the question begins with '**Why**', it is actually asking '**How**' or which **mechanism** is causing this discrepancy.

A **poor applicant** may take a number of approaches unlikely to impress the interviewer. The first and most obvious of these is to say "We never learned about colour-blindness in school" and make no attempt to move forward from this. The applicants who have done this only make it worse for themselves by resisting prompting as the interviewer attempts to pull an answer from them, saying "fine, but I'm not going to know the answer because I don't know anything about this", or an equally unenthusiastic and uncooperative response.

Another approach which is unhelpful in the interview is the 'brain dump', where instead of engaging with the question, the applicant attempts to impress or distract with an assortment of related facts: "Colour-blindness mainly affects men. You can be completely colour-blind or red-green colour-blind. Many animals are colour-blind, but some also see a greater number of colours." Having gotten off to this start isn't as impressive as a more reasoned response, but the interview can be salvaged by taking the interviewer's feedback on board. Many of these facts could start a productive discussion which leads to the answer if the applicant listens and takes hints and suggestions from the interviewer.

151) *How much does the Earth weigh?*

Don't be perturbed, if you're applying to study medicine at Oxbridge, you will be expected to be able to answer this question (especially if you have studied maths or physics at A-level/IB).

This is a fantastic illustration of the power of simplifying assumptions. It is possible to **get extremely close to the correct answer with no specialist knowledge**. Consider this approach:

Method 1:

I'm going to use $Mass = Density \; x \; Volume$
The interviewer would tell you that the Earth's radius is approximately 6,000 Km.

Thus, Volume of the Earth $= \frac{4}{3}\pi r^3 = \frac{4}{3} \; x \; \pi \; x \; (6,000,000)^3$
You can approximate π to 3 to give: $V = 4 \; x \; 216 \; x \; 10^{18} \approx 10^{21} \; m^3$

The majority of the Earth core is made up of iron and since that is very dense, it probably contributes the most to the Earth's average density. I know that the density of water is 1,000 kg/m^3 and I'll assume that iron is 10 times as dense as water.

Thus, the average density of Earth $\approx 10^4 \; kg/m^3$
Therefore, the Mass of the Earth $\approx 10^{21} \; x \; 10^4 = 10^{25} kg$

Method 2:

A good physics student should also be able to use the fact that the Moon orbits the Earth to calculate its mass.

Since the Moon is approximately the same distance away from the Earth during its orbit, the **resultant force acting on the moon must = 0.** Thus:

Gravitational Attraction between Moon and Earth = Centripetal Force

$$\frac{Gm_1m_2}{r^2} = \frac{m_2v^2}{r}$$

$$\frac{Gm_1}{r} = v^2$$

Therefore, Mass of the Earth, $m_1 = \frac{v^2 r}{G}$

At this point, the interviewer would probably stop you as the only thing stopping you from proceeding is knowing the moon's velocity and the distance between the Earth and Moon. A harsh interviewer may not give these to you immediately in which case you might have to use some general knowledge- e.g. it takes light one second to travel from the Moon to Earth.

Thus, $r = 1 \; x \; 3 \; x \; 10^8 = 3 \; x \; 10^8 m$. If you assume that the Moon has a circular orbit, you could also use this to calculate the Moon's velocity:

$$Orbital \; Velocity = \frac{Orbital \; Distance}{Time \; for \; one \; Orbit} = \frac{2\pi r}{1 \; month}$$

$$v = \frac{6 \; x \; 3 \; x \; 10^8 \; metres}{1 \; x \; 30 \; x \; 24 \; x \; 60 \; x \; 60 \; seconds} = \frac{1.8 \; x \; 10^9}{2.6 \; x \; 10^6}$$

$$= 0.7 \; x \; 10^3 = 700 \; ms^{-1}$$

Finally: $m_1 = \frac{v^2 r}{G} = \frac{(700)^2 x \; 3 \; x 10^8}{6.67 \; x \; 10^{-11}}$

$$m_1 = \frac{4.9 \; x \; 10^5 x \; 3 \; x 10^{19}}{6.67} = \frac{15 \; x \; 10^{24}}{6.67}$$

$$= 2.25 \; x \; 10^{24} kg \; [\text{Real Answer: } 6 \; x \; 10^{24} kg]$$

152) *Which of the two molecules below is more acidic? What factors make this the case?*

$$\text{(A)} \quad -OH \quad \text{vs.} \quad \text{(B)}$$

This question is introducing the candidate to the idea that the **concept of acidity** can be applied to more molecules than just the classic "acids" you learn at school.

A good candidate would first define acidity:

$$HA \rightleftharpoons H^+ + A^-$$

Then need to **highlight the key reactive areas** on each of the molecules and assign how each of the molecules would behave when behaving as an acid. In this case, both molecules form $RO^- + H^+$ as the products. The crux of this problem is that the stability of MeO^- is greater than $(Me)_3CO^-$ which is because the O^- is more stable in A.

Methyl groups are electron donating groups and in molecule (B) there are three Me groups pushing onto the carbon bonded to the oxygen, therefore, this carbon is more electron rich than molecule (A) so destabilises the O^-. Therefore, the equilibrium for molecule (B) in water is more shifted towards ROH rather than RO^- so molecule A is more acidic than molecule B. A good candidate will also then link this to equilibrium constants.

$$K_a = \frac{[H_3O^+]_{eq}[A^-]_{eq}}{[HA]_{eq}}$$

This question should not be too difficult - good students would be expected to give a comprehensive answer that synthesises multiple chemistry principles from the A-Level syllabus. This question tests how comfortable people are with these principles and if they can use them in different scenarios.

EXAMPLE INTERVIEWS

Remember that you're unlikely to be asked a random string of questions. In most interviews, there will be a natural sequence of questions rather than a haphazard disordered barrage. Ultimately, the medical school interview is an intellectual conversation, so your answers will often lead to related follow-up questions rather than just being ignored.

To illustrate this, we've included transcripts of two example interviews here. Videos of these can also be found on YouTube (search *UniAdmissions* Medical School Interview).

Mock Interview: Weak Applicant

Interviewer:	Hello. How do you do?
Applicant:	*I'm fine, thank you very much.*
Interviewer:	We're here to find out a bit more about you. Now, why have you applied for medicine?
Applicant:	*My parents are doctors and I've seen a lot of medicine in the past. I was interested and did a lot of science at school. Medicine seems very interesting, worthwhile.*
Interviewer:	So what kind of medicine are you interested in?
Applicant:	*For my work experience, I spent a week in GP and a week in a hospital in clinics.*
Interviewer:	What did you see specifically?
Applicant:	*In neurology, I saw patients with Parkinson's disease, motor neurone disease, neurological problems, and patients with facial problems. That's really interesting.*
Interviewer:	So you've applied for a course in medicine. Why not nursing?
Applicant:	*I just feel that doctors have a bit more of an interesting job and they make more of the decisions in hospitals. I think they are a bit…more involved really.*
Interviewer:	Do you not think nurses are involved?
Applicant:	*They are definitely involved, but I just think doctors' roles are a bit more interesting as they do a little bit more in hospital and make a lot of the decisions. It seems though it would be a more interesting job.*
Interviewer:	Fine. So what in particular are you interested in, I am not sure I understand?
Applicant:	*I was really interested in science.*
Interviewer:	Why didn't you apply to be a scientist?
Applicant:	*I think medicine seems like an interesting application. I enjoyed my work experience, I've seen lots of things in medicine and I would like to really help people.*
Interviewer:	Right, let's move on. I was looking through your personal statement and see you do a bit of music. Tell me a bit more about that?
Applicant:	*I have been singing in choirs and performing in orchestras a few times a week for a while. We've performed around the UK in a lot of different cathedrals and it's really interesting. I've been with my group for four and a half years now. I've performed in some really interesting pieces, and really enjoy piece learning. We go through the repertoire really quickly, learn a lot of new pieces, and perform in interesting places. It's really enjoyable.*
Interviewer:	What have you learned from it?
Applicant:	*When you're involved in a music group, it's a lot about teamwork and I've learned about the music skills themselves.*
Interviewer:	So tell me about a situation where you've shown good communication skills.

Applicant:	*For instance, I did Duke of Edinburgh Gold and we had a few days' expedition in hills. The weather there was really wet and it required someone to organise the teams, get everyone motivated and get everyone's morale up because some people were struggling with fitness.*
Interviewer:	I asked for communication skills, not leadership.
Applicant:	*I guess... In Duke of Edinburgh as well, I did a first aid course and you had to be really clear with talking, expressing what it is you need to do. You need to be able to let someone know very clearly who you are, what you're doing, why you're there. You need to be able to get information from them about what has happened. That's the type of communication skills that are very important.*
Interviewer:	Hmmm…What other skills do you think are important for a doctor?
Applicant:	*I think knowledge is obviously really important. Whether you have the right knowledge and are able to apply it, and whether you are able to work in a team. Obviously, different doctors understand that the patients have different problems. Doctors need to talk to each other to make sure they all understand each other.*
Interviewer:	So do you think it's more important for a doctor to have good communications or to have good knowledge?
Applicant:	*I think knowledge is more important because...without knowledge, you couldn't be a safe doctor. Without communication skills, you wouldn't be such a good doctor but you'd be safe because you knew the right things. I think they're both important but I think the knowledge is probably a little bit more important.*
Interviewer:	Fair comment. And how do you cope with emotional difficulty or stress?
Applicant:	*Well...I think, having a work-life balance is important. If your work is stressful, you could go away from work and know you've got something different to do like a lot of music. It's a chance to refresh yourself and to mix with different people who aren't in the same position and...have a life away from it as well.*
Interviewer:	Fine. Let's move on to a few scenarios that you may encounter if you become a junior doctor. Imagine you're now the Health Minister and you have one million pounds surplus. You can choose to spend that on an MRI machine. Are you aware of what an MRI machine is?
Applicant:	*Yes, they used it when I was...in neurology. They'd have MRI scans.*
Interviewer:	Good, you can buy the MRI machine or you can use it to fund fifty liver transplants, but the caveat with that is that these liver transplants are for people who have alcohol-induced cirrhosis. What would you do? Who would you give it to?
Applicant:	*...you said the liver transplants are alcohol induced? Probably the MRI machine.*
Interviewer:	Right. And say you're a junior doctor in A&E and you are busy on a shift. A 16-year-old girl comes in. She's lost a lot of blood and needs a blood transfusion. It transpires that she's also a Jehovah's Witness and refuses the transfusion. What do you do?
Applicant:	*She refuses the transfusion... I guess that's the patient's choice. Is 16 old enough to choose? You can consent to treatment at 16, so if she wants to refuse the treatment then she can. Obviously, you'd want to make sure that she understood that it was serious. But if she decided that's what she wanted to do then you'd have to respect her choice.*
Interviewer:	Fair enough. You're actually slightly wrong in the sense that at 16 you can consent to treatment, but you can't refuse it. It's a grey area. But what if she was 28? She could definitely refuse treatment then. Would you still respect her decision?
Applicant:	*I'd be very reluctant and I'd really want to make sure that she understood. It's only a good decision if she understands what it means. If she thinks it's something unimportant, but she decides it, then it wouldn't be a fair decision. She needs to understand the consequences of her decision. But if she understood the consequences of the decision then...*
Interviewer:	Well, we'll leave it then. Thank you very much for your time. We'll be in touch soon.
Applicant:	*Okay.*

FEEDBACK

Interviewer:	How did you get on?
Applicant:	*I felt some of the questions were really difficult. There were things I wasn't really expecting, so it took me a while to think what was the best example or...the best thing to say. It took me a little bit of time to think really and I felt I was a little bit slow.*
Interviewer:	I want to pick up on what you said. You weren't really expecting these types of questions. What type of questions were you expecting?
Applicant:	*I guess I was expecting questions like 'why medicine? Why would you like to come here?'*
Interviewer:	It was phrased slightly differently but…
Applicant:	*I guess I wasn't expecting you asking so much about work experience because I thought 'Well, I've written it in my personal statement. Maybe I wouldn't need to talk about it here as well.'*
Interviewer:	I think every question I asked you is very fair. They've all come up in previous interviews before. I kind of got the impression actually that you hadn't prepared as much as you probably think you had. Is that a fair comment?
Applicant:	*I think so. I felt before the interview… I was probably well prepared, but in the interview, I just felt that I wasn't. I hadn't really thought what I'd say to these types of questions.*
Interviewer:	Absolutely. I got the impression you knew what you wanted to say, but it just wasn't coming out right. The only way you can improve with that is just practising. That doesn't mean you turn to a robot and start rehearsing thing by rote, but it does mean that you practice to improve your fluency and confidence.
	In particular, there were certain things which I think you need to address. For example, in the ethics question, I asked you which option would you choose? You gave me an answer straight away which was "I'd choose the MRI," whereas you really need to work out an answer and explain why you chose this. You have to go through a scenario: If we buy the MRI and we don't do the transplants, these 50 people may die. If we do the transplants, the MRI machine cannot be used. You need to be a little more aware of the ethical principles. It's very simple: do no harm and do good. You may also want to refer to something called utilitarianism - 'the greatest amount of good for the greater amount of people'.
Applicant:	*Okay. Anything else?*
Interviewer:	In terms of the situational question, when I asked you for a time when you'd shown good communication skills, you gave me a time when you'd shown good leadership. I thought "Oh well, he's not answering my question." I think you need to be a bit more specific with your answers.
	That's not to say it was a terribly bad interview. I think you can just improve a lot with not that much work actually.
Applicant:	*I just got a letter through recently, my first interview is in three weeks' time.*
Interviewer:	That's plenty of time to prepare. Make sure you go through the common questions, practice properly and then you'll be amazed at how much better it goes. I can guarantee if we run this again in a week's time, if you prepare at least two hours a day, you'd be a lot, lot better.
Applicant:	*Okay, I had a question about the ethical questions… It's difficult to think of all the options and to me, it made sense at the time. When to know whether you answer quickly or whether you should give a description.*
Interviewer:	I think with anything where you're given a choice, you should always discuss both options and the arguments for and against both options and finally, if you're pushed to come to a conclusion, then give an answer.
	For something like, "would you kill a patient?", it's obvious what you would do, but with quite complex scenarios, yes, I would take my time over it.
	The correct answer is not **your answer**. The correct answer is **your explanation**.
Applicant:	*Okay. Thank you.*
Interviewer:	No problem. It's been great speaking to you. Best of luck for your interview.

Mock Interview: Strong Applicant

Interviewer:	Hello. How do you do?
Applicant:	*Very well, thanks. Nice to meet you.*
Interviewer:	Excellent. How was your journey today?
Applicant:	*It was good, thanks.*
Interviewer:	Good. I'd like to get to know you a bit better. Why do you want to do medicine?
Applicant:	*Well, it's something that I've thought of for quite a number of years. I'm really interested in science and in doing some of the practical applications of science. I've done a lot of work experience recently and I've really enjoyed all the different parts of medicine that I've seen. So it's really just reinforced that idea.*
Interviewer:	Tell me about this work experience. You seem to have enjoyed it.
Applicant:	*Well, I've done quite a few different things... I was in hospital for a bit of time with the surgical team in ENT.*
Interviewer:	What did you see?
Applicant:	*Oh, quite a lot really, and the team was really good. They gave me a chance to get involved, go to theatre and see some of the procedures, see some patients going through the clinic and then watch what happened to them.... I could see the difference it made and it seemed really interesting. It was interesting going through the procedure and see how it would work; I did a lot of theory behind it.*
Interviewer:	Good. So you were with the ENT team learning, but were you actually doing anything?
Applicant:	*Not really. It was very much risk observation, to be honest. They were always trying to involve me: answer my questions and talk about it. I didn't really get the chance to do anything practical so to speak.*
Interviewer:	So that's something you'd be interested in as a career?
Applicant:	*Possibly, yes. It's still early to say, I want to make sure I've seen a good sample of everything first. But it's definitely something, from what I've seen so far, I'd be interested in. It was a really fascinating speciality.*
Interviewer:	So would you ever consider other specialities, such as nursing for example?
Applicant:	*Well, I haven't so much thought about nursing.*
Interviewer:	Why is that?
Applicant:	*It's a really worthwhile job, nurses are hugely important.*
Interviewer:	Absolutely.
Applicant:	*But I'm bridging on from the scientific ends, I'd like a bit more of an intellectual challenge.*
Interviewer:	But why not be a scientist?
Applicant:	*It's a fair career path, but from what I've seen from my work experience, I'd like to work in a hospital. It seems really a worthwhile thing to do.*
Interviewer:	Good. And so why have you applied here specifically?
Applicant:	*Well, there are a few reasons. I'd really like to do the integrated course with early patient contact. That's something that really appeals to me, especially having been through my work experience: being with patients and seeing the clinical side of things... I think it is a long time to wait...two or three years of just doing science. I really want to get a bit of experience with patients early on.*
Interviewer:	That's a very fair comment. What disadvantages do you think this course has?
Applicant:	*I guess from the patient integration point of view, you'd need to approach patients with some knowledge, good background knowledge, so I guess that's something to take into consideration... I think on balance, I would probably like to see patients as early as possible. So I have to learn those skills as early as possible.*
Interviewer:	So do you think it's more important for a doctor to be knowledgeable or good with patients?

Applicant: *I'm not sure ... A good doctor needs to be both from what I've seen. All of the doctors I've been most impressed with in work experience are those people who you can tell they're really knowledgeable, but the patients seem to connect with them as well. So I think they're both really important.*

Interviewer: Do you think you can learn to be a good communicator? Or are you born with it?

Applicant: *I really don't know. Some people find it easy- they're just naturals with people and it comes more easily. And again, I'm sure it's something that you can learn...I've seen some of the ways that doctors approach consultations and these really impressed me. So I'm sure they're skills that over time, with the right kind of training, you can improve upon.*

Interviewer: Absolutely. Here we do emphasise on communication skills. You get quite a lot of teaching about it.... Obviously, medicine is an excellent profession, but what do you think are some of the disadvantages?

Applicant: *I guess it can be quite stressful at times. In my work experience in the medical teams, I was in geriatrics and that seemed quite difficult at times. Some of the patients are quite ill and there are also quite difficult family circumstances. It can be quite emotionally difficult and quite stressful.*

Interviewer: Did you find it emotionally difficult?

Applicant: *A little bit. I wasn't as directly involved, but I could see I would be if I was actually the person responsible, and it did have an effect on me.*

Interviewer: Well, in 20 years you may be responsible for these people's care. How would you deal with it? How do you deal with stress at the moment?

Applicant: *I think it's good to have something else as well as work. For example, at the moment I do quite a lot of music. I sing with my choir and I perform in an orchestra. I think it's important having something where you can go relax and take some time away from your work. That can be helpful. I keep things in perspective and approach each thing fresh and ready.*

Interviewer: Yes, I was looking through your personal statement. I noticed you do quite a lot of music. Is that something you're quite passionate about?

Applicant: *It's something I really enjoy. I'd like to keep it going as long as possible because I think having another interest on the side is useful to have. Having the music has helped... I do a lot of church pieces and I've performed in a lot of cathedrals around the UK. We occasionally do an overseas performance as well.*

Interviewer: Interesting - Tell me about a situation where you made a difference to the team?

Applicant: *Music's one of those things where you do notice, especially as a team, everyone needs to be performing together. There are certain times when someone, like a soloist, for example, has a lot resting on them because if it's quite a long solo, no one else has to prepare or practice to the same extent. They've got to make sure they're there on time and they are fit and ready to sing. There can be a bit of pressure for that because you know a lot of people are counting on you being able to perform and no one else can step in. So I think it makes a big difference to the team.*

Interviewer: So what did you do in that situation? How did you make a difference?

Applicant: *When you're in that position, it's all about preparation. It's knowing that you can't just turn up and expect things to go well. You've got to make sure you learn the part.*

Interviewer: Is there any specific instance you're thinking of?

Applicant: *Well, there was quite a big performance, for instance... in St Paul's Cathedral six to seven months ago now. I had a solo part for that but it was going to be eight or ten minutes of music to learn, which was quite a lot.*

Interviewer: Absolutely. That's not really a team exercise. What would you say to that?

Applicant: *I think it's a good exercise in the sense... that you're playing one important part of the team as a whole. It's not all about you: it's about you, the other soloists, the whole choir in total, the accompanists, and when you have an important role, you have to do your job well but your job alone doesn't make it. It's how it all fits in and making sure you're prepared so you don't let the team down, making sure that everything fits together. No wrong notes!*

Interviewer:	Obviously, you've been doing that for a few years now. Is that right?
Applicant:	*Yes.*
Interviewer:	That's great. I want to talk a bit about the ethical situations you may come across when you become a junior doctor. Now, recently there's been a lot of NHS reforms made. Do you know anything about the NHS reforms?
Applicant:	*Well, from what I understand, there's a lot more controls being given to GPs. They are getting more responsibilities on how they allocate funds, what treatments are funded, and what treatments aren't funded. That's my understanding from the general practice point of view.*
Interviewer:	I was thinking of the overall aims of these reforms, what we're trying to do with them.
Applicant:	*A lot of it is because they need to save money.*
Interviewer:	Yes. So imagine, for example, you've been made the Health Minister and you've found a surplus of one million pounds. Now you've got the choice of spending that on an MRI machine. Do you know what an MRI machine is?
Applicant:	*Yes, I saw them last week in ENT - they use it for some of the imaging.*
Interviewer:	Exactly. Or you can use that one million to perform a few operations, specifically liver transplants. The caveat for those is that they'll only be used for patients who are suffering from alcohol-induced liver cirrhosis.
Applicant:	*Okay.*
Interviewer:	And it's your choice now whether you choose to spend that on the MRI machine or the fifty liver transplants. What would you do?
Applicant:	*So ... it's either an MRI machine in a hospital and are there any upkeep costs in that or...?*
Interviewer:	Yes. They'll be maintained by the NHS Trust.
Applicant:	*So it's...having an MRI machine or you don't have it and you do the operations?*
Interviewer:	Yes. What would happen if you didn't do the operations? Do you know anything about people who have liver failure?
Applicant:	*To the extent that it can regenerate...*
Interviewer:	In these cases, people who require liver transplants will almost inevitably die if they don't get that transplant. So, what would you do?
Applicant:	*Well, I guess I would probably think in terms of a time scale... It would concern me to neglect the transplants that need doing because that's 50 lives that would be lost if we didn't go that route. But then again, you do have to consider how many people the MRI machine could help. It would help far more. Would it have such a big influence? And if you go with the transplants, you'd save 50 people directly.*
	I guess it comes down to how useful the MRI machine is. Obviously, it would be a huge patient group, but how much difference would it make to each one? You need to balance the benefits, which one would give more benefit overall.
Interviewer:	What do you think?
Applicant:	*It's hard to say really. I'm always concerned to neglect people who need operations. I'd be swinging towards doing the operations, thinking that for those people it's really important. They're specific people whereas for the MRI machine, it's a futuristic sort of thing. Maybe there could be some other way of diagnosing. Obviously, it is very hard to say, but maybe I'd lean towards the operations as a more direct way of doing good to people.*
Interviewer:	There was a caveat to that question. These people are alcoholic so one could argue it's self-induced. Would you still do it?
Applicant:	*It is self-induced, but it's a really difficult line to draw. If you say, it's self-induced, that person doesn't deserve treatment then where do you draw the line? What about...smokers? It could be anyone, someone that doesn't have a good diet or someone that had a sporting injury. I just think it's really dangerous to go down this route. Would it be relevant? I feel that it shouldn't be.*

Interviewer:	So do you think it's fair that we discriminate or should we aim to treat everyone equally?
Applicant:	*It seems to me it's fairer to treat people based on what they need rather than on the basis of who deserves it.*
Interviewer:	Yes. I guess that's what the reforms are all about. Let's move on to the second scenario which is not an uncommon situation. You're a junior doctor on call in a busy A&E shift. An ambulance brings in a 16-year-old girl. She's lost a lot of blood because she was involved in a road traffic accident and she needs a blood transfusion urgently. As a good doctor, you start the transfusion only to hear her say that she's a Jehovah's Witness and doesn't want the blood transfusion. What would you do?
Applicant:	*How old is she? She's 16?*
Interviewer:	Yes. She's 16.
Applicant:	*She needs the transfusion but she's refusing it?*
Interviewer:	Yes.
Applicant:	*So...Are the parents around?*
Interviewer:	The parents are on their way but they're not here. They'll be about half an hour by which time it may be too late.
Applicant:	*She's still a child but... is 16 old enough to make those decisions? I know you can consent to treatment without your parents knowing about it... So I guess she can refuse if she wanted to.*
Interviewer:	Yes, it's strange, isn't it? The way you said it made perfectly logical sense. If you can consent at 16, you can't refuse treatment if it's in their best interest and there's no other person around.
	So in that case, it would be fairly straightforward. You would transfuse. Obviously, try and find out and let the parents know.
	This becomes slightly more complicated if they're 28 years old, for example. What would you do then?
Applicant:	*Well, I guess they do have the right to refuse treatment if they didn't want it. But to make the decision, they'd have to understand the situation and what the problem is. If for instance, they thought it was a minor thing and they're refusing it when actually it was a really important thing which could potentially have an influence on their life, it wouldn't then be a valid decision. I guess they could refuse it, though. If she knew the consequences of not having the transfusion and she decided that she didn't want it, then she would have the right to refuse it surely.*
Interviewer:	Possibly. That's all we've got time for. Thank you very much for coming down.
Applicant:	*Thank you.*

FEEDBACK

Interviewer:	How was that?
Applicant:	*It was quite tough actually. I thought things started okay because I was prepared for those sorts of questions. I was expecting to be asked why I had applied here, but when it came down to the ethical types of situations, I found that really hard. They were very tough decisions and I didn't know how best to approach it.*
Interviewer:	Yes, they are tough questions. I think I would agree with you. You started off very well. If anything, you were almost too quick to answer some of the questions. I thought you could take slightly longer.
Applicant:	*Okay.*
Interviewer:	We were speeding through a lot of the questions initially and it almost gave me the impression you'd rehearsed these a few times too much. But in general, your answers were very well constructed and quite personal to you, which was very good... you're quite well spoken.
	I asked you to tell me about a time when you've worked in a team well, showed good teamwork, how did you think you answered that question?
Applicant:	*Well, I was trying to think of the right circumstance...I do a lot of music and it's teamwork, there's that balance between individual and teamwork. The more of a team it is, potentially the less of a role each individual has. Everyone has the solo parts. I wanted to try and think of something where it was about everyone, but where I had a particular responsibility for a particular role. That's why I tried to focus it on when I was in St Paul's Cathedral.*
Interviewer:	Do you think it was quite focused or you could have done better?
Applicant:	*I took a while to...*
Interviewer:	You did. I felt you were rambling for the first part and not giving me an answer.
	There's a really simple thing you should do with these. You should set the scene: say -this was my role and this is where I was and this is how I made a difference, and the final points would be what you learned from it for the future.
	I did eventually get all the information, but it was all over the place. I think something just more structured would have been better.
Applicant:	*Yes, I felt that if I had a better-structured approach then maybe it would have flowed a bit better. So I should start by setting the scene...*
Interviewer:	Yes.
Applicant:	*And then talk about the situation itself? What I actually did and then how it made a difference.?*
Interviewer:	How it improved, what the result was. You can apply that framework for all of them, to tell me about good leadership, good communication skills, how it made a difference in the team.
	That's really again a complex example of what you did, then all of these are actually very valid.
	Let's talk about the ethics. Now, I personally thought you tackled the first ethics very well. I liked how you got more information out of me - that was very well done. How do you think it went after though?
Applicant:	*For the second one, I don't think I knew exactly the legal stance. I knew about consenting to treatment but in terms of refusal, I didn't know exactly where the legal stance stands.*
Interviewer:	Well, this was a hybrid ethical situation question and before we go on to the Jehovah's Witness question, I want to go back to the MRI machine. There are a few ethical principles you must know, and if you know those, you can answer 95% of ethical questions that you'll get.
Applicant:	*I think I did read something actually.*
Interviewer:	Yes, it's a paper written by Tom Beauchamp and James Childress in 1979. The important thing is there are four key principles you need to know. Have you heard of

	them?
Applicant:	*To do good is better.*
	To avoid harm.
	The patient has the right to choose.
	And then the final one is about justice.
Interviewer:	For those, the best way to do is to think about which ethical principles are valid. So, which one do you think was the most important there?
Applicant:	*I guess it's avoiding harm.*
Interviewer:	Possibly more important?
Applicant:	*Justice?*
Interviewer:	Yes. You don't harm them explicitly but I think if you use that framework, you're likely to cover all your bases. Here's a really useful tip: try and collect as much information as you can, pros and cons using the ethical framework and then finally give your own opinion, which you did at the end.
	Then with the Jehovah's Witness, you fell into a trap because you assumed that because they were a Jehovah's Witness they couldn't have a blood transfusion. Can you think of any reasons why they wouldn't want a blood transfusion?
Applicant:	*Could it be due to a lack of understanding about the procedure? It could be that they don't understand it's important, and they think it's unnecessary...*
Interviewer:	Absolutely, when you've lost a lot of blood, you could be quite dizzy or disorientated. You could be very confused or have a fear of needles.
	Don't fall into these traps that are scattered around. But in general, I thought it was quite a strong interview. Obviously, the first half was stronger than the second, but the second half even then wasn't by any means weak. But you've still got things to work on.
Applicant:	*Okay.*
Interviewer:	Any questions?
Applicant:	*No, thank you - that was really helpful.*
Interviewer:	No problems. Thank you for coming and best of luck.
Applicant:	*Thank you.*

FINAL ADVICE

Some DOs:

✓ **DO** speak freely about what you are thinking and ask for clarifications
✓ **DO** take suggestions and listen for pointers from your interviewer
✓ **DO** try your best to get to the answer
✓ **DO** have confidence in yourself and the abilities that got you this far
✓ **DO** a dress rehearsal beforehand so that you can identify any clothing issues before the big day
✓ **DO** make many suggestions and have many ideas
✓ **DO** take your time in answering to make sure your words come out right
✓ **DO** be polite and honest with your interviewer
✓ **DO** prepare your answers by thinking about the questions above
✓ **DO** answer the question the interviewer asked
✓ **DO** think about strengths/experiences you may wish to highlight
✓ **DO** visit www.uniadmissions.co.uk/example-interviews to see mock video medical school interviews
✓ **DO** consider attending an interview course: www.uniadmissions.co.uk/medical-school-interview-course

Some DON'Ts:

✕ **DON'T** be quiet – even if you can't answer a question, how you approach the question could show the interviewer what they want to see

✕ **DON'T** be afraid to pause for a moment to gather your thoughts before answering a question. It shows confidence and will lead to a clearer answer

✕ **DON'T** give them attitude or the feeling you don't want to be there

✕ **DON'T** rehearse scripted answers to be regurgitated

✕ **DON'T** answer the question you wanted them to ask – answer the one that they did!

✕ **DON'T** lie about things you have read/done (and if you already lied in your personal statement, then read/do them before the interview!)

Interview Day

➢ Get a good night's sleep
➢ Take a shower in the morning and dress at least smart-casual. It is probably safest to turn up in a suit
➢ Get there early so you aren't late or stressed out before the interview even starts
➢ Don't worry about other candidates; be nice of course, but you are there for you. Their impressions of how their interviews went have nothing to do with what the interviewers thought or how yours will go
➢ It's okay to be nervous – they know you're nervous and understand, but try to move past it and be in the moment to get the most out of the experience
➢ Talk slowly and purposefully; avoid slang and not use expletives.
➢ Try to convey to the interviewer that you are enjoying the interview
➢ It is very difficult to predict how an interview has gone so don't be discouraged if it feels like one interview didn't go well – you may have shown the interviewers exactly what they wanted to see even if it wasn't what you wanted to see. Indeed, many people who are given an offer after their interview had felt that it had not gone well at all
➢ Once the interview is over, take a well-deserved rest and enjoy the fact that there's nothing left to do
➢ Above all, smile

Afterword

Remember that the route to success is your approach and practice. Don't fall into the trap that *"you can't prepare for medical interviews"*– this could not be further from the truth. With targeted preparation and focused reading, you can dramatically boost your chances of getting that dream offer.

Work hard, never give up, and do yourself justice.

Good luck!

Acknowledgements

I wish to thank the many tutors for their help with compiling this mammoth book – it wouldn't have been possible without you all. I'm hopeful that students will continue to benefit from your wisdom for many years to come.

About UniAdmissions

UniAdmissions is an educational consultancy that specialises in supporting **applications to Medical School and to Oxbridge**.

Every year, we work with hundreds of applicants and schools across the UK. From free resources to our *Ultimate Guide Books* and from intensive courses to bespoke individual tuition – with a team of **300 Expert Tutors** and a proven track record, it's easy to see why *UniAdmissions* is the **UK's number one admissions company**.

To find out more about our support like intensive **courses** and **tuition**, check out **www.uniadmissions.co.uk**

YOUR FREE BOOK

Thanks for purchasing this Ultimate Guide Book. Readers like you have the power to make or break a book – hopefully you found this one useful and informative. If you have time, *UniAdmissions* would love to hear about your experiences with this book.

As thanks for your time we'll send you another ebook from our Ultimate Guide series absolutely <u>FREE</u>!

How to Redeem Your Free Ebook in 3 Easy Steps

1) Find the book you have either on your Amazon purchase history or your email receipt to help find the book on Amazon.

2) On the product page at the Customer Reviews area, click on 'Write a customer review'

Write your review and post it! Copy the review page or take a screen shot of the review you have left.

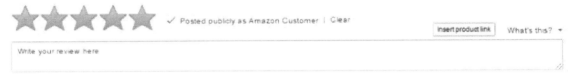

3) Head over to www.uniadmissions.co.uk/free-book and select your chosen free ebook! You can choose from:

➢ The Ultimate UKCAT Guide – 1250 Practice Questions
➢ The Ultimate BMAT Guide – 600 Practice Questions
➢ The Ultimate TSA Guide – 300 Practice Questions
➢ The Ultimate LNAT Guide – 400 Practice Questions
➢ The Ultimate NSAA Guide – 400 Practice Questions
➢ The Ultimate ECAA Guide – 300 Practice Questions
➢ The Ultimate ENGAA Guide – 250 Practice Questions
➢ The Ultimate PBSAA Guide – 550 Practice Questions
➢ The Ultimate FPAS SJT Guide – 300 Practice Questions
➢ The Ultimate Oxbridge Interview Guide
➢ The Ultimate Medical School Interview Guide
➢ The Ultimate UCAS Personal Statement Guide
➢ The Ultimate Medical Personal Statement Guide
➢ The Ultimate Medical School Application Guide
➢ BMAT Past Paper Solutions
➢ TSA Past Paper Worked Solutions

Your ebook will then be emailed to you – it's as simple as that!

Alternatively, you can buy all the above titles at **www.uniadmisions.co.uk/our-books**

UKCAT INTENSIVE COURSE

If you're looking to improve your UKCAT score in a short space of time, our **UKCAT intensive course** is perfect for you. It's a fully interactive seminar that guides you through all 5 sections of the UKCAT.

You are taught by our experienced UKCAT experts, who are Doctors or senior medical tutors who excelled in the UKCAT. The aim is to teach you powerful time-saving techniques and strategies to help you succeed on test day.

➢ Full Day intensive Course
➢ Copy of our acclaimed book "The Ultimate UKCAT Guide" (RRP £30)
➢ Full access to extensive UKCAT online resources including:
➢ 2 complete mock papers
➢ 1200 practice questions
➢ Fully worked answers to all questions
➢ Online *on-demand* lecture series
➢ All resources fully up-to-date for major test changes in 2016
➢ Ongoing Tutor Support until Test date – never be alone again.

Timetable:
➢ **1000 – 1030:** Registration
➢ **1030 – 1100:** Introduction
➢ **1100 – 1230:** Section 1
➢ **1230 – 1300:** Section 2
➢ **1300 – 1330:** Lunch
➢ **1330 – 1445:** Section 3
➢ **1445 – 1600:** Section 4
➢ **1600 – 1700:** Section 5
➢ **1700 – 1730:** Summary
➢ **1730 – 1800:** Questions

The course is normally £195 but you can **get £10 off** by using the code "*BKTEN*" at checkout.

www.uniadmissions.co.uk/ukcat-crash-course

£10 VOUCHER:
BKTEN

BMAT INTENSIVE COURSE

If you're looking to improve your BMAT score in a short space of time, our **BMAT intensive course** is perfect for you. It's a fully interactive seminar that guides you through sections 1, 2 and 3 of the BMAT.

You are taught by our experienced BMAT experts, who are Doctors or senior Oxbridge medical tutors who excelled in the BMAT. The aim is to teach you powerful time-saving techniques and strategies to help you succeed on test day.

➢ Full Day intensive Course
➢ Copy of our acclaimed book "The Ultimate BMAT Guide" (RRP £30)
➢ Full access to extensive BMAT online resources including:
➢ 4 complete mock papers
➢ 600 practice questions
➢ Fully worked solutions for all BMAT past papers since 2003
➢ Online *on-demand* lecture series
➢ Ongoing Tutor Support until Test date – never be alone again.

Timetable:

➢ **1000 – 1030:** Registration
➢ **1030 – 1100:** Introduction
➢ **1100 – 1300:** Section 1
➢ **1300 – 1330:** Lunch
➢ **1330 – 1600:** Section 2
➢ **1600 – 1700:** Section 3
➢ **1700 – 1730:** Summary
➢ **1730 – 1800:** Questions

The course is normally £195 but you can **get £10 off** by using the code "*BKTEN*" at checkout.

www.uniadmissions.co.uk/bmat-course

£10 VOUCHER:
BKTEN

MEDICINE INTERVIEW COURSE

If you've got an upcoming interview for medical school – this is the perfect course for you. You get individual attention throughout the day and are taught by Oxbridge tutors + senior doctors on how to approach the medical interview.

➢ Full Day intensive Course
➢ Guaranteed Small Groups
➢ 4 Hours of Small group teaching
➢ 2 x 30-minute individual Mock Interviews + Written Feedback
➢ Full MMI interview circuit with written feedback
➢ Ongoing Tutor Support until your interview – never be alone again

Timetable:
➢ **1000 – 1015:** Registration & Welcome
➢ **1015 – 1030:** Talk: Key to interview Success
➢ **1030 – 1130:** Tutorial: Common Interview Questions
➢ **1145 – 1245:** 2 x Individual Mock Interviews
➢ **1245 – 1330:** Lunch
➢ **1330 – 1430:** Medical Ethics Workshop
➢ **1445 – 1545:** MMI Circuit
➢ **1600 – 1645:** Situational Judgement Workshop
➢ **1645 – 1730:** Debrief and Finish

The course is normally £295 but you can get £35 off by using the code "*BRK35*" at checkout.

www.uniadmissions.co.uk/medical-school-interview-course

£35 VOUCHER:
BRK35

NOTES

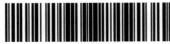

Printed in Great Britain
by Amazon